discussions of ethics and consent, therapeutic relationship, safe and mindful physical touch, music, the multiplicity of the psyche, numinous mystical experience, psychedelic group therapy, and the immense importance of integration following psychedelic experiences. Case examples bring these discussions to life. This is a valuable resource for therapists and anyone else interested in psychedelics."

Michael Mithoefer, MD, Senior Medical Director for Medical Affairs, Training and Supervision, MAPS Public Benefit Corporation

"This book arrives at a critical time in the evolution of psychedelic therapy as it articulates the challenges, mystery, and beauty of the psychedelic renaissance. The authors include diverse voices, each with their own sensitivities and refreshing perspectives, blending science, theory, ethics, and heart within broader societal forces. Being of service in partnership with compassion and ethical care are at the heart of each chapter. This book offers a wealth of information from practitioners with extensive clinical and research experience that is fresh, relevant, and culturally responsive."

Marcela Ot'alora G., LPC, Principal Investigator, MDMA-AT, and **Bruce Poulter,** MAPS MDMA Researcher, Trainer, and Supervisor

I0130960

"The wild and wooly field of psychedelic-assisted psychotherapy is in need of expert guidance and this edited book offers a lot of it from a diverse group of experienced practitioners and researchers, who cover everything from the somatic to the spiritual and social activist sides of this important movement. I am honored that Bob Grant contributed a clear and practical chapter on integrating ketamine with my Internal Family Systems (IFS) approach. My personal and clinical experience with this combination has been amazing, and Bob's guidelines are extremely valuable. His personal journey is also inspiring."

Richard C. Schwartz, PhD, Developer of the IFS Model and Adjunct Faculty, Harvard Medical School

"*Integral Psychedelic Therapy* is a cutting-edge exploration of psychedelic-assisted therapy by some of the top therapists and researchers in the field, providing an abundance of essential insights that are foundational to this work. This is a core text for practitioners looking to develop their skills as well as anyone interested in psychedelic healing."

Rick Doblin, PhD, Founder and Executive Director, Multidisciplinary Association for Psychedelic Studies (MAPS)

"This is a multi-faceted gem of a book! *Integral Psychedelic Therapy* is practical, necessary reading for anyone looking to understand the psychedelic revolution underway in psychotherapy and psychiatry."

Julie Holland, MD

"Psychedelics occasion a state of consciousness of immense therapeutic power and at the same time extraordinary vulnerability. Guidebooks are important, and this one, written by thoughtful and skillful practitioners, is a must-read for therapists who wish for these medicines to serve both personal healing and the greater good of society."

David E. Presti, University of California, Berkeley

"Within this wondrously evolving field of psychedelic medicine, we are discovering that the therapeutic envelope is more important, and potentially more meaningful, than the molecule. This book provides an elegant compendium of innovations, and deepens our shared understanding of expanded states. For clinicians and explorers alike."

Brian Richards, PsyD, Sunstone Therapies, The Johns Hopkins Center for Psychedelic and Consciousness Research

"This timely collection, produced by clinicians and researchers at the forefront of the psychedelic movement, is a must-read for both newcomers and experts. It combines clinical inquiry and a humanistic approach, weaving in social justice and respect for Indigenous traditions. As regulation by the FDA, decriminalization, and mainstreaming advance globally, it's urgent to cultivate a thoughtful understanding and culture around these powerful substances. This book goes beyond mere glorification, alarmist calls for 'ethics' and 'safety,' or empty tokenization to dive deep into nuanced and complex discussions around psychedelic-assisted therapies."

Bia Labate, PhD, Executive Director, Chacruna Institute

"The prevalence of mental health conditions and the speed at which psychedelics look set to be incorporated into mainstream medicine means there will need to be many more specially-trained therapists in the very near future. This will be a steep learning curve and we will need to carefully combine elements from conventional psychiatry with knowledge learned from Indigenous and underground practitioners. This book does just that—providing an excellent, multidisciplinary education covering the techniques used."

Amanda Feilding, Founder and Executive Director of the Beckley Foundation, Oxford, UK

"This book is a treasure trove of ideas and practical tips, refreshingly and importantly foregrounded in acknowledgement of the debt owed to indigenous plant medicine using traditions, and the impact of colonization, patriarchy, white supremacy, and corporate greed on the trajectory of psychedelic healing traditions. The subsequent chapters offer many different types of gifts; particular key issues, such as consensual touch, are considered from different viewpoints, as well as so many other important topics for anyone working with these healing modalities. For those who feel familiar with the 'basics' of 'prep-session-integration', this book delves deeper into some of the complexities, mysteries, nuanced applications, and ethical questions. The chapter on 'Decolonizing Psychedelic-Assisted Therapy' by Danielle Herrera, MFT was a wake up call for me, and is, I feel, a must-read for our community."

Rosalind Watts, PhD, Founder and Co-Director of Acer Integration

"*Integral Psychedelic Therapy* brings needed attention and wisdom to a range of the most important aspects of working with psychedelics. At a time of rapid progress in clinical research, this book is a welcome reminder of the cultural context surrounding these medicines, including the history of psychedelics, the debt owed to indigenous wisdom and the tragic damage the 'War on Drugs' has done to marginalized communities and to the advancement of health care and individual freedom. The more clinically oriented chapters remind us not to lose sight of the 'core, human elements of the work' and the richness and depth of the human healing process. The authors draw on their own clinical experience to offer informed and insightful

Integral Psychedelic Therapy

Integral Psychedelic Therapy is a groundbreaking, evidence-based collection that explores how psychedelic medicine can be incorporated into contemporary psychotherapy.

This book builds on current psychedelic research by providing an in-depth articulation of the practice of psychedelic therapy, weaving together a variety of complementary therapeutic frameworks, case examples, and practical guidance for cultivating a highly effective, ethically grounded, integral approach. Chapters by a diverse set of practicing psychotherapists and leading researchers aim to provide practitioners with a method that centers liberation of all dimensions of being through intersectional, client-centered, trauma-informed, and attachment-focused practices, alongside thoughtful attunement to the relational, somatic, imaginal, cultural, and transpersonal dimensions of healing.

Integral Psychedelic Therapy will be essential reading for psychotherapists in practice and in training as well as those seeking personal healing and holistic transformation.

Jason A. Butler, PhD, is a clinical psychologist, a psychotherapist and supervisor at Sage Integrative Health; an associate professor in the Integral Counseling Psychology department at the California Institute of Integral Studies; and a therapist and trainer for the MAPS MDMA-assisted therapy program.

Genesee Herzberg, PsyD, is a clinical psychologist and co-founder and director at Sage Integrative Health, a holistic health and psychedelic therapy clinic in Berkeley, California. She is also a therapist, trainer, and supervisor for the MAPS MDMA-assisted therapy program.

Richard Louis Miller, MA, PhD, is a clinical psychologist, founder of Cokenders Alcohol & Drug Program and Wilbur Hot Springs Health Sanctuary, and host of the Mind Body Health & Politics radio show and podcast.

Integral Psychedelic Therapy

The Non-ordinary Art of
Psychospiritual Healing

Edited by Jason A. Butler, Genesee
Herzberg and Richard Louis Miller

Routledge
Taylor & Francis Group

LONDON AND NEW YORK

Designed cover image: Gina Tuzzi

First published 2024
by Routledge
4 Park Square, Milton Park, Abingdon, Oxon OX14 4RN

and by Routledge
605 Third Avenue, New York, NY 10158

Routledge is an imprint of the Taylor & Francis Group, an informa business

British Library Cataloguing-in-Publication Data
A catalogue record for this book is available from the British Library

ISBN: 978-0-367-76641-2 (hbk)
ISBN: 978-0-367-76642-9 (pbk)
ISBN: 978-1-003-16797-6 (ebk)

DOI: 10.4324/9781003167976

Typeset in Times New Roman
by Apex CoVantage, LLC

Contents

Contributors

Brian T. Anderson, MD, MSc, is an assistant clinical professor in the Department of Psychiatry and Behavioral Sciences, University of California, San Francisco (UCSF) Weill Institute for the Neurosciences, and he is an attending in the Psychiatric Emergency Services at Zuckerberg San Francisco General Hospital. His research has included both ethnographic studies of religious practitioners who use psychedelics in community settings and clinical trials of psychedelic therapies. In 2018, he conducted a pilot study of psilocybin-assisted group therapy for demoralization in older, long-term AIDS survivor men. He is a co-founding member of the University of California, Berkeley Center for the Science of Psychedelics. Currently, his research focuses on the development of 1) novel interventions to address psychological distress in patients with serious medical illness and 2) training and safety standards for psychedelic guiding.

Jason A. Butler (he/him), PhD, is a licensed clinical psychologist, a psychotherapist, and supervisor at Sage Integrative Health; an associate professor in the Integral Counseling Psychology department at the California Institute of Integral Studies (CIIS); and a therapist with the MAPS MDMA-assisted psychotherapy expanded access program. Jason is white, queer, and gender fluid. He is a passionate teacher and stands proudly in a long maternal line of school teachers. His therapeutic approach weaves together archetypal, relational, somatic, and liberation frameworks.

Shanna Butler (she/her), PhD, is a depth and somatic-oriented psychologist, psychedelic psychotherapist, professor, ritual and magic maker living and practicing in the unceded lands of the Pomo and Miwok peoples. Shanna identifies as white, queer, and genderqueer, and she centers intersectional feminism, social justice, decolonization, and allyship in her personal and psychotherapy practices.

Shirley Dvir (she/her), LMFT, is the founder and lead teacher of Relational Somatic Healing and a licensed marriage and family therapist. For over 10 years, she taught as a certified Hakomi teacher at the Hakomi Institute of California; John

F. Kennedy University; California Institute for Integral Studies; and Shiluv Center in Tivon, Israel. She has also supervised associates pursuing marriage and family therapy licensure and currently mentors licensed practitioners. Her main work today focuses on healing relational wounds with safe embodied touch. Her spiritual practice and meditation support how she holds her work and her teaching.

Gisele Fernandes-Osterhold (she/her), LMFT, is a licensed psychotherapist, clinical supervisor, psychology professor, and psychedelic therapy researcher. Her work is trauma informed and culturally aware, rooted in somatic, humanistic–existential, and transpersonal psychologies. Gisele's personal approach to healing is embodied spirituality, inspired by her practices of yoga, dance, and traditions of her native Brazil. Gisele is the director of facilitation for psychedelic therapy studies in the Translational Psychedelic Research Laboratory at UCSF and mentors at the Center for Psychedelic Therapies and Research at CIIS. She maintains a private practice and lives with her husband and children in Berkeley, California.

Veronika Gold, LMFT, originally from the Czechia, has an expertise in the treatment of trauma. Veronika is a co-founder of Polaris Insight Center, a therapist, consultant, and trainer for MDMA-AT and ketamine-assisted psychotherapy (KAP). She is a training facilitator for the EMDR Humanitarian Assistance Program, a certified Somatic Experiencing practitioner, and a Realization Process Teacher. Veronika advocates for accessibility of PAT, fair compensation for providers, and integrity in PAT and training. In her free time, you will find her in hot springs or in nature, studying transpersonal and contemplative traditions.

Robert M. Grant, MD, is a medical doctor specialized in pulmonary medicine, a professor of medicine at the UCSF, and a certified IFS practitioner. He completed the Certificate in Psychedelic Therapy and Research at the California Institute of Integral Studies in 2016, its inaugural year, where he continues to mentor students. He co-founded Healing Realms Psychotherapy in San Francisco, which offers ketamine-assisted IFS therapy. He has led MDMA research. He teaches psychedelic-assisted psychotherapy at University of California, Berkeley.

Danielle M. Herrera (she/her), LMFT, is an Ohlone Land (Oakland)-based psychotherapist providing psychedelic-assisted psychotherapy, psychedelic integration, and harm reduction psychotherapy. She is a Queer, detribalized mixed-Indigenous woman from Chiricahua, Yaqui, Chicana, and Filipina descent. Her culture and her background working within harm reduction treatment for unstably housed communities, individuals, and families inform her warm and emotion-focused decolonized framework, with attunement to systemic oppressions and violences that impact the individual within a complicated ecosystem. Danielle enjoys working with spiritual emergence; Queer, Black, Indigenous, and People of Color; people who use drugs; and others outside of the mainstream.

Genesee Herzberg, PsyD, is a clinical psychologist from the California Bay Area. She is co-founder of Sage Integrative Health, a holistic psychedelic clinic, and Alchemy Community Therapy Center, a sliding-scale psychedelic clinic and internship training center. Genesee is a therapist, supervisor, and trainer in ketamine- and MDMA-assisted therapy (MDMA-AT) with Sage and MAPS. She is passionate about making psychedelic medicine accessible, developing innovative body-centered approaches to psychedelic healing, and promoting ethics and integrity as psychedelics go mainstream. Genesee is a lover of hot springs, dance, magic, plants, and feminist sci-fi.

Jacki Hull, MFT, is a licensed marriage family therapist with a Master's in Counseling from the Institute of Transpersonal Psychology. She is a core faculty member and developer at Relational Somatic Healing, a somatic-based therapy that includes the therapeutic relationship and safe, ethical touch as interventions toward healing. Today, her work focuses on therapeutic relationship, relational touch, and ketamine-assisted therapy to address developmental trauma and attachment ruptures. She is passionate about working with those affected by cancer, grief, and loss. Jacki has been in private practice since 2011. Her practice is based in Berkeley and Fairfax, California, and online.

Jessica Katzman, PsyD, is a queer Canadian clinical psychologist who studied integrative and transpersonal approaches to psychotherapy at the California Institute of Integral Studies in San Francisco, California. She is the co-founder of Healing Realms, a depth-oriented KAP practice, and offers harm reduction therapy and psychedelic integration in her private practice. She is passionate about supporting people from various subcultures and the Lesbian, Gay, Bisexual, Transgender, Queer, Questioning, Intersex, Allies, Asexual, and Pansexual communities with social justice-oriented and trauma-informed care. She is fascinated by creative expression (writing, dance, and art), as well as deepening her connection to the natural world.

Emma Knighton, MA, LMHC, is a white, queer, able-bodied femme with ancestral lineage rooted in Celtic Druidry. She is a somatic trauma therapist, psychedelic integration therapist, psychedelic educator, and conscious organizer and leader. In their clinical work, Emma works at the intersection of complex post-traumatic stress disorder (PTSD) from childhood abuse, queer identity development, and consciousness exploration. Her clinical and leadership approach is grounded in queer, consent, feminist, and liberation theories. Emma teaches courses on integrating trauma-attuned consent practices into psychedelic-assisted therapy (PAT) and strives to be in service to the psychedelic space with integrated mind, body, spirit, and community.

Richard Louis Miller, MA, PhD, is a clinical psychologist for 61 years. He is the founder of Cokenders Alcohol & Drug Program and Wilbur Hot Springs Health Sanctuary; host of the Mind Body Health & Politics; author of *Psychedelic Medicine, Psychedelic Wisdom* (2022) and *Sexual Medicine* (2023); consulting psychologist at Haight Ashbury Medical Clinic, California State Assembly, and U.S. Department of Justice; advisor on the President's Commission on Mental Health and the California Governor's Council on Wellness and Physical Fitness; and a member of the National Board of Directors, Marijuana Policy Project. He is Ukranian and a pansexual, with five evolved, contributing, adult children and one granddaughter. He is an endurance athlete, an existentialist, a political and social activist, and a vegan, whose life is significantly enhanced by his ever-patient and beautiful wife, Jolee.

Karen Peoples, PhD, is a clinical psychologist in private practice for 40 years. She is a personal/supervising analyst and faculty at the Psychoanalytic Institute of Northern California. She is currently an associate supervisor for MAPS and was a therapist for MAPS Phase 3 study of MDMA-AT at UCSF. In her free time, Karen savors the contemplative practice of yoga, exploring subtle forms of learning through sacred relationship, hiking among the redwoods, and devotional singing. One of her greatest joys has been swimming in the wild with dolphins.

Camara Rajabari (she/her), LMFT, is an intuitive, arts-based, ancestral psychotherapist practicing in the unceded lands of the Chochenyo and Ohlone peoples in Oakland, California. She assists Black, Indigenous, and People of Color experiencing anxiety, depression, and intergenerational trauma to reconnect to their power, restore their sense of self, and trust in their divine inner wisdom. Ritual is an essential resource in her practice to support her clients in disrupting cycles of grief, trauma, and systemic oppression.

Harvey Schwartz, PhD, is a licensed clinical psychologist in private practice in San Francisco, California since 1985 and is a co-founder of and lead trainer at Polaris Insight Center, San Francisco. He is also a sub-investigator and therapist on MAPS MDMA-assisted psychotherapy phase 2/3 clinical trials and serves as a clinical supervisor and trainer for MAPS. Throughout his career, Dr. Schwartz has specialized in and is the author of two major books on treating complex PTSD and severe dissociative disorders. His approach blends relational psychoanalytic, archetypal/transpersonal, and existential therapy traditions. His professional interests include grief, shamanism/transpersonal psychotherapy, transference/countertransference, and working with non-ordinary states of consciousness (NOSC) and training the next generation of psychedelic psychotherapists. He loves literature, music, redwood trees, hot springs, dogs, mysticism, and foreign languages.

Eric Sienknecht, PsyD, is a co-founder, psychologist, and lead trainer at Polaris Insight Center, a KAP clinic and training center in San Francisco, California. He has undergone training with the Ketamine Training Center and MAPS, and he is a sub-investigator, study therapist, and supervisor on the Phase 3 MDMA-AT clinical trials for treatment of PTSD. His professional interests include psychoanalysis, psychedelic and NOSC research, and transpersonal psychology.

He is passionate about the therapeutic potential of music and psychedelics, and he enjoys creating playlists for psychedelic journeys.

Evan Sola, PsyD, is a licensed clinical psychologist in private practice in Oakland, California. He is a researcher in the MAPS-sponsored clinical trials for MDMA-AT for PTSD, and a passionate teacher, trainer, and supervisor in this field. He has worked with various ketamine clinics in the bay area, including Sage and Polaris Insight Center. His special interests include working with children in play therapy, men's issues and military-related trauma, and using psychedelics to explore psychological growth in neurodivergent populations when co-occurring with depression and trauma.

Christopher Stauffer, MD, is a queer and non-binary psychiatrist, addiction specialist, and clinical researcher at the VA Portland Health Care System and Oregon Health & Science University. They are the director of the Social Neuroscience and Psychotherapy Lab (www.chrisstauffermd.com), which aims to maximize the benefits of therapeutic alliance in individual and group psychotherapy through the adjunct use of social psychopharmacology, such as oxytocin, MDMA, and psilocybin. Dr. Stauffer serves as a supervisor for MAPS MDMA Therapy Training Program and is principal investigator of the first clinical trial of MDMA-assisted group therapy for PTSD.

Foreword

The invitation to write a foreword for this book came at a propitious moment in the development of the field of psychedelic-assisted therapy, amid the emergence of the future iteration of mental health services, delivered by the promises of the *psychedelic renaissance*. Also alive in this context are the substantial individual, social, and cultural repercussions of a global pandemic on mental health and human behavior. A growing body of research shows encouraging clinical results in the treatment of trauma, depression, demoralization, end-of-life existential issues, addiction, and eating disorders using MDMA, psilocybin, ketamine, and other psychedelic medicines. Meanwhile, the field of psychedelic-assisted therapy has gained accelerated support from donors, the medical establishment, and corporate investors in recent years. Alongside the excitement, recognition, funding, and media coverage directed toward psychedelic-assisted therapy, ethical standards; the lack of proper training; and issues of accessibility, sustainability, diversity, and inclusivity are increasingly becoming part of the foreground of the movement. These gaps in the burgeoning field highlight the need for further guidance and structure around ethical, clinical, and social considerations for these groundbreaking treatments.

This book may serve as a cornerstone to the psychedelic-assisted therapy field at this time. This essential contribution offers a depth-oriented, somatic, and relational therapeutic approach emphasizing the imperative of ethical standards, the relevance of the therapeutic use of touch, the significance of the unconscious in symbolic meaning making and intersubjective processes, and the necessity of trauma-informed approaches, all while centering liberation psychology and decolonial practices. The topics addressed in this book and the themes embraced by the authors are of great relevance and not yet comprehensively articulated in existing publications on psychedelic-assisted therapy.

The diverse authors of this book approach their chapters grounded in their diverse social and cultural identities, as well as their extensive clinical experience providing psychedelic-assisted therapy in government-approved clinical research, private practice, and non-profit organization settings. Their contributions are aimed toward a vision of psychedelic-assisted therapy centered in decolonial practices, attuned to the somatic, imaginal, cultural, and relational dimensions of being, allowing the emergence of transpersonal processes. Each chapter elaborates on practical and theoretical aspects of this treatment modality through a unique theoretical framework, providing inspiration and guidance to readers working in this field as well as those compelled toward psychedelic work for personal transformation.

The editors of this book have been dedicated to this offering for years in their engagement with the development of the psychedelic-assisted therapy field as clinicians, researchers, educators, and visionaries.

I worked alongside Dr. Jason A. Butler as core faculty in the Integral Counseling Psychology (ICP) program at the California Institute of Integral Studies in San Francisco. I had been teaching in ICP for seven years when he joined the department, bringing his inspired contributions from depth and transpersonal psychology, with a social justice focus and a special attention to the body and to community. Dr. Butler had published about social and cultural considerations in psychedelic-assisted therapy and was about to launch a pioneer clinic, Sage Institute, in partnership with his wife Dr. Genesee Herzberg. Dr. Herzberg had been involved in conducting research in the Multidisciplinary Association for Psychedelic Studies (MAPS) clinical trials using MDMA for the treatment of PTSD, as well as manifesting her entrepreneurial prowess in opening her clinic for integrative health and psychedelic-assisted therapy, Sage Integrative Health in Berkeley.

In 2019, Jason and Genesee's vision led to the creation of Sage Institute, the first clinic to provide low-fee psychedelic-assisted therapy to underserved communities in Oakland, California. Their pioneering work encompassed not only providing accessible psychedelic-assisted therapy but also creating a training institute, where a relational and depth-oriented approach to psychotherapy would be the clinical foundation for treating depression, anxiety, trauma, and interpersonal wounding via altered states of consciousness. I still remember the excitement in the room during a fundraising event before the opening of Sage Institute. The building in Oakland where the clinic was to be located, known as The Haven, was also a home for offices of MAPS, Decriminalize Nature Oakland, the San Francisco Psychedelic, and other community organizations active in the psychedelic movement in the San Francisco Bay Area. It appears that the dream of psychedelic therapy pioneer Stan Grof, to one day offer these treatments at local mental health clinics, is finally coming to fruition. Now, this book offers the insights of the dedicated therapists who contributed to the manifestation and operation of this unique mental health clinic, as well as those of close colleagues working alongside them in the field.

Since March 2020, the world has been dealing with a pandemic that has devastated families, communities, and industries, changing how people socialize, how they work, and how they relate to life in general. It has been a systemic change that initiated a whole new reality permeated by virtual relationships and consumerism via technology in an unprecedented and magnified way. Today, as psychedelic-assisted therapy finds its second wave of clinical research and practice and inches closer toward legalization and medicalization, it is possible to download an app on a cell phone and purchase psychedelic medicine for an in-home experience guided in a virtual therapy session, or without a guide at all. Sadly, these types of automated and technological applications to psychedelics are often not grounded in a model of depth and relational psychotherapy, and these do not take into consideration the potential that symbolic, intersubjective, somatic, and transpersonal experiences can offer in this treatment. Automatization, virtualization, and commodification, in the wake of pandemic realities and emerging investment opportunities, do not consider what this book dares to put forward: a comprehensive and holistic approach to psychedelic-assisted therapy. This book is an invitation to pause, slow down, and contemplate important deeper clinical and social issues that may otherwise be lost in the frantic pace and narrow focus of commercial interests and instant access.

In recent years, another shadow within the developing psychedelic field has come to light, as scandals around ethical transgressions and violations have erupted and shaken the foundation of psychedelic therapy, bringing to the surface sexual and emotional abuse of clients, covered up or minimized within cult-like community behavior. The core of the motivation that leads people to pursue psychedelic therapy is in many cases the fact that multiple attempts toward healing have been unsuccessful. The vulnerability of such wounded seekers paired with careless, unsupervised, poorly trained, inflated, or even ill-intentioned psychedelic guides has brought forth devastating stories of pain and suffering in the United States and abroad. This book provides a foundational grounding in ethics and standards of care that protect the client against these harmful boundary violations.

This volume is launched in the context of significant advances in medical research leading toward the promise of groundbreaking treatments while the field is also facing tremendous challenges related to rapid growth, commercialization, unethical behavior, unsustainability of natural resources, lack of cultural diversity, and major obstacles to accessibility. Once Food and Drug Administration approval is granted for the use of specific psychedelic medicines for various mental health ailments, it will be imperative that an ethical, sustainable, and accessible model is created, beyond the shadows of the underground, the reductionistic narrowness of research studies, and especially the capitalist commodification of psychedelics. The field needs more of what this book provides: an approach that integrates supporting evidence from medical research with contemporary psychotherapeutic theory and practice, valuing trauma-informed in-depth psychological explorations in a relational, somatic, transpersonal, archetypal, and socially just framework to ethically and effectively unlock the multitude of possibilities that these treatments offer to best serve all those who can benefit.

May it be so.

Gisele Fernandes-Osterhold

Acknowledgments

This book was initially dreamed into being at Wilbur Hot Springs, where the healing and generative mineral waters inspired extensive reflection and conversation about how to move the psychedelic therapy field forward. A chance meeting with Dr. Richard L. Miller in the dining hall sparked a lively discussion about the psychedelic field and our many areas of shared interest, leading to a fast friendship and a shared vision of hosting an event at Wilbur bringing together a group of experts in the field to learn from one another; cross-pollinate; and refine best practices in depth-oriented, trauma-informed, and socially just psychedelic therapy. Joining in collaboration with our dear friends Veronika Gold and Harvey Schwartz, we planned a conference to occur in May 2020, hosted at Wilbur Hot Springs, entitled "Seeing Clearly Council." We were in the final stages of preparation when the Covid pandemic hit, and we were forced to cancel the in-person gathering. In place of the conference, we invited the presenters to collaborate in the collective writing of this book. We are deeply grateful for the contributors' dedication, flexibility, and patience through a three-year journey of shifting gears, changing timelines, multiple rounds of edits, and all the lessons learned through editing our first book.

The collaborative and co-creative spirit present within this group of authors, friends, and colleagues has been an essential resource amid the recent accelerated expansion and mainstreaming of the psychedelic movement. Through deep experiences and study with the authors of this compilation, we have collectively explored the healing power of psychedelic medicine and refined our ideas and approach. Those of us who learned about ketamine-assisted therapy from Raquel Bennett and the KRIYA Institute went on to form a consultation and study group, while the San Francisco contingent of the MAPS Phase 3 therapists developed an ongoing learning and practice community. Both of these groups have served as invaluable sources of personal and professional support, as we each developed our models and protocols and went on to launch psychedelic clinics in the San Francisco Bay Area (Polaris Insight Center, Healing Realms, Temenos, Sage Integrative Health, and Sage Institute). This book is yet another manifestation of the supportive and collaborative energy that we all hold dear—the quality of thinking in this book is evidence of the beauty that is born when we work together.

In the process of writing this book, we have been consistently nourished and inspired by our vibrant learning communities: the team of devoted practitioners and staff at Sage Integrative Health; the network of Sage Institute teachers and supervisors; and the faculty, staff, and students in the Integral Counseling Psychology department at the California Institute of Integral Studies.

Alongside the extensive peer support that has been a foundation for our learning and contributions to the psychedelic field, we are deeply grateful for the invaluable guidance and mentorship of our teachers and the pioneers who courageously came before us in moving this field forward amid a very different political climate. We extend tremendous gratitude to our mentors Michael and Annie Mithoefer, Marcela Ot'alora, Bruce Poulter, Karen Peoples, Harvey Schwartz, Raquel Bennett, Celina De Leon, Sandra Mederos, Joy Quevedo, Steve Jenkins, Vivian Dent, Kaisa Puhakka, Frank Echenhofer, Gary Bravo, David Presti, Kristi Panik, and Patricia James. We have also learned a great deal from the early pioneers of the Western psychedelic movement, including although not limited to Maria Sabina, Stan Grof, Ralph Metzner, Ann and Sasha Shulgin, Claudio Naranjo, George Greer, Requa Tolbert, Charles Grob, Alicia Dansforth, Julie Holland, Francoise Bourzat, Phil Wolfson, Eli Kolp, and Evgeny Krupitsky. Finally, this field would be in a very different place if it were not for Rick Doblin's tireless, dedicated, passionate work to legalize psychedelic medicine while generously making himself available for ongoing guidance, support, and solidarity.

This book would not be possible without the deep holding and healing offered by our medicine communities: Healing the Healers, Starbeings, Circle of Sacred Nature, and Star Circle, as well as the generosity, patience, flexibility, and understanding of our friends, families, and especially the Sage Integrative Health co-founder Julie Megler, as we moved through the all-encompassing rabbit hole of creating this book.

We are grateful to those who work tirelessly to move the psychedelic field forward toward a more equitable and just future while generously supporting us on our path of creating innovative and accessible models and treatment settings for psychedelic-assisted therapy, including Bia Labate, Gisele Fernandes-Osterhold, Lia Mix, Emma Knighton, Bennet Zelner, Jennifer Jones, Dave McGaughey, Derek Razo, and David Bronner.

We thank Leonard Cetrangolo, Karen Peoples, Harvey Schwartz, Amanda Khan, Laya Jamali, and Laura Neil for their generosity and brilliance in editing various chapters. We also thank Dr. Rupa Marya and Terry Cross for the use of their diagrams.

Lastly, we offer our deep appreciation to the clients and research participants who entrusted themselves in our care and helped shape this approach to psychedelic therapy through their courageous engagement with healing.

Chapter 1

Introduction

Jason A. Butler and Genesee Herzberg

Entheogenic plant medicine healing practices have been central to a variety of ancient and contemporary global traditions. For centuries, Indigenous and Pagan healers have carefully safeguarded the medicinal use of entheogenic plants, despite the oppressive forces of colonization and religious persecution. These traditions have demonstrated the inextricable and ever-mysterious connection between matter and spirit, between medicine and mind, and between plants and consciousness.

The current era has been described as the "psychedelic renaissance," characterized by a resurgence of these medicines in research, clinical, spiritual, and community settings, as well as the media and popular culture. Psychedelic-assisted therapy is now in a critical stage of development, as the field evolves toward a broad adaptation of these practices into Western medicine. There is great potential for psychedelic medicine to become widely available to the public, thanks to widespread efforts toward medicalization, legalization, and decriminalization. We are witnessing an upsurge in novel research investigating a broad range of psychedelic compounds to treat a variety of indications, alongside the rapid proliferation of psychedelic clinics and training programs. Amid this rapid expansion, there is a strong need for further development of therapy models, such as those featured throughout this book, which can help usher the field of psychedelic therapy toward a thoughtful integration of time-tested therapeutic paradigms and trauma-informed, culturally attuned practice, providing an integral framework for holistic healing with psychedelic medicines.

As the field grows, there are a number of notable risks at play. Psychedelics are frequently framed as a "cure" or "silver bullet," setting the stage for opportunistic exploitation, misinformed expectation, and the resulting significant disappointment—with the potential to cause harm to participants who do not understand the risks involved or the effort necessary to obtain lasting results. We are also witnessing the commercialization of the industry in such a way that prioritizes profit maximization over human benefit, as illustrated through numerous publicly traded psychedelic companies that have burst forth in the past few years to take advantage of the shift in tides of public opinion and policy. As psychedelic medicine scales, corporate interests have a strong potential to obscure the core, human elements of the work; it is becoming increasingly commonplace to extricate the therapist from

DOI: 10.4324/9781003167976-1

the practice of psychedelic therapy to reduce costs and increase profitability. Furthermore, the traditionally competitive spirit of corporatization has the potential to drive small-scale, client-centered, purpose-driven clinics that prioritize the therapeutic relationship out of business.

In response to the potential harms caused by the corporatization of psychedelics, this book aims to model an alternative. The collection of authors contributing to this volume are leaders in the field, many of whom have built or work for a variety of psychedelic therapy and training centers throughout the West Coast of the United States, each valuing individualized, person-centered, holistic, depth-oriented approaches to psychedelic therapy. The deep, supportive, cooperative relationships among us demonstrate an alternative to extractive capitalism—a "psychedelic approach" to business—in which individuals and organizations technically in "competition" with one another work in collaboration, learn from each other, offer complementary services, and cultivate right relationship to psychedelic medicines and the field as whole. As we demonstrate through this volume, coming together in this way can create a whole greater than the sum of its parts. Furthermore, this collaborative approach sets the foundation for the commercialization of psychedelics to reach its highest potential—a world in which psychedelic clinics exist in every neighborhood, built and run for and by the local community, alongside a network of psychedelic practitioners and trainers who rely on one another for support, collaboration, professional development, mutual accountability, shared learning, and innovation.

Despite significant recent shifts away from misguided perspectives on psychedelics and oppressive drug policy, we are still profoundly impacted by the nearly global prohibition of psychedelic medicines over the past half century. The War on Drugs has caused significant harm to countless people, contributing to mass incarnation, a major upsurge in violence, and the destruction of communities—particularly communities of color. Simultaneously, the reactive criminalization of scientific study and therapeutic practice with psychedelic medicines slowed the advancement of mental health care by hampering the investigation of the therapeutic potential of these promising medicines, relegating practice to primarily underground and Indigenous contexts, putting practitioners who continue to offer these treatments at risk, and impinging on the integration of psychedelic medicines with contemporary approaches to psychotherapy.

Prior to the criminalization of psychedelics, a multitude of articles were published, tracking the efficacy of psychedelic-assisted therapy. The resurgence of research on psychedelic medicines in the last two decades provides growing evidence supporting the safety and efficacy of psychedelic-assisted therapy for a variety of conditions. This book builds on current psychedelic research by providing an in-depth articulation of the practice of psychedelic therapy—weaving together a variety of complementary therapeutic frameworks, case examples, and practical guidance for cultivating a highly effective, ethically grounded, integral approach to psychedelic therapy. The primary aim of this text is to provide practitioners of psychedelic therapy with a method that centers liberation of all dimensions of being through intersectional, client-centered, trauma-informed, and attachment-focused practices, alongside thoughtful attunement to the relational, somatic, imaginal, cultural, and transpersonal dimensions of healing through psychedelic therapy. In these pages, you will find a practical vision that aims to steer the burgeoning field of psychedelic-assisted therapy toward its development as a powerful model of holistic healing.

Psychedelic-assisted therapy is a gem with many facets. Each chapter in this book is a refraction of light through the facets we hold as most central to this work:

- Deep understanding of the historical, cultural, political, and systemic antecedents to the current psychedelic landscape
- Cultural humility, reciprocity, accessibility, intersectional awareness, and socially just practices
- Safety, strong ethical standards, and ongoing informed consent
- The essential role of the therapeutic relationship in healing developmental trauma
- Attending to trauma held in the body and facilitating its release
- The power of therapeutic touch, and essential ethical considerations regarding its application in psychedelic therapy
- Reconnecting to the healing intelligence of the dreaming psyche
- Mystical experience, archetypal energies, and the subtle body
- Creating a sacred container of ritual and intention
- The multiplicity of the psyche and integrating dissociated parts of self
- The power of group psychedelic therapy for personal, interpersonal, and collective healing
- The challenges and opportunities of integrating non-ordinary states

This book gathers a community of practitioners who have been conducting groundbreaking work with psychedelic-assisted therapy in research, community mental health, and private practice settings. We weave together depth, relational, somatic, trauma-informed, Internal Family Systems, and liberation therapies, each of these voices working in harmony to create a comprehensive approach to psychedelic therapy. When taken together as parts of a whole, these distinct but highly compatible approaches to healing provide an integral framework for facilitating transformative therapeutic work with psychedelic medicines.

In service of preparing the reader for the nuanced exploration of psychedelic-assisted therapy through the different lenses offered in this book, we will now provide an overview of what you can expect from the following chapters.

To make psychedelic therapy accessible, equitable, and culturally informed, practitioners need to be well grounded in the historical conditions that surround and inform our conscious and unconscious relationships to psychedelic medicines and the mental health system in general. The history and underlying intent of the War on Drugs is essential context for anyone interested in psychedelic therapy. In the second chapter of this volume, Richard Louis Miller provides an overview of the devastating impact of this unjustifiable "war," particularly for Black, Indigenous, and Latinx communities. Miller's detailed historical account highlights the racist motivations behind the establishment and enforcement of drug policy in the United States. Miller then offers a brief history of psychedelic research and encourages ongoing political vigilance to ensure that psychedelic medicines are no longer barred from scientific inquiry and personal, communal, and therapeutic use.

For centuries, colonialist powers, like the U.S.A., have been using drug policy as a tactic of oppression "to control and sanction Indigenous populations in conquered lands and deny their ancestral practices" (Fordham, 2021). In Chapter 3, Danielle M. Herrera responds directly to the damage wrought by the ongoing impact of colonization and the structural oppression embedded in many psychotherapy models. Weaving together a dialogue between post-colonial studies, liberation psychology, and psychedelic-assisted therapy, Herrera provides key considerations and practical guidance pertaining to the dismantling of neo-colonial practices in the field and broadening the accessibility of psychedelic healing. Herrera offers the reader a foundational framework for attuning to the manifestations of systemic oppression on both cultural and individual levels, assisting clients in metabolizing cultural trauma, and opening expanded pathways toward collective liberation through psychedelic-assisted therapy.

One of the most complex and important conversations about ethics in psychedelic-assisted therapy centers on is the process of client consent. In Chapter 4, Emma Knighton draws together the elaborate and well-established guidelines around consent developed within queer and kink communities and applies them to psychedelic therapy. She provides a model for working with power dynamics, establishing embodied consent, creating soft and hard boundaries, and cultivating aftercare practices in psychedelic-assisted therapy.

In Chapter 5, Genesee Herzberg and Jason A. Butler weave together relational psychoanalytic theory and technique with contemporary psychedelic research and clinical experience to articulate a model for relational psychedelic therapy. The authors give specific attention to the process of healing the relational wounds of developmental trauma through attunement to the unconscious interpersonal dynamics that emerge between client and therapist in psychedelic-assisted therapy.

In Chapter 6, Veronika Gold offers a foundational somatic and trauma-informed framework for the practice of psychedelic-assisted therapy. She begins by providing the reader with a description of perinatal and developmental trauma and how post-traumatic stress impacts the nervous system. Continuing the conversation from Chapter 4, Gold explores considerations for facilitating a thorough process of informed consent in preparation for the use of therapeutic touch. Throughout the chapter, she provides a wealth of practical guidance and multiple case examples to illustrate somatic approaches in psychedelic therapy.

Weaving together several foundational elements articulated in the previous two chapters, in Chapter 7, Shirley Dvir and Jacki Hull illustrate their approach for facilitating safe, ethical, and relationally attuned touch in psychedelic-assisted therapy. They highlight the essential nature of touch in human development, outline the impact of trauma on the body, and provide an overview of the history and practice of therapeutic touch in psychotherapy. Through multiple case examples and thoughtful articulations of theory, Dvir and Hull describe their model of Relational Somatic Healing in conjunction with ketamine-assisted therapy as an effective approach for healing developmental trauma.

In Chapter 8, Jason A. Butler and Evan Sola provide a framework for working with the symbolic images, visions, inchoate sensations, intense emotions, and archetypal energies consistently evoked by psychedelics. The authors weave together Jungian and psychoanalytic theory and technique with psychedelic research and practice to articulate an imaginal model for psychedelic therapy. Using illustrative case examples from ketamine- and MDMA-assisted therapy, the authors provide elaborate descriptions of the psyche's innate intelligence, as expressed through dreams and the dreamlike nature of psychedelic experience.

In Chapter 9, Karen Peoples weaves together contemporary Jungian (CJ) and psychoanalytic conceptualizations of the "infinite unconscious" to provide a framework for working therapeutically with mystical and non-ordinary states of consciousness (NOSC). She offers the reader numerous considerations for containing archetypal energies, working with the subtle body to facilitate sensory–energetic transformations in consciousness and navigating the tensions between non-conceptual awareness and associative play in psychedelic therapy.

In Chapter 10, Shanna Butler and Camara Rajabari offer recommendations for cultivating client-centered, culturally sensitive ritual in psychedelic-assisted therapy. The authors thoughtfully describe the impact of colonization, white supremacy, and cultural appropriation on psychedelic-assisted therapy. Speaking from within their own experiences of ritual as a practice of social justice, they bring forward a vision for "invoking the numinous"—using ritual, psychedelic medicines, and magic to facilitate personal, cultural, and ancestral healing.

In Chapter 11, Robert M. Grant provides an overview of psychedelic-assisted Internal Family Systems therapy. Grant outlines the IFS model, describes the common principles and values shared between psychedelic therapy and IFS, and articulates his understanding of how psychedelic medicines can facilitate effective therapy within an IFS approach. Grant offers the practices he has developed and lessons he has learned from his years of experience facilitating ketamine-assisted IFS treatments. He concludes his chapter with a statement about how IFS fits within a social justice framework.

In Chapter 12, Eric Sienknecht offers the reader an in-depth exploration of music in psychedelic therapy. His chapter points to music as an essential component of psychedelic therapy that can potentiate transformative therapeutic outcomes. Sienknecht offers practical guidance for helping clients "listen *into* music," which can provide significant support for accessing NOSC and peak experiences, emotional expression and catharsis, imaginal material and processing of memories, as well as states of ease and relaxation. The emotionally attuned and client-centered approach he articulates provides the reader with a strong foundation for skillfully integrating the powerfully therapeutic influence of music in psychedelic therapy.

In Chapter 13, Christopher Stauffer and Brian T. Anderson provide key insights and frameworks derived from their experience facilitating psychedelic-assisted group therapy. Stauffer and Anderson summarize the existing research on this modality and describe the model they have used for preparation, medicine sessions, and integration in a group format. Stauffer and Anderson bring the chapter to a close with a vision for psychedelic-assisted group therapy as a method for ushering in individual and societal transformation through communal healing.

In Chapter 14, Jessica Katzman and Harvey Schwartz provide a history and overview of psychedelic integration, including the immense value of intentional practices, as well as the most common obstacles to successful outcomes. This chapter provides essential frameworks for addressing the challenges and expanding the opportunities for healing and spiritual development through the careful integration of psychedelic experiences. Katzman and Schwartz illustrate how setbacks, detours, and "zigzags" in the process of integration are loaded with healing potential when navigated with creativity, mutuality, and wisdom.

A New Paradigm

The field of psychedelic therapy is in its infancy, and there is much we have yet to learn about how these medicines work, which medicines are most effective for which individuals and symptom profiles, and how best to make use of them for lasting individual and societal healing. As the field matures, there will surely be a blossoming of novel modalities and significant evolution in how we conceptualize best practices. We see great promise in the incorporation of more body-based practices, including integrative health modalities, such as bodywork, acupuncture, naturopathic medicine, nutrition, and dance/movement. These practices have strong potential to complement the naturally embodying effects of many psychedelic compounds. As humans become increasingly disembodied, we are in dire need of effective methods to bridge the divide between psyche and soma, body and mind, and matter and spirit. We offer here a rigorous yet approachable model for psychedelic therapy, built from the creative contributions of practicing psychedelic therapists at this early phase in the modern iteration of the field. We hope this volume can serve as a foundation upon which the non-ordinary art of psychospiritual healing can continue to develop.

Psychedelic therapy, at its best, is a deeply integrative approach, weaving together the multiplicity of influences from traditional wisdom and contemporary psychotherapy, integrating psyche and body, ethics and cultural context, relational and spiritual development, and individual and collective liberation. As we face the most significant extinction event in the history of the Earth alongside the increasingly insidious enactment of systemic and overt oppression, massive wealth inequality, and a crumbling mental health safety net, there is an unprecedented urgency to develop healing modalities that are effective, expedient, and accessible to all. Psychiatric medication and standard psychotherapy, although helpful, have not been effective enough to mitigate the mental health crisis. The integral approach to psychedelic-assisted therapy outlined throughout this book helps practitioners—as well as those seeking personal healing—actively engage the full spectrum of consciousness and initiate holistic transformation. Psychedelic therapies, held in such a framework, have the potential to be an essential component in shaping a new paradigm of individual, interpersonal, cultural, and ecological healing.

Reference

Fordham, A. (2021, June 29). How the United States fueled a global drug war, and why it must end. *Open Society Foundations*. www.opensocietyfoundations.org/voices/how-the-united-states-fueled-a-global-drug-war-and-why-it-must-end

Chapter 2

The Attack on Psychedelic Therapy and Its Slow Recovery

Richard Louis Miller

Psychedelic compounds found in plants, fungi, and animal secretions have been used as tools for healing in Indigenous and Pagan cultures across the globe for centuries. Psychedelic therapy was among the first uses of these consciousness expanding tools in the modern Western world after they were discovered, synthesized, or appropriated from Indigenous communities in the mid-20th century (Smith, 1958). These compounds showed great medicinal promise in the Western context. Nonetheless, the U.S.A. and many countries across the globe outlawed most of the well-known psychedelics after many were distributed and used recreationally on a mass scale during the 1960s, 1970s, and 1980s. Prohibitions suffocated once promising research into the medicinal effects of psychedelics, and psychedelic therapy overwhelmingly moved underground. Meanwhile, U.S.A.'s half-century-long "War on Drugs" has demolished communities while putting a dramatically disproportionate number of Black and Brown people in prison. This widespread prohibition of psychedelics played a major role in institutionalizing racism and other forms of oppression while ironically criminalizing these powerful medicinal tools capable of healing the emotional and physical pain caused by trauma, including trauma resulting from living in systems of oppression.

When we heal, the effects ripple outward. Psychedelic medicines are uniquely capable of producing expanded states of consciousness that allow dissociated parts of the psyche to be reclaimed, cared for, and integrated into a patient's sense of wholeness. What would the world look like today had we spent that past 50 years effectively helping people heal through expanded states of consciousness? How can we ensure scientific research remains free to explore, study, and safeguard breakthrough tools for humanity?

As a practicing psychologist who was once able to legally use psychedelics in my clinical practice, I observed the type of profound healing that ripples through the generations. Can you imagine the tension of committing your life to helping people and not being able to legally offer a treatment you know to be safe and highly effective to those who come to you for care? People are dying because they cannot access these prohibited medicines; the system forces you to be complicit in harm.

DOI: 10.4324/9781003167976-2

Lysergic acid diethylamide (LSD) was criminalized in 1967, the same year I was licensed to practice clinical psychology. A chemical compound known to have monumental effects on human consciousness—one that is linked to significant medical and psychological benefits—is a therapist's dream. This dream of transformative healing halted abruptly when LSD was outlawed by the United States government. By government decree, LSD research and therapy in both academic and private settings virtually ended. My faith in my country was shattered. Outlawing a valuable medicinal substance was a major affront to our constitutional rights and to my chosen field of practice. This was the same government that experimented, from 1953 to 1973, on unknowing U.S. citizens—predominantly people of color, those with a history of psychosis, and other vulnerable populations—by giving them LSD and other psychedelics to explore their potential usefulness as chemical weapons and to find out if they were a form of truth serum. This program was called MK-Ultra. While all tools can be used for good or bad, we lost access to some of the most powerful tools for healing.

In 1965, I looked down at a handful of small black seeds. These unpretentious seeds were a gift from nature that I purchased when I was completing my doctorate in psychology. Timothy Leary and Richard Alpert's (1964) book, *The Psychedelic Experience*, inspired the purchase through their discussion of psychedelics. This text opened my eyes to the potential of healing through expanded states of consciousness in ways I had never explored or learned about while training to be a psychologist at an elite institution. If this text's wisdom held true, then following it would challenge, push, and expand the set of tools and principles I had been taught to promote emotional and mental health. I purchased thousands of Heavenly Blue and Pearly Gates morning glory seeds. These seeds contain lysergic acid hydroxyethyl amide, a less potent relative of LSD; my closest friend, Alan Pinsince, and I each ingested 400 seeds, while two friends agreed to sit for us.

My life was changed for the better forever. The experience was also so frightening for our sitters that they swore never to sit for a psychedelic journey again. Yet, what appeared to them surely as psychosis was instead the expression of repressed material. Witnessing emotional processing on rocket boosters is no easy task, and I am grateful to our sitters to this day. As an experienced psychedelic therapist, I am aware of the gravity of such a role. Part of my experience was a "bad trip;" I started imagining that people were banging on the walls with hammers and got scared; sure I was losing touch with reality, as, of course, I was. Fortunately, I opened my eyes and looked out the window, and there were two telephone repair men hammering. I laughed until I cried. What I then saw during the many hours that followed was the history of humanity.

I watched humankind's progression from apes to humans, from caves to skyscrapers, and from tribes to cities to countries and ultimately to one world. I saw the progression of commerce from trading to using stones, to gold, to paper as currency. I watched the pyramids being built in Egypt and the aqueducts being built in Rome. I saw that everything we need to know about guiding our behavior was to be found within. I learned that each of us arrives with all the information we need on how to conduct our lives, embedded as part of who we are. We arrive, ready made, with an internal how-to-live guidebook. All we need to do is learn how to read it. These therapeutic tools put me in touch with myself in a way that life itself had not taught me. My path of academic prestige and outside validation shifted toward one of service and purpose through this experience, limiting the weight of outside influences.

I had the summer of 1967 off from teaching at the University of Michigan and found my way to the Esalen Institute in Big Sur, California. I was Esalen's first resident scholar; Esalen co-founder Dick Price offered me a place to live in a lovely round house over a creek, facing the Pacific Ocean. My friend, Lionel Bloom, flew in from Paris and brought with him some "Sandoz LSD!"—the purest of the pure; we ingested it. During that journey, I had the experience of listening and under-standing people's communications through their voice tones while hardly hearing the words they used. My life was changed again by LSD. From then on, I heard verbal utterances as lyrics and music, with each communicating the intended mes-sage. Bodies of research on communication are dedicated to teaching this skill of understanding non-verbal communication. What I could have intellectualized quickly in a classroom but struggled to put into practice was instead deeply felt, understood, and embodied in my practice after a single session with LSD. These potent molecules bring with them so much hope for what is possible and have thus inspired exceptional innovation and creativity.

These powerful tools—capable of accelerating learning and initiating profound healing—seemed incapable of being kept from beneficial use. Then, in 1969, a University of Michigan student, John Sinclair, was caught with two marijuana cigarettes and sentenced to ten years in prison.[2] I looked with dismay at the pieces of my shattered respect for our government. What values must a government hold to crush a student's life for possessing a plant? This psychoactive plant contain-ing tetrahydrocannabinol causes virtually no deaths, yet is still federally illegal.[3] Meanwhile, tobacco causes 480,000 deaths per year and has never been criminal-ized ("Tobacco Related Mortality," 2020).

Such a misguided policy is infuriating to rational thought; it is not rooted in medical research and is counterproductive to the falsely stated objective of sup-porting public health. Good students of history know that alcohol prohibition created the largest illegal drug cartel in history and did not decrease alcohol con-sumption. Bootleg alcohol was more dangerous to people's health, at times even causing death or blindness. Instead of learning from the American social policy disaster of prohibition, our government has continued to make illegal that which it fears: a challenge to the maintenance of power. At the time of this writing, United States federal law continues to criminalize the possession of marijuana, psilocybin, LSD, and MDMA. Thus, licensed clinicians are banned from using these powerful medicines as tools in psychotherapy, and tens of millions of people suffering from mental illness in the U.S.A. alone are denied their remarkable healing potential. What does a government gain, and what do its citizens lose, by making these medi-cines illegal?

The Racist History of the War on Drugs

The U.S. government's history of suppressing certain mind-altering substances is intricately intertwined with institutionalized racism and other systems of oppression. President Nixon's so-called war on drugs was actually a war against Chinese and Latin American immigrants, Black, Indigenous, and other Americans of color, as well as the white counterculture. In the following pages, we will take a detailed look at how this unfolded. This section contains racist statements made by the U.S. government, political leaders, and the media. Although these statements are at times difficult to read, they are important to name as a way of elucidating the institutional racism that was and continues to be enacted through drug policy in the U.S.A.

The early conversation on drug policy centered around race, not health. Racism was prioritized over national health as a means of exerting a false sense of superiority and creating a power hierarchy that benefits some citizens while suppressing others. History reveals drug policy's evolution as a racist tool rather than a safeguarding measure. Throughout the 1800s, opiates and cocaine were largely unregulated drugs. In the 1890s, the Sears & Roebuck catalog, distributed to millions of American homes, sold a syringe and a small amount of cocaine for $1.50 (Richter, 2020). Then, in 1900, the *Journal of the American Medical Association* published an editorial stating, "Negroes in the South are reported as being addicted to a new form of vice—that of 'cocain sniffing' or the 'coke habit'" (The Cocain Habit, 1901). Some newspapers falsely claimed cocaine use caused Black men to rape white women.

Meanwhile, Chinese immigrants were attacked and blamed for importing opium to the U.S.A. In 1902, the American Pharmaceutical Association's Committee on the Acquirement of Drug Habits declared, "If the Chinaman cannot get along without his dope, we can get along without him" (as cited in Newton, 2016, p. 41). This committee blatantly overlooked the fact that upper- and middle-class white women—prescribed morphine or other opioids by their doctors—made up most of opiate addicts in America at the time (Trickey, 2018).

New legislation followed as government leadership used fear tactics conflating drug use by immigrants and people of color with crime. The Pure Food and Drug Act of 1906 required labeling of patent medicines that contained opiates, cocaine, alcohol, cannabis, and other intoxicants. Then, in 1908, President Theodore Roosevelt appointed Dr. Hamilton Wright as the first "Opium Commissioner" of the United States. Wright (1909) repeated the false notion that, "it has been authoritatively stated that cocaine is often the direct incentive to the crime of rape by the negroes of the South" (p. 24). He also made the inflammatory statement that, "one of the most unfortunate phases of the habit of smoking opium in this country is the large number of women who have become involved and [are] living as common-law wives or cohabitating with Chinese" (p. 25).

The rhetoric framing immigrants and people of color under the influence of drugs as criminals led to harsher and harsher policies culminating in the criminalization of recreational drug use (Bancroft, 2012). In 1914, Rep. Francis Burton Harrison of New York pushed through Congress the Harrison Narcotics Tax Act—the first federal criminal law in the US regulating the non-medical use of drugs, specifically opium and coca products. Dr. Wright testified at a hearing for the Harrison Act that drugs gave Black people uncontrollable, superhuman powers and made them rebel against the authority of white people (Cockburn, 1998). The head of the State Pharmacy Board in Pennsylvania was quoted during the testimonies saying that, "Most of the attacks upon the white women of the South are the direct result of a cocaine-crazed Negro brain" (Cockburn & St. Clair, 1998, p. 32). Just before the Harrison Act was passed, *The New York Times* published an article entitled, "Negro Cocaine 'Fiends' Are New Southern Menace" (Williams, 1914).

The trend of regulating mind-altering substances—paired with false and inflammatory racist statements intended to perpetuate systems of oppression—continued to expand in its scope and choke hold to the benefit of capitalists and politicians. The federal government began regulating marijuana in 1937 when Congress passed the Marihuana Tax Act. Just as the Harrison Act used taxation and regulation to effectively prohibit heroin, cocaine, and other drugs, the Marihuana Tax Act of 1937 effectively outlawed the possession or sale of marijuana. Politicians exploited old-fashioned racism and fear of immigrants to drive marijuana prohibition. State and national media tried to turn public opinion against Mexican and other Latin American immigrants by branding these communities as violent, lazy criminals bent on destroying the American way of life.

Political support for the prohibition of marijuana was driven by wealthy tycoons with a vested interest in outlawing hemp, led by Andrew Mellon, America's wealthiest man of the time and the Secretary of the Treasury. Andrew Mellon had a significant investment in the DuPont company, which had developed nylon in the 1930s. Hemp fiber threatened to be a significant rival to nylon, so it benefitted DuPont and Mellon to remove the cannabis plant as a potential competitor. Mellon appointed his nephew, the notorious racist Harry Anslinger, as chief of the Federal Bureau of Narcotics. Anslinger went on a 30-year binge prosecuting people of color.

William Randolph Hearst, the media magnate, had made a fortune in the logging and timber industry. He feared that hemp could be a cheaper and more effective substitute for paper pulp. Not knowing that hemp lacks the cellulose concentration to be an adequate substitute for paper, Hearst was concerned that his assets would take a significant hit. He used the power of his publishing empire to wage a propaganda war on marijuana. His newspapers and other media told stories about how cannabis made people go crazy and murder their families. The 1936 release of the movie *Reefer Madness* demonstrated the same kind of propaganda as entertainment. Such reports were complete fiction, but they had the desired effect of creating negative public perception around mind-altering substances, which persisted through the 1970s and beyond.

Business incentives to curb market adoption of these substances—alongside legislation as a tool for imposing power politics—led to more stringent measures. In

1952, the Boggs Act provided stiff mandatory sentences for offenses involving a variety of drugs, including marijuana. The legacy of mandatory minimums continues to this day to fill American prisons disproportionately with people of color, despite legalization of marijuana in the same states where these sentences are still being served. Richard Nixon continued to use drug laws to criminalize and control minorities—and to neutralize the impact of the civil rights movement of the mid-1960s—throughout his tenure in Congress and the White House. To understand Nixon's position on the drug war, we need only listen to the words of his closest advisor, John Ehrlichman:

> We knew we couldn't make it illegal to be either against the war or blacks, but by getting the public to associate the hippies with marijuana and blacks with heroin, and then criminalizing both heavily, we could disrupt those communities. We could arrest their leaders, raid their homes, break up their meetings, and vilify them night after night on the evening news. Did we know we were lying about the drugs? Of course we did.
>
> (LoBianco, 2016)

In 1970, Congress passed the Controlled Substances Act (CSA), which established categories or "schedules" in which individual drugs were placed depending on their perceived medical usefulness and potential for abuse. Schedule 1, the most restrictive category, contains drugs that the federal government deems to have no valid medical use and a high potential for abuse. The act placed marijuana into Schedule 1, along with heroin, LSD, and psilocybin. This act reflects President Richard Nixon's racism and animus toward the counterculture, rather than scientific, medical, or legal opinion. The 1972 Shafer Commission, an investigative body appointed by Nixon, recommended that marijuana be decriminalized and thus removed from Schedule 1. Nixon vehemently rejected his own commission's report; it reflected scientific expertise, and not power politics.

What happens when power politics infringe on public health and scientific inquiry? The Schedule I designation made it difficult for physicians or scientists to procure marijuana for research purposes. Defining marijuana as medically useless and restricting research access created major barriers to its development for medicinal use through normal medical, scientific, and pharmaceutical protocols. Our body's endocannabinoid system—our natural pain relief system that works seamlessly with the cannabinoids found in marijuana—became off limits for scientific research.

Over time, laws became stricter and included mixed incentives to catalyze state lawmakers toward supporting the federal agenda. The 1990 Solomon–Lautenberg amendment urged states to suspend the driver's license of anyone who commits a drug offense. Several states passed laws in the early 1990s complying with the amendment to avoid a penalty of reduced federal highway funds. Once encroached upon, it grew increasingly difficult to liberate scientific inquiries once more. Multiple efforts to reschedule cannabis under the CSA failed; the U.S. Supreme Court ruled in 2001 that the federal government has a right to regulate and criminalize cannabis, even for medical purposes.

Cultural critics spoke out against the conflation of drug policy with racial politics as a tool of oppression. James Baldwin, acclaimed Black author and activist and a contemporary of Nixon, commented that, "the drug laws can be used selectively and sporadically, against the poor or the otherwise undesirable, which is by no means incidental. Their enforcement is a tremendous political and economic weapon against what we call the Third World" (as cited in Lee, 2013, p. 271). Today, this legacy continues as prisons across America are disproportionately filled with people of color serving mandatory minimums.

It is no secret that racism continues to influence the enforcement of drug laws. Jill Soffiyah Elijah, then an instructor at Harvard Law School's Criminal Justice Institute, wrote in the Boston Globe in 2002:

> Today, African Americans make up nearly two-thirds of those sent to state prison for drug offenses, according to Human Rights Watch. This, even though white drug users outnumber African Americans by more than five to one. In 1996, African Americans were 33 times more likely to go to jail for drug offenses than whites; African American youths were 55 times more likely than whites to be sent to adult prisons for drug offenses.
>
> (p. 88)

More than a decade later, according to a 2013 American Civil Liberties Union report, Black people were nearly four times more likely to be arrested for marijuana possession than whites despite their similar rates of usage (Ezekiel et al., 2020).

As a result of the War on Drugs, many have lost faith in the American criminal justice system; too many citizens experience it as a system of oppression rather than an institution promoting justice. This is especially true in minority communities, although not just because of the drug war. Numerous videos of police shooting unarmed Black people have created increased concern regarding the quality of policing, the training of police, and fairness in enforcement of the law overall. Yet, drug laws specifically have been highly effective in decreasing opportunities for Black and Brown Americans. They have drained tax funds away from education and mental health, instead directing them toward building and staffing the police force and prisons. The enormous expenditure of government funds dedicated toward our dysfunctional drug policy is hardly improving.

It is time to recognize not only that Black lives matter, but that drug laws and the insidious systemic racism that fuels the prison industrial complex have contributed to a toxic stew that divides police and vulnerable communities. The government has failed communities of color miserably—communities that make up a critical portion of our population, soon to be the majority by 2050. The drug war carries an inter-generational legacy of oppression harming the bodies and minds of our societies. Why are we still fighting this so-called war? Alcohol prohibition lasted 13 years. The drug war overshadows this era as a blip in history—now in effect for over half a century. The drug war has caused immeasurable harm to countless people, to the United States as a whole, and to the values for which it stands.

History of Psychedelic Research

Now, let us turn to an examination of psychedelics, their medical promise, and their prohibition. Sandoz Laboratories began widespread distribution of LSD to researchers and psychotherapists in 1949, six years after Albert Hoffman discovered its psychoactive properties. Throughout the 1950s and 1960s, scientists in several countries conducted extensive research into therapeutic uses of psychedelics. Psychedelic medicine showed promise for treating trauma, substance use disorder, obsessive compulsive disorder, and other ailments. Six international conferences and dozens of books were released, alongside over a thousand peer-reviewed clinical papers published by the mid-1960s detailing the use of psychedelic compounds, administered to approximately 40,000 patients. Early studies by leading intellectuals, such as Humphrey Osmond, Betty Eisner, and others, examined the potential for psychedelic therapy to treat alcoholism and other substance use disorders.

Bill Wilson, founder of Alcoholics Anonymous (AA), participated in medically supervised experiments in the 1950s on the effects of LSD on alcoholism. Bill is quoted as saying:

> It is a generally acknowledged fact in spiritual development that ego reduction makes the influx of God's grace possible. If, therefore, under LSD we can have a temporary reduction, so that we can better see what we are and where we are going—well, that might be of some help. . . . So, I consider LSD to be of some value to some people, and practically no damage to anyone.
>
> (Alcoholics Anonymous, 1984, pp. 370–371)

Wilson felt that regular use of LSD in a carefully controlled, structured setting would be beneficial for many recovering alcoholics. In 1957, he wrote, "I am certain that the LSD experiment has helped me very much. I find myself with a heightened colour perception and an appreciation of beauty almost destroyed by my years of depression" (as cited in Hill, 2012). Most AA members were strongly opposed to his experimenting with a mind-altering substance, and Wilson eventually dropped LSD advocacy with AA despite its scientific promise. Early studies of alcoholics who underwent LSD treatment reported a 50% success rate with quitting drinking after a single high-dose session (DiVito & Leger, 2020). The individual case reports are often dramatic in their narrative illustration of how behavioral change is made possible through transcendent therapeutic experience.

Researchers, like Timothy Leary, felt psychedelics could alter the fundamental personality structure or subjective value system of an individual to great potential benefit. Beginning in 1961, Leary conducted research with volunteers who were currently incarcerated in Massachusetts Correctional Institution at Concord, in an attempt to reduce recidivism through short, intense psychotherapy sessions.

Participants were administered psilocybin during these sessions, with regular group therapy in between. The rate of new crimes was reduced by 50% (Leary & Metzner, 1968). In his follow-up study, Doblin (1998) highlighted that the treatment approach in this study lacked ongoing support post-release. Doblin stresses the importance of further study using a revised approach that includes psilocybin-assisted group psychotherapy and post-release programs.

During this period, psychedelic therapy was also researched in several other specific populations, including patients with neurosis, schizophrenia, and psychopathology; children with autism; and persons with terminal illnesses (Costandi, 2014; Sigafoos et al., 2007; Byock, 2018). In 1955, anesthesiologist Eric Kast used LSD as an active placebo in his study of analgesics among patients with terminal cancer. As Passie (2021) highlights in his review of this study, Kast found that "patients who received LSD reported a decrease in pain and a more relaxed attitude toward death, along with deepened self- and situational insight" (p. 101).

Throughout the 1960s, concerns about the use of psychedelic drugs within the counterculture resulted in the imposition of increasingly severe restrictions on medical use and psychiatric research of psychedelics. Many countries either banned LSD outright or made it extremely scarce, and Sandoz halted production of LSD in 1965. During a congressional hearing in 1966, Senator Robert Kennedy questioned the shift of opinion, stating, "Perhaps to some extent we have lost sight of the fact that LSD can be very, very helpful in our society if used properly" (When Bobby Kennedy defended LSD, 2012).

Studies on medicinal applications of psychedelics ceased to a halt in the United States when the CSA was passed in 1970. Despite objections from the scientific community, authorized research into the therapeutic potential of psychedelics was discontinued worldwide by the 1980s. This act changed the course of history. Healing does not exist in a vacuum. Psychedelic-assisted therapy can take people from a contracted state into one of human flourishing. Healed people are better friends, neighbors, siblings, and parents; they have the emotional resources to nourish others beyond themselves. Imagine how different the world would look today had we been able to support deep healing through psychedelic medicine over the past half century, rather than just treating symptoms.

During this era, disincentives for those championing healing through psychedelics grew increasingly extreme. In 1968, Charles C. Dahlberg and colleagues published an article in the *American Journal of Psychiatry* detailing various forces that had successfully discredited legitimate LSD research. The essay argued that individuals in the government and pharmaceutical industry sabotaged the psychedelic research community by canceling studies with strong potential while labeling genuine scientists as charlatans (Dahlberg et al., 1968). Despite broad prohibition, some psychedelic researchers and therapists found ways to continue their work in the following decades, albeit at a slower pace. Some therapists took advantage of windows of opportunity preceding the scheduling of particular substances, or alternatively, developed non-drug techniques to enter altered states of consciousness, such as Holotropic Breathwork.[4] Meanwhile, psychedelic therapy was conducted clandestinely in underground networks consisting of licensed therapists and others within the community.

In the early 2000s, there was a surge of renewed interest in the therapeutic use of psychedelics—led by Dr. Rick Doblin and MAPS—contributing to an increase in clinical research focused on the psychopharmacological effects and the safety and efficacy of these substances. Advances in science and technology allowed researchers to collect and interpret extensive data from animal studies, and the advent of new technologies, such as positron-emission tomography and magnetic resonance imaging scans, made it possible to examine the sites of action of psychedelics in the brain. Retrospective studies involving users of illicit drugs as voluntary subjects were conducted, allowing data to be collected on the effects of psychedelics on the human brain while simultaneously sidestepping bureaucratic difficulties associated with providing illegal substances to human subjects.

The new century also ushered in a shift in political attitudes toward psychedelic medicine—specifically within the FDA. Curtis Wright, deputy director of the FDA Division of Anesthetic, Critical Care, and Addiction Drugs from 1989 to 1997, explains a motivation for this change, "The agency was challenged legally in a number of cases and also underwent a process of introspection, asking 'Is it proper to treat this class of drugs differently?'" (Williams, 1999). These shifts in political attitudes sparked a new era of clinical research. Significant clinical research has been conducted with psilocybin and MDMA in the United States since the turn of the century, with special permission and breakthrough therapy designations by the FDA, while other studies have investigated the mechanisms and effects of ayahuasca and LSD (Mithoefer et al., 2016; Nielson & Megler, 2014; Oram, 2018).

Modern research indicates beneficial effects of psychedelic medicine for treating a range of ailments when used in the right therapeutic set and setting. MDMA-assisted psychotherapy is being actively researched by MAPS; clinical trials led by Dr. Michael and Annie Mithoefer and colleagues, conducted between 2004 and 2010, report an overall remission rate of 66.2% and low rates of adverse effects for the 20 participants with treatment-resistant PTSD who volunteered for the study (Emerson, 2016). In 2018, MAPS published the results of another trial investigating the efficacy of MDMA-assisted therapy for chronic PTSD in 26 participants and found that "PTSD symptoms were significantly reduced at the 12-month follow-up compared with baseline" (Mithoefer et al., 2016, p. 486). This research has been instrumental in moving MDMA into Phase III trials toward approval as a prescription medication (Mithoefer et al., 2019).

In a 2016 study, Dr. Robin Carhart-Harris, current head of the University of California, San Francisco's Psychedelic Division, led a team of some 26 researchers who produced the first images of the brain on LSD (Carhart-Harris et al., 2016). They compared brain activity on LSD to a normal, non-tripping baseline and concluded that LSD leads to a large increase in "connectivity"—neurons talking to one another—giving credence to the long-held idea that an acid trip can lead to new ideas (Schwartz, 2017).

In 2016, both Johns Hopkins University (Griffiths et al., 2016) and New York University (Ross et al., 2016) conducted small randomized, placebo-controlled studies with psilocybin. These were among the first controlled trials measuring the effects of psilocybin and psychotherapy on depression and anxiety in patients with life-threatening cancer. Across clinician ratings and self-ratings, the psilocybin treatment produced statistically significant decreases in anxiety and depression for at least six months. No drug-related serious adverse effects were noted. In a one year follow-up of the Johns Hopkins study of Dr. Roland Griffiths, there were "substantial and sustained" improvements in levels of depression as measured by pre- and post-testing. Compared to taking a selective serotonin reuptake inhibitor (SSRI) every day, this administration of a psychedelic was groundbreaking (Griffiths et al., 2016).

This treatment paradigm can potentially replace ongoing psychotropic prescriptions, but how? Carhart-Harris (2020) describes the potential for psychedelic therapy as follows:

> The impact of successful psychedelic therapy is often one of revelation or epiphany. People speak of witnessing "the bigger picture," placing things in perspective, accessing deep insight about themselves and the world, releasing pent-up mental pain, feeling emotionally and physically recalibrated, clear-sighted, and equanimous. This is very different from people's descriptions of the effects of SSRIs, where a contrasting feeling of being emotionally muted is not uncommon.
>
> (para. 9)

In recent years, the resurgence of psychedelic research has peaked public interest, generated by a spike in media attention. Many are calling this new era the "psychedelic renaissance." Alongside the proliferation of research, the field of psychedelic therapy has exploded in the past decade. Psychedelic clinics are popping up all over the world, currently offering ketamine-assisted therapy and setting themselves up to offer other psychedelics as they become legal. Psychedelic retreat centers have sprouted in almost every country that has more relaxed laws around psychedelic use. Psychedelic therapy training programs now abound. Psychedelic drug development companies are raising millions of dollars in investment funds, and there are over 50 publicly traded psychedelic companies. The market for psychedelic drugs is projected to grow to $10.75 billion by 2027 (Phelps et al., 2022). Despite significant financial investment in the field, access remains a major issue. In 2019, Sage Institute in Oakland took strides toward addressing the question of accessibility by becoming the country's first low-fee psychedelic therapy clinic.

Nonetheless, in 2022, at the time of this writing, research continues to be significantly hampered by the fact that LSD, psilocybin, MDMA, marijuana, and other psychedelic substances remain illegal at the federal level and, with a few exceptions, at the state level as well. Furthermore, millions of users of these substances are breaking the law and risk imprisonment. When so many people break the same laws, it becomes evident that the government is suffering from sociocultural lag whereby its laws conflict with the behavior of its citizens in the same way they did during prohibition of alcohol in the 1920s. This time, however, licensed therapists who guide their patients in psychedelic experiences risk losing their license and possible criminal prosecution. How can medical providers who have committed to supporting people in healing deny their clients modalities known to be effective without experiencing great ethical dilemmas? Given these limitations, the public is being deprived of information about, and access to, an entire class of medicines with dramatic potential for healing as well as creativity.

Together, we can continue to create a future in which the scientific study of all substances is legal—one in which no scientific inquiry is criminalized. As good citizens, we need to stay vigilant in our critiques of our government, given that even when striving to do good, governments can do harm. I hope that this book, and others like it, will help make it possible for researchers and therapists to work openly with psychedelics and make their results available to all those who can benefit. Our mission is to recognize our government's history of making illegal that which it fears as a challenge to the maintenance of power, and to help our government understand that human flourishing is achieved by aligning each citizen with their most powerful self, their most healed self, ultimately building a more harmonious, innovative, and flourishing society.

Notes

1   Sandoz was the laboratory where Albert Hoffman first synthesized LSD in 1938.
2   Sinclair was released after two years in prison when his 10-year sentence was overturned by the Michigan Supreme Court; then 50 years later, in 2019, he was among the first people to purchase recreational marijuana in Michigan.
3   A study of adverse events reported to the FDA from 1997 to 2005 found zero deaths caused primarily by cannabis and an average of 31 deaths per year in which cannabis was a contributing factor (Deaths from marijuana, 2019).
4   Holotropic Breathwork is a therapeutic technique developed by Stanislav Grof for achieving altered states of consciousness through rapid breathing over an extended period. It is said by its adherents to facilitate emotional healing and personal growth.

References

Alcoholics Anonymous. (1984). *"Pass it on:" The story of Bill Wilson and how the A.A. message reached the world.* Alcoholics Anonymous World Services.

Bancroft, C. (2012). Emplotting immigration: The rhetoric of border narratives. *Cognitive Semiotics, 4*(2), 40–56. https://doi.org/10.1515/cogsem.2012.4.2.40

Byock, I. (2018). Taking psychedelics seriously. *Journal of Palliative Medicine, 21*(4), 417–421.

Carhart-Harris, R. L. (2020, June 8). We can no longer ignore the potential of psychedelic drugs to treat depression | Robin Carhart-Harris. *The Guardian.* Retrieved March 17, 2022, from www.theguardian.com/commentisfree/2020/jun/08/psychedelic-drugs-treat-depression

Carhart-Harris, R. L., Muthukumaraswamy, S., Roseman, L., Kaelen, M., Droog, W., Murphy, K., Tagliazucchi, E., Schenberg, E. E., Nest, T., Orban, C., Leech, R., Williams,

L. T., Williams, T. M., Bolstridge, M., Sessa, B., McGonigle, J., Sereno, M. I., Nichols, D., Hellyer, P. J., . . . Nutt, D. J. (2016). Neural correlates of the LSD experience revealed by multimodal neuroimaging. *Proceedings of the National Academy of Sciences, 113*(17), 4853–4858. https://doi.org/10.1073/pnas.1518377113

The cocain habit. (1901). *JAMA: The Journal of the American Medical Association, 36*(5), 330. https://doi.org/10.1001/jama.1901.02470050034011

Cockburn, A., & St. Clair, J. (1998). *Whiteout: The CIA, drugs and the press.* Verso.

Costandi, M. (2014). A brief history of psychedelic psychiatry. *The Guardian.* Retrieved November 3, 2022, from www.theguardian.com/science/neurophilosophy/2014/sep/02/psychedelic-psychiatry

Dahlberg, C. C., Mechanek, R., & Feldstein, S. (1968). LSD research: The impact of lay publicity. *American Journal of Psychiatry, 125*(5), 685–689. https://doi.org/10.1176/ajp.125.5.685

Deaths from marijuana vs. FDA-approved drugs—medical marijuana—procon.org. (2019, October 17). *Medical Marijuana.* Retrieved March 17, 2022, from https://medicalmarijuana.procon.org/deaths-from-marijuana-vs-fda-approved-drugs/

DiVito, A. J., & Leger, R. F. (2020). Psychedelics as an emerging novel intervention in the treatment of substance use disorder: A review. *Molecular Biology Reports, 47*(12), 9791–9799. https://doi.org/10.1007/s11033-020-06009-x

Doblin, R. (1998). Dr. Leary's concord prison experiment: A 34-year follow-up study. *Journal of Psychoactive Drugs, 30*(4), 419–426. doi: 10.1080/02791072.1998.10399715

Elijah, J. S. (2002, October 13). Casualties of the war on drugs. *The Boston Globe.*

Emerson, A. (2016, November 3). Treating PTSD with MDMA-assisted therapy (2016): Multidisciplinary association for psychedelic studies. *MAPS.org.* Retrieved March 17, 2022, from https://maps.org/news/bulletin/mdma-ptsd-2016/

Ezekiel, E., Greytak, E., Madubuonwu, B., Sanchez, T., Beiers, S., Resing, C., Fernandez, P., & Galai, S. (2020, April 20). A tale of two countries: Racially targeted arrests in the era of marijuana reform. *ACLU.org.* Retrieved March 17, 2022, from www.aclu.org/report/tale-two-countries-racially-targeted-arrests-era-marijuana-reform

Griffiths, R. R., Johnson, M. W., Carducci, M. A., Umbricht, A., Richards, W. A., Richards, B. D., Cosimano, M. P., & Klinedinst, M. A. (2016). Psilocybin produces substantial and sustained decreases in depression and anxiety in patients with life-threatening cancer: A randomized double-blind trial. *Journal of Psychopharmacology, 30*(12), 1181–1197. https://doi.org/10.1177/0269881116675513

Hill, A. (2012, August 23). LSD could help alcoholics stop drinking, AA founder believed. *The Guardian.* Retrieved March 17, 2022, from www.theguardian.com/science/2012/aug/23/lsd-help-alcoholics-theory

Leary, T., & Alpert, R. (1964). *The psychedelic experience: A manual based on the Tibetan book of the dead.* Penguin.

Leary, T., & Metzner, R. (1968). Use of psychedelic drugs in prisoner rehabilitation. *British Journal of Social Psychiatry, 2*(27).

Lee, M. A. (2013). *Smoke signals, a social history of marijuana.* Scribner.

LoBianco, T. (2016, March 24). Report: Aide says Nixon's war on drugs targeted blacks, hippies | CNN politics. *CNN.* Retrieved March 17, 2022, from www.cnn.com/2016/03/23/politics/john-ehrlichman-richard-nixon-drug-war-blacks-hippie/index.html

Mithoefer, M., Feduccia, A. A., Jerome, L., Mithoefer, A. T., Wagner, M., Walsh, Z., et al. (2019). MDMA-assisted psychotherapy for treatment of PTSD: Study design and rationale for Phase 3 trials based on pooled analysis of six Phase 2 randomized controlled trials. *Psychopharmacology* (Berlin), *236*, 2735–2745.

Mithoefer, M., Grob, C., & Brewerton, T. (2016). Novel psychopharmacological therapies for psychiatric disorders: Psilocybin and MDMA. *The Lancet Psychiatry, 3*(5), 481–488.

Newton, D. E. (2016). Hamilton Wright (1867–1917). In *Prescription drug abuse: A reference handbook*. Essay, ABC-CLIO, LLC; an imprint of ABC-CLIO, LLC.

Nielson, J., & Megler, J. (2014). Ayahuasca as a candidate therapy for PTSD. In *The therapeutic use of ayahuasca* (pp. 41–58). Springer.

Oram, M. (2018). *The trials of psychedelic therapy: LSD psychotherapy in America*. JHU Press.

Passie, T. (2021). History of the use of hallucinogens in psychiatric treatment. In C. Grob & J. Grigsby (Eds.), *Handbook of medical hallucinogens* (pp. 95–120). Guilford Press.

Phelps, J., Shah, R. N., & Lieberman, J. A. (2022). The rapid rise in investment in psychedelics: Cart before the horse. *JAMA Psychiatry, 79*(3), 189–190. doi: 10.1001/jamapsychiatry.2021.3972

Richter, D. (2020, January 12). When Sears sold cocaine. *Commercial News*. Retrieved March 17, 2022, from www.commercial-news.com/community/richter-when-sears-sold-cocaine/article_18040136-33bf-11ea-a4f4-fb8171cc1262.html

Ross, S., Bossis, A., Guss, J., Agin-Liebes, G., Malone, T., Cohen, B., Mennenga, S. E., Belser, A., Kalliontzi, K., Babb, J., Su, Z., Corby, P., & Schmidt, B. L. (2016). Rapid and sustained symptom reduction following psilocybin treatment for anxiety and depression in patients with life-threatening cancer: A randomized controlled trial. *Journal of Psychopharmacology, 30*(12), 1165–1180. https://doi.org/10.1177/0269881116675512

Schwartz, C. (2017, May 6). Molly at the Marriott: Inside America's premier psychedelics conference. *The New York Times*. Retrieved March 17, 2022, from www.nytimes.com/2017/05/06/style/psychedelic-drug-resurgence-daily-life.html

Sigafoos, J., Green, V. A., Edrisinha, C., & Lancioni, G. E. (2007). Flashback to the 1960s: LSD in the treatment of autism. *Developmental Neurorehabilitation, 10*(1), 75–81.

Smith, C. M. (1958). A new adjunct to the treatment of alcoholism: The hallucinogenic drugs. *Quarterly Journal of Studies on Alcohol, 19*(3), 406–417. https://doi.org/10.15288/qjsa.1958.19.406

Trickey, E. (2018, January 4). Inside the story of America's 19th-century opiate addiction. *Smithsonian.com*. Retrieved March 17, 2022, from www.smithsonianmag.com/history/inside-story-americas-19th-century-opiate-addiction-180967673/

U.S. Department of Health & Human Services. (2020, April 28). Tobacco-related mortality. *Centers for Disease Control and Prevention*. Retrieved March 17, 2022, from www.cdc.gov/tobacco/data_statistics/fact_sheets/health_effects/tobacco_related_mortality/index.htm

When Bobby Kennedy defended LSD: Multidisciplinary association for psychedelic studies. (2012, July 12). *MAPS*. Retrieved March 17, 2022, from https://maps.org/news/media/3152-when-bobby-kennedy-defended-lsd

Williams, E. H. (1914, February 8). Negro cocaine "fiends" are new Southern menace. *The New York Times*, p. 12.

Williams, L. (1999, April 1). Human psychedelic research: A historical and sociological analysis: Multidisciplinary association for psychedelic studies. *MAPS*. Retrieved March 17, 2022, from https://maps.org/1999/04/01/human-psychedelic-research-a-historical-and-sociological-analysis/

Wright, H. (1909, February 1–26). *Report of the international opium commission, Shanghai, China*. Rep. Shanghai: North-China Daily News & Herald, 1909. Archive.org, 17 March 2010. Web. 17 August 2014. https://archive.org/details/cu31924032583225

Chapter 3

Decolonizing Psychedelic Therapy

A Prayer for Awareness, Call for Commitment, and Offering of Applications

Danielle M. Herrera

This chapter will focus on fostering dialogue between post-colonial studies and the field of psychedelic-assisted therapy with the intention of generating questions and animating practices related to decolonizing the work. The author will provide key considerations and points of inquiry pertaining to the amelioration of neo-colonial practices in the field—allowing clinicians, educators, and students of psychedelic therapy to adopt a framework that is attuned to systemic oppression that impacts the individual and perpetuates colonization within the treatment and society as a whole.

A Decolonized Introduction and Intention: Part 1

May I begin this chapter with a blessing, to that which is in you, dear reader, which will receive that which is in me. Thank you for your openness. May this be an offering to the medicines, peoples, lands, and Spirit that have entrusted upon me this voice. In reciprocity, we return our graces with the decolonial embodied—offerings through language and form, to empower the ancient new world, who is already on her way.

> COLONIALISM. Definition: turning bodies into cages that no one has the keys for.
>
> (Billy-Ray Belcourt, 2015, para. 10)

Disclaimers

We could explore this topic in great depth beyond these pages, so it becomes necessary to begin with a few tender disclaimers. A full review of the historical context of Western colonialism and decolonial efforts is beyond the scope of this chapter. Building on the tremendous work of post-colonial studies, intersectional feminism, critical race theory, harm reduction therapy, and liberation psychology, this chapter will provide practical applications clinicians can utilize to integrate a decolonial commitment and approach into their therapy practice, most specifically, in psychedelic therapies. Because this topic is vast and complex, I encourage you to explore

DOI: 10.4324/9781003167976-3

beyond these pages (for further discussion of Western colonialism and decolonial approaches to psychotherapy, see Duran, 2019; Watkins & Shulman, 2008; Comas-Díaz & Rivera, 2020).

What Is Decolonization?

Decolonization is the process of undoing colonialism. Decolonization has no synonym; it is a distinct project separate from civil and human rights or social justice endeavors. It is not about "fixing" colonial institutions. It is not reform. Decolonization is not a metaphor (Tuck & Yang, 2012); rather, it is what Eric Ritskes (2012) calls a "tangible unknown," a goal but never an endpoint, an ideal decolonized sovereign nation future to be navigated toward, albeit a place we cannot truly return to, as the colonized cannot ever be truly decolonized. Decolonization is what Corntassel (2017) calls "everyday acts of resurgence," which regenerate Indigenous knowledge, epistemologies, and ways of life. Indigenous knowledge is always adapting, always creating, and always moving forward. Decolonization is an action, a practice, and often as necessarily dangerous, violent, and unsettling as settling itself was and remains today.

A critical reminder here as we traverse further into our discussion of decolonizing psychotherapy: paradoxically, psychotherapy cannot ever be decolonized. A decolonized academia is a contradiction; it is not honest. We can be in action, but we must admit to who/what we are and how/why we are situated with the privileges afforded to us through engaging with academia on Indigenous land. Much like Ibram X. Kendi's (2019) central message in his bestseller *How to Be an Anti Racist* that the opposite of "racist" is not "not racist" but more truly, "anti-racist"—the opposite of "colonized" is not "decolonized" but rather in action: decolonial, decolonizing, and anti-colonial. And as to not undermine true Indigenous activist work, you may consider using words, such as decenter, disinvest, or the like to capture more appropriately the work you *are* doing, at least until you are truly willing and able to *not use decolonization as a metaphor* (Tuck & Yang, 2012). Utilizing Kendi's framework, undoing colonialism thus involves constantly identifying and describing the colonial and then actively dismantling it. This allows for flow of learning and unlearning in these unfixed identities. As much as one can be racist one minute and an anti-racist the next, our minds and practices can be colonial in one minute and decolonial in the next. Thus, a commitment to undoing colonialism is a commitment to radical transformation of the psyche, all while acknowledging the harms done to and by us as individuals and community.

Speaking to those of us in the field of Western mental health, no matter our embodied role: there is blood on our hands. Despite our purest intentions to provide space for various forms of healing, historical harms cannot be undone. Nor shall they be forgotten. While I will name some examples of these harms throughout this writing, know this is but a scratch on the surface of the deep intergenerational and transgenerational wounding that has resulted from colonialism within the field. While taking care to not reclaim and appropriate

Indigenous practices, we are initiated with the complex task of reanimating and honoring Indigenous ways of being for all, as colonialism—and its embeddedness in structures and systems that sustain us—harms us all.

It feels appropriate here to thank you, reader, for holding this grief so far. May we promise purpose in the grief, as it is grief that compels us to do something, to love more. Judith Butler (2004) argues that grief furnishes "a sense of political community of a complex order and it does this first of all by bringing to the fore the relational ties that have implications for theorizing fundamental dependency and ethical responsibility" (p. 22). Collectively, we show up, in honor of this grief. Thank you for being here. And so our grief becomes an invitation to this community and the practice of decolonizing.

Colonization is the birthplace of supremacy and capitalism, and the byproduct of supremacy and capitalism is trauma. This is captured brilliantly in Figure 3.1 created by Rupa Marya, MD.

As you land on the demarcation of "Trauma" in this flowchart, I ask you to breathe into the sense of "you are here," in acknowledgment of both your own traumas and the traumas of clients you may serve. Notice how this is experienced in your body, for the holding of the self and your clients. Note how, in modern Western medicine, the healers of trauma are those designated therapists. The new age of trauma therapy thus demands an engagement with decolonial perspectives and

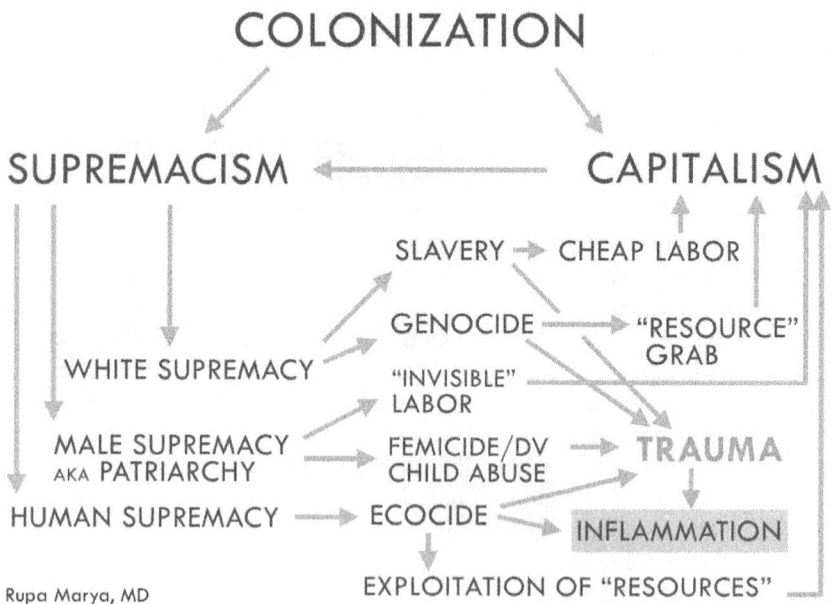

Figure 3.1 Colonization (Marya, 2018)

practices toward an abundant unknown that we feel within our bones—our internal and inexplicable knowing of another possible world. In the liminal space with our clients in this work, we build this world. In this community with our clients, we reimagine our futures.

The epistemological, ontological, and cosmological relationship that Indigenous peoples have with the land moves toward restoration in the practice of decolonization. What is demarcated in the structure of colonialism as "pre-modern" or "savage" is destroyed. In Indigenous time that is not linear but more circular in its pattern, decolonial efforts heal actively and impact the present moment. Through this work as an overarching therapeutic practice, lineages and futures are healed.

A Decolonized Introduction and Intention: Part 2

And so we begin again, now with an alternative offering to habitual colonial communication within an academic setting. Instead of the verbal curriculum vitae that perpetuates hierarchy, I will introduce myself through lineage and story, prioritizing a reciprocal relationship through the written word. Acknowledging: that which *is* in you can only hear that which *is* in me when we both exist beyond our limited titles and names. I encourage a similar practice in how you tell your story to colleagues, friends, clients, and communities alike.

Thank you for being here, my name is Danielle, or Dani. I love people for a living. I am the daughter of Lisa, who is mothered by my Chiricahua Apache and Mexican Grandmother and fathered by my Filipino Grandfather. I am the daughter of John, who is mothered by my Mestiza Grandmother and my Pascua Yaqui Grandfather. I come from a lineage of medicine people and mystics, often lacking the container in which to thrive; I come from a lineage of drug users, sex workers, and hard workers. I grew up in various hoods of Los Angeles, primarily the southernmost port-town of Tongva territory, "San Pedro"—far from my ancestral roots. I am a sister, an auntie, a friend, a lover, and a poet. I am forever learning. I show up for everyday practices of decolonization in my chosen forms of art and loving. I embody the role of a psychotherapist now; this is my art and my loving. I am accountable to the harms done by and to my ancestors. I am accountable to my community. I write to you from the unceded land of the Chochenyo Ohlone, otherwise known as "Oakland," California. This land is graciously cultivated by the rematriation efforts of Sogorea Te' Land Trust.[1]

I was raised separated from many aspects of my people and my culture due to a history of forced assimilation, colonialism, and genocide. I am a queer, detribalized, mixed-Indigenous woman. While I have been blessed to be raised with many rich elements of connection to my ancestry, I have also embodied countless internalized teachings of colonialism throughout my being. To this day, and tomorrow, I will continue in practices of healing this soul wound. This soul wound has led me to my work. As I work to reclaim my Indigeneity, I seek to understand what right relationship looks like. I know nothing but the truth of an ancestor's demand for me to continue in their lineage of medicine work. In this time, in this context, and in my heart, this is most possible within the field of psychedelic-assisted therapies. I believe psychedelic therapists are often spiritual healers in hiding. I believe these healers can work in ways that do not perpetuate colonial harm or replicate capitalist frameworks. I believe another world is possible and collectively we find our way.

An Introduction to Decolonizing Psychedelic Therapy

The field of psychotherapy is ripe with colonial mentality. Racism and supremacy are woven into the founding ideas of psychology; Stanley Hall's belief in "adolescent races" and Erick Erikson's individualist and sexist stages of development are just a couple examples. Any introductory course on psychology will reveal an entrenchment of colonial mentality, a history that is undeniable in its impact on treatment for individuals and communities today—often despite the best of intentions.

For example, Dr. Cindy Blackstock (2011) asks us to consider the much-revered Maslow's hierarchy of needs—where extreme individualism is idealized as ultimate self-development—which in reality contributes to social injustices and environmental exploitation. Blackstock identifies how this iconic structure prioritizes the individual as removed from the context of community and spirituality and instead offers an alternative: the embracing of Blackfeet Nation beliefs of community, ancestral knowledge, spirituality, and multiple dimensions of reality. In Blackstock's model, Maslow's triangle becomes a tipi, with self-actualization at the base of the tipi, and thus, the foundation on which community actualization is built. Native American scholar and child welfare expert Terry Cross (2007) reimagines the hierarchy as non-hierarchical, with spirituality at the center. With these reimaginings of an otherwise unquestioned psychological groundstone, we cannot help but wonder: *What other foundational psychologies are entrenched in colonization? Which psychologies delegate us with the task of reimagining from the perspective of a decolonized mind?*

The field of psychedelic therapies, while young and much more alternative than its traditional ancestor, remains guilty (on multiple counts) of colonial entrenchment. Although many protocols for psychedelic therapies are adapted, by design, from Indigenous practices, we find these adaptations often leaning more toward appropriation than a truly reciprocal or right relationship. For example, some psychedelic therapy training programs encourage intention-based ritual and spiritual elements learned from Indigenous cultures. This might include prayer, energetically cleansing the therapy room with herbs, calling in the directions, or engaging in song. Some of these practices may be mindlessly borrowed by Western-trained therapists who received limited exposure to spiritual facilitation, have a limited understanding of cultural appropriation, and do not acknowledge or give back to the culture(s) they borrow from. The true teachings of integrity around cultural ritual and ceremony are then lost, and therapists risk losing the very spirit of medicine work itself.

In August 2019, MAPS invited a cohort of clinicians of color to train in the first-ever MDMA Therapy Training Program for Communities of Color. The intention

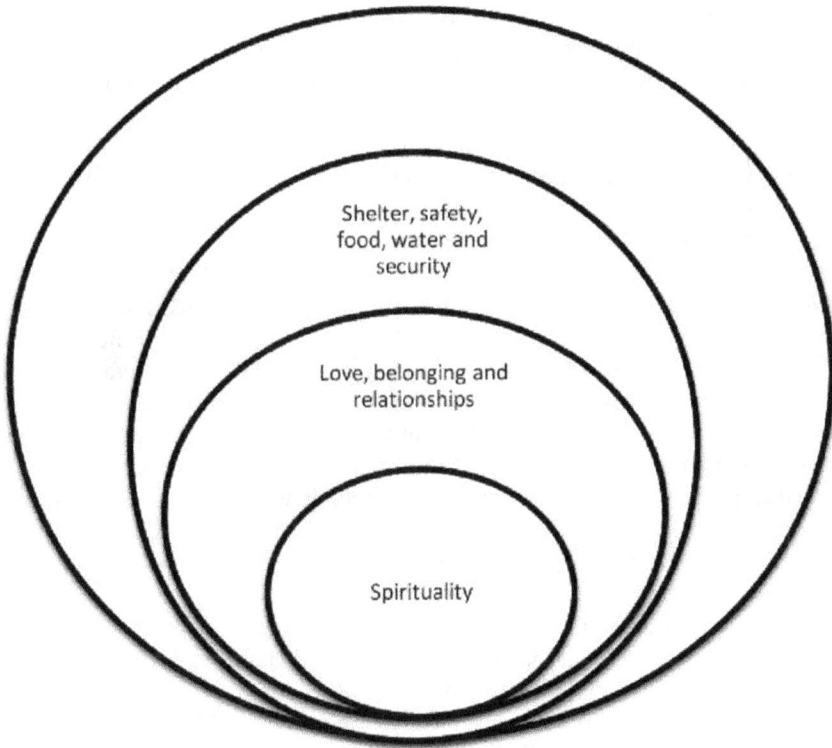

Figure 3.2 Cross (2007) reinterprets Maslow's hierarchy of needs through Indigenous eyes

of this training was primarily to respond to the fact that the field of psychedelic therapy is predominantly white. This predominance, MAPS acknowledged, would undeniably result in issues of access for non-white participants, particularly those seeking support for racialized traumas. In a follow-up statement after the training, Shannon Carlin (2020), MAPS chief of therapy training, addressed one of the harms that had taken place at the training that led to significant rupture followed by a demand for repair. Moving forward, as Carlin names, "required re-establishing the container, this time co-created by the community of the cohort" itself. As a member of this cohort, I found that the most memorable teaching moment of this event occurred when the baton was passed to the wisdom in the room, and the decree of "Spirit First" was made by Belinda Eriacho, MPH of Zuni and Diné lineage, who had taught earlier in the session on intergenerational trauma and its legacy for Native Americans. "Spirit First" was embraced by the cohort, who built an altar of sassafras, flowers, candles, medicines, oracle, and texts of wisdom. The energy of the training room, cohort, and community noticeably shifted by following the intention of prioritizing Spirit—the medicine; the Great; and everything above, below, between, and unseen. I offer this memory as a lesson and a blessing: may we learn from the grace that is masked by these experiences of discomfort. May we intimately know that Spirit must be prioritized in this evolution of medicine work—in psychedelic therapy. Misattunement to this teaching is an invitation to rupture—ruptures that we want to carefully prevent in the holding of those beautiful beings landing on the demarcation of trauma.

Franz Fanon (1963), a psychiatrist and decolonial theoretician, speaks of the notable group of "colonized intellectuals" bred from colonialism, who struggle in their desire to relate to culture under colonialism while fighting colonialism. Are psychedelic therapists, researchers, and educators, with their academic degrees and board licenses, akin to these colonized intellectuals? Are those in this field exempt from replicating harm, even when we fight for social justice and practice from systemic or feminist theoretical frameworks, cultural sensitivity and humility, and decolonial application? Absolutely not. Thus, Fanon speaks to the undeniable need to radically transform the curriculum. Applying this theory to the field of psychedelic therapy, just an infant at the time of this writing, we hold her like so: demanding radical protection from the very indoctrination and socialization that breeds supremacy and capitalism—colonization, under our noses. When not protected, often without our consent or awareness, our ability to rethink alternatives and what could be possible is foreclosed. The work of psychedelic therapy must remain committed to representing the truth, not a facsimile, of what decolonization of therapy looks like. This line of work is a return.

And so we ask, what is it that we bring to the collective table in this practice? A pill? A lozenge? A silver bullet? Or an entirely new approach to psychospiritual healing? If nothing more convinces you of the need to prioritize a decolonized lens in the field of psychedelic therapy, let it be this: there is a moment when the relationship between an individual and a medicine offers an opening, an opportunity for a changed narrative. In this moment, an orchestrator of space provides a set and setting that resurrect Spirit and ritual. This moment calls into question belief systems that position healing as passive and purchased (capitalism), isolated (individualist over communal), occurring solely through talking rather than being (cognitive over embodied/emotionally expressive), and separated from the divine (personal rather than transpersonal). In this moment, entire cultures are remembered. Culture is medicine. Medicine is culture.

Decolonizing psychedelic therapy thus begins with Spirit. Spirit as in the ineffable, as in the nameless thread of everything that is. This is the first of all practical considerations, and everything else follows. And everything else must be enrobed in it.

In this chapter, we seek to prioritize the intention of being accessible, thus offering techniques in language that feel digestible to all, regardless of education and ability to digest academic media. While decolonizing therapy is a topic in infancy at the time of this publication, much has been explored in the epistemology of decolonial theory, which can be applied to our topic of interest. For example, one may benefit wildly from utilizing the framework of the *Processes of Decolonization* by Poka Laenui (2006), which is written through the author's observations based on her personal experience with colonization of Hawai'i: I find her work to be deeply relevant and applicable to client work. Laenui suggests five phases of decolonization:

1. Rediscovery and recovery
2. Grieving
3. Dreaming
4. Commitment
5. Action

There are no clear demarcations between the steps, nor must they be held to strict completion; the specificity of Leanui's steps may be incredibly helpful for minds across the range of neurodiversity who benefit from distinct phases in a clear sequence.

Similarly, Quijano's (2000) seminal article offers a lens through which we can identify coloniality, thus offering a framework for the decolonial. Quijano describes the colonial matrix of power as occurring in four interrelated domains:

1. Control of economy (land appropriation, exploitation of labor, and control of natural resources)
2. Control of authority (institution and army)
3. Control of gender and sexuality (family and education)
4. Control of subjectivity and knowledge (epistemology, education, and formation of subjectivity)

A therapist can be aware of these domains and collaboratively engage with the client to identify where colonial control impacts them. Collaboratively exploring a client's suffering through a lens that understands the all-pervasive structures of colonialism provides opportunities for personal and cultural healing and empowerment.

For example, a client may express tension in their experience of gender binaries and another day describe challenges accessing nutrient-dense foods. Both of these scenarios could be approached by holding space for the ambiguous yet profound grief of colonialism—the forgotten celebrations of gender expansion and the loss of biodiversity of Indigenous plants. Violence and all, how liberating it can feel to hear, "It makes so much sense that you are feeling this way when your context is a colonial structure that continues to harm you." Compare this to the basic reflection "you are hurting," or tone-deaf reframing, "Well, things are looking up regarding gender!," or solution, "I wonder if you can order some supplements online?" Postcolonial frameworks, like Quijano's, offer a way of thinking that can be applied to therapy and support the movement toward individual and collective liberation. We move toward, and outward—far from systems that otherwise feel like an inevitable perpetuation of colonial traumas—an ongoing practice for dismantling systems of oppression. So, where can we start when the language and access to these theories feel distant?

Practical Applications of Decolonizing Work in Psychedelic Therapy

Decolonizing the Psyche (Your Psyche, First)

Chicana cultural theorist Gloria Anzaldúa's (1987) decolonial magnum opus, *Borderlands/La Frontera* is ripe with offerings for overpowering coloniality. Anzaldúa focuses on the inner life and consciousness of the mestiza to suggest that the most critical decolonial efforts occur within the psyche, emphasizing the danger of internalized colonialism and its ability to strip our sense of self. To Anzaldúa, "the struggle has always been inner, and is played out in the outer terrains" where "nothing happens in the 'real' world unless it first happens in the images in our heads" (p. 109). Anzaldúa suggests that no decolonial progress can be achieved in the physical realm without first occurring in the liminal space of the psyche, without first involving abolishment of internalized colonialism.

Here. In your body, first. With consent from our ancestors. Listen to the land of your inner and outer being. To commit to decolonizing psychedelic therapy, you must first name your intention to do so and begin with your own intergenerational and ancestral trauma work. Decolonizing our psyches starts by reconnecting to our roots. Where are your roots? How are they interconnected? With whom do they connect you? Ask. Ask elders, ask mentors, ask psyche. Your own psychotherapy. Your own healing practices. Your own decolonial research. Your own rematriation of nature, land, community, and Spirit. However, this may look for you. However it looks, notice. Ask yourself and your kin some important questions, expand.

- Where have I created false binaries? Where have I mislabeled myself or others?
- What embodiments of mine have been in reaction to violent systems?
- What ancestral wounds do I hold in my body? When and where have I reacted from my ancestral wounds?
- What do my practices of decolonization look like now? What does my decolonization work look like moving forward?
- What are the evaluative criteria I check in with before I react, share, and respond?
- How can I react, share, and respond from a place of already being liberated from oppressive systems—even if I am not fully liberated?
- How can I engage in dialogue that is mutually reinforced by the motivation for collective liberation, rather than to protect or serve my ego?

In your body. Remembering to tend to the grief that emerges in our bodies when we initiate a healing process upon the land of a colonial culture. Remembering Spirit and the senses, bringing rest and spaciousness to the mind. When we embrace our somatic awareness, we become embodied, and this welcomes embodiment in others. Through our connection to our body and its relationship to other bodies, including the natural world around us, we are unable to forget our role in a system that functions through interconnectedness and collectively. Here, we cannot be alone. Here, we are embraced by ecosystems and ancestors and resourced through wisdom and strength that do not end at our own fingertips. Here, we can access spiritual elements that live beyond the periphery of the skin. Here, we offer embodied medicines to clients. Here, we breathe, and we ask about colonialism:

- How does colonialism show up in my own daily rituals and ceremonies?
- How does colonialism show up in the clinical work I do?
- How might I lean into hierarchies without awareness?
- How might I overvalue the written word?
- How might I overvalue the individual and dismiss the collective in my approach?
- How do I panic or move to "fix;" how do I try to make something or someone "better"?
- How might I prioritize logic and reason over what is happening in the body?
- How do I place value on colleagues and clients based on their education and wealth?
- How do I navigate the guilt and shame that come up when doing this work?
- How do I navigate my own imposter syndrome?

This work will look different for each of us, as we are all unique and all have a colonizer within. This is nothing to be ashamed of, just something to be aware of and to respond to in the promise of liberation. Just keep showing up. Do not forget, we are making this up as we go. Deeper and deeper, into the tangible unknown.

Decolonizing the Process

Traditional schools of counseling theory hold an underlying assumption that people are independent and individualistic, and often neglect to look at how individuals are impacted by the wider culture, systems of oppression, and access to privilege and power. Psychological symptoms resulting from systemic oppression and violence are often pathologized as individual faults—failures to "adjust" to or "function" within "mainstream society"—rather than seen for what they are: psychological manifestations of the multifaceted struggles that many face navigating oppressive institutions and macrosystems. American Indians and Alaskan Natives, for example, experience significantly higher rates of mental health problems than the general population of the United States due to their long history of colonization, genocide, systemic oppression, and resulting cultural and intergenerational trauma (American Psychiatric Association, n.d.). When this population enters a traditional psychotherapy treatment with rightful difficulty in adjustment, anger, or depression, they will likely have their struggles framed through an individualist lens, be it cognitive errors, maladaptive behaviors, or their limited ability to cope. Moreover, there is a good chance that their collectivist culture and lifestyle may be misunderstood or even pathologized. A shift to a decolonizing approach to therapy requires a shift away from the focal point of individualism, which breeds oppression and perpetuates trauma in the very populations most in need of mental health services.

In a Rewire article on the topic of decolonizing therapy, Dr. Jennifer Mullan, a clinical psychologist who utilizes Instagram for her platform @decolonizingtherapy, explains "decolonizing therapy involves looking at how the mental health industrial complex continues to inflict a lot of harm on people because it chooses to remain apolitical" (Varanasi, 2021). Mullan speaks to the overdiagnosis of Black, Indigenous, and People of Color children, when the stigmatization of black and brown skin occurs alongside the stigma of a mental illness diagnosis, ultimately risking funneling these children into the school to prison pipeline and juvenile justice system. When attempting to write about intergenerational trauma and racism in her dissertation, Mullan notes that she felt discouraged, as psychologists are "not supposed to be political." Thus, she posits that while traditional therapy can be beneficial, it may just be inadequate for folks who need an oppression-focused approach. As practitioners of psychedelic therapy, we must commit to cultivating a decolonized lens in the service of being not just adequate or "good enough," but *exceptional* when it comes to our attunement to the systemic oppression and violence that impact our clients and communities within complicated and historically harmful ecosystems.

How do we learn from other psychotherapy theorists other than Sigmund Freud and Carl Jung? Or even from psychedelic therapy theorists other than Stanlisov Grof and Ralph Metzner? How can we remember that these healing traditions are millennia old? How might we look back into our own ancestral lineages for wisdom on individual and collective healing through plant medicine? Can our collective imagination, guided by the wisdom of our ancestors, be a primary source of the evidence in evidence-based practice? Can we respect the value of practice-based evidence? Perhaps our ancestors have already completed the research and engaged in generations of peer review. Can we trust our intuitive sense? The blueprints of these practices are inscribed in our bodies and emerge into consciousness as an offering—may we receive.

Decolonizing the Medicine

Psychedelic therapists must develop respectful relationships to the medicines we use and through this process reanimate medicines as entities with Spirit, rather than laboratory-designed drugs. When we invite a client into a relationship with a medicine, we are given the opportunity to offer not only a psychoactive molecule or a novel experience but an entirely new way of being. Language holds the power to cast spells for healing. When we shift away from the materialist language of Western science and rename a drug as "medicine," we give the body space to expand into healing, rather than contract into the many stigmas, biases, and cultural traumas associated with the term "drug." Beyond the name, we are invited to consider the origin story of our medicines, back to their plant ancestors. For example, MDMA, designated a breakthrough treatment when combined with psychotherapy, is the descendant of *Sassafras albidum*, a genus of a tree native to eastern North America and eastern Asia. When we name and honor this tree in our medicine work, we reanimate a lineage of healing and re-invite Earth into the therapeutic container.

We may consider having an actual representation of the plant ancestor—its bark, oil, or leaf, on an altar or in the session room, and we may make offerings to these living symbols. We may be intentional about the containers that hold our medicines, considering the energies held in plastics, for example, compared to materials of the earth. We may serve medicines using materials that are designed with care and story, heirloom spoons, or crafts of local tribes. Depending on how appropriate it is with individual clients, we may write to, sing with, speak among, or invoke the spirits of these medicines and the medicine's own ancestors, guardians, and guides. We may even make space to acknowledge, if appropriate and beneficial to the client, the profound privilege it is to heal with the help of these medicines, and even name and honor the stories of individuals and communities whose lives have been harmed or lost by the War on Drugs. We may keep a symbol on the altar to apologize for these systematic harms and injustices, and hold those impacted in memory.

In a similar vein, we may work with the grief and loss that exist on the trail toward this psychedelic renaissance we now find ourselves in. We can acknowledge the mistakes we have made in our journey toward recognizing the transformative power of these medicines, and the ignorances and biases in our relationships to drugs, drug culture, and people who use drugs. We must not miss the opportunity to name the harms done by psychedelic exceptionalism—the belief that psychedelics are "good" drugs and non-psychedelics and therefore their users are "bad." Psychedelic therapists and the community that surrounds this work hold a depth of power and responsibility to change the narrative around all drugs. They can use their platform to retell the stories of drug use toward its truth of being overwhelmingly positive and life enhancing with tremendous potential for healing, as opposed to perpetuating the stigma, policy, and war that have resulted in epidemic levels of criminalization and death.

In his book, *Drug Use for Grown-Ups*, renowned professor and neuroscientist Dr. Carl L. Hart (2021) argues that the greatest damage from drugs flows from their being illegal. He identifies that much of our perceptions of drugs has little to do with the psychoactive chemicals themselves, and much more to do with our deeply internalized racism and discriminations against the user and the body they inhabit. Dr. Hart—along with communities of harm reductionists, drug policy leaders, clinicians, and drug users alike—are demanding decriminalization and de-stigmatization of all drugs, not just those currently in the form of "nature." This retelling honors the stories of the bodies who have lost their freedoms or their lives in the very search for expanded consciousness that we hail as "breakthrough therapy." If decolonization is an act of resurgence, may we bring back the dead and abolish the systems that unjustly allow drug use to be healing for one and fatal to another.

Practicing decolonial medicine work is harm reductionist in nature, that is, we acknowledge the relationship between the user and the drug as just that—*a relationship*. One in which both bodies are powerful, and neither more powerful than the other (as opposed to the traditional 12-step model where admitting power-lessness is the first step in healing). We also acknowledge the ability of the user to reduce the risks associated with a drug as well as to maximize the benefits.

Decolonizing the Setting

The process of decolonizing means we are always examining, noticing, and ask-ing why. Why do therapists' counseling rooms and websites look the way they do? What creates the essence of comfort? For whom? Why? Decolonizing the therapeutic space, especially in psychedelic therapy, demands intention and ani-mistic relationship with every aspect of the room. How do we embrace the perspec-tive that everything we are in relationship with is alive and possesses a spiritual essence—and is therefore reciprocally in relationship with us? What can we offer the container that has so generously provided our clients with profound opportuni-ties to be held? What does environmental holding and a well-attuned setting look like across cultures and identities?

The setting in which psychotherapy occurs needs to be intentionally client centered, as any one-size-fits-all approach risks upholding a colonial mentality. Some clients may experience a higher capacity for healing in an outdoor envi-ronment, perhaps better able to process stimuli when moving. Some clients may prefer being indoors during therapy, but still benefit from access to elements and materials that represent the natural world. As we consider this, we might notice how these suggestions conflict with traditional psychotherapy teachings. Can therapy occur outside? Why not? Can I bring a bowl of water into therapy for a client who I feel may benefit from connecting with this element in session? Can I accept an offering of food? If no, why not? Do we give ourselves permis-sion to have art supplies if we are not trained art therapists? How might we bring music into psychedelic therapy in a way that enhances our clients' healing? Do we feel the freedom to have music in sessions that are not medicine sessions? Do we allow ourselves to have decor or art on the walls that expresses our beliefs? Where are our limits in regard to disclosure, and how much permission do we feel to share? Do we notice how these questions sound akin to self-policing, the cop in our head, the colonizer?

If you share community or connection with somebody who identifies as Indig-enous to Turtle Island, you may have heard the demand for "land back." Much like decolonization, this is no metaphor. Still, I call upon those who are committed to decolonizing therapy to view decolonizing the setting as a practice of "land back." While not enough, while never replicating the true, necessary return of physical land, here we are, at the very least, reclaiming a healing space as a space for radi-cal liberation. Beyond empty land acknowledgments and performative practices of cultural sensitivity, the space of psychedelic therapy becomes an offering to re-indigenize. It is a reclamation of the reciprocal relationship. What I give I receive in return.

Decolonizing the Therapeutic Relationship

The relationship between a therapist and a client is sacred; it is a third entity born from the cumulation of interactions between the two individuals—magic in all senses of the word. An agreement mutually held with the intention to heal. This space, this exchange, this dance is nothing less than a radical expression of hope in commitment to healing: an interactional, alchemical process designed for impact, designed for resilience.

Or, is it flatly a provider being matched with a patient, in the interest of leveraging control over symptoms? Is it a transactional relationship in the interest of receiving a diagnosis or psychiatric drugs to become a more valuable member of society? To "work" more "efficiently"?

Mary Watkins (2015) describes the necessity of decolonization efforts that cultivate interpersonal practices between practitioners and their clients, providing a relational and ethical foundation for joint inquiry, restorative healing, and transformative action. Born from liberation theology then migrating into psychology, Watkins (2015) offers a critical paradigm shift through the concept of *acompanamiento* (accompaniment), in which a reorientation is made by the accompanier (in this case, the therapist): the therapist stands alongside the client and offers listening, witnessing, advocacy, space to develop critical inquiry, and joint action to address desired and needed changes. Jeannie Little of Harm Reduction Therapy Center refers to this stance as "meeting people where they are at" (J. Little, personal communication, 2020). Standing alongside and opening space for folks who need witnessing and advocacy help the collective recover lost memory, awareness, and *conocimiento* (consciousness). Walking with, therefore, becomes the central foundation not only for healing at the individual level but also for collective liberation and decolonization.

By embodying this approach in psychedelic therapy, we reimagine who serves and who heals. The relationship thus gains a newfound quality of reciprocity—a mode of relation central to many Indigenous communities. In a reciprocal dynamic, balance in power is restored and a deep potential for healing becomes accessible. Consider, for example, a reciprocal therapeutic relationship, where both bodies are healing one another, where both therapist and client make offerings and receive gifts. How might this promote healing? How might this cause harm?

There are countless ways therapists are taught to remain professional and private. While many of these practices are critical to maintaining an ethical therapeutic relationship, other practices have become unquestioned tradition and may uphold colonial mentality. When considering psychotherapy ethics and practices, such as professional boundaries, I encourage a reflexive pause. This pause allows clinicians to orient their commitment to decolonization to the concepts of dual/multiple relationships; self-disclosure; inviting a client's loved ones into session; dress/attire; promoting self-care; manner of speech and language; and even the inclusion of divination, ritual, ceremony, and magic within the therapy. How were you introduced to these concepts in your education? How does your relationship to these practices promote healing? How might these practices cause harm? Who benefits? Who is left out? Can you imagine a client who might benefit from a shift in your way of enacting these practices? What does a reciprocal therapeutic relationship mean to you? What might that look like?

Decolonizing Access

It would be irresponsible not to name the need to prioritize accessible psychedelic therapy when discussing decolonizing in this field. "If it is not accessible to the poor, it is neither radical nor revolutionary" (Herrera, n.d.). I admit to struggling to feel balanced when offering psychedelic therapy without an equal commitment to offering lower-threshold services to underserved communities. To achieve accessibility of this modality, it is important for every clinician to consider how to find such a balance in their practice.

Psychedelic therapy must not remain a luxury commodity only for those with enough privilege to afford the high cost of treatment and see it as a viable option. There is much to be said about what makes some cultures and communities feel psychedelic therapy is a safe, viable option, while others do not. Who is psychedelic therapy designed to speak to? Think culture, class, age, gender, sexuality, body, ability, relationship structures, and even symptoms. Who is likely to feel safest with psychedelic therapy in the way it exists today? Who is currently left behind? What changes can clinicians and organizations make to communicate an intention to leave no one behind?

Share this work—may knowledge be accessible beyond academia, beyond continued education units and certificates, and beyond workshops and retreat centers that can feel as if they are invitation only to those with significant wealth. The instructions for how to do this work do not reside in the references. No, the instructions are commonly found in that invisible thread between therapist and client, therapist and therapist, client and client, and all to the soil, to the water, to the sky. Steal this work. May the PDFs fly free. May there be no barriers to our collective healing.

Clinical Considerations for Decolonizing Psychedelic Therapy

Confronting the Mystical

One of the key ways that colonization impacts our inner experience—our relationship to ourselves—is through severing our sense of oneness or union with the Divine (The Creator, Great Spirit, God, etc.). An event as horrifying as colonization can be embodied as a spiritual or religious trauma. The distortion of spiritual relationship under colonialism was an intentional effort to control the masses. When a specific few within a society are named initiates into an intimate relationship with the Divine (for example, a prophet), only a limited number of people, the chosen ones, need to be influenced. The harrowing result then is a few sovereign individuals with markedly disparate power compared to the general population, leaving this latter group with a profound sense of separation from divinity—the original imposter syndrome. The "I am not enough for the divine to commune with me."

Offering recommendations for women of color living "in the borderlands," Gloria Anzaldúa (1987) suggests that one may begin to decolonize their psyche by accessing the spiritual and supernatural. She notes that this key process is precluded by a Western colonial mindset that emphasizes "rationality." In her book *Sacred Instructions*, Sherri Mitchell (2018) notes that "reestablishing an immediate connection to our Creator is one of the most important steps that we can take in ending the hold of colonization in our lives" (p. 95). What does this mean for psychedelic therapists committed to decolonizing themselves, the work, the field? What does this mean for psychedelic therapists whose graduate training may have ignored or even discouraged incorporating divinity, mysticism, and faith into the treatment approach? What does this mean for the work we do with our clients, who courageously embrace the unknown through NOSC with the intention of healing? It would be remiss for me to suggest anything other than an undeniable evolution of this work: psychedelic therapies must embrace the mystical. Of course, spirituality must be held in a client-centered framework—integrated if and when the client desires and consents, never pushing the spiritual, and instead meeting the client where they are at. Psychedelic therapies are decolonial when they embrace the spiritual, as it presents itself, and when they welcome our connection to greater consciousness, from which we are not separate.

At a practical level, it is common for people to have what they would describe as "spiritual" or "mystical" experiences while on psychedelics, even when going into the journey with a staunchly atheist or agnostic belief system. In an article on the topic, Shayla Love (2021) shares the story of a client, Kevin, who held a firm conviction against spirituality in his treatment for opiate dependency. Yet, in his work with the psychedelic medicine ibogaine, Kevin experienced "a power greater than [himself], the nature of the cosmos—nothing supernatural." When working with a therapist to integrate a mystical experience, the meaning a client makes of their experience is greatly impacted by the metaphysical beliefs their therapist holds. In order for experiences, such as Kevin's, to reach their full transformative potential, they must be met with openness; acknowledgment; and reflection of their depth, power, and value.

Matthew Johnson (2021), associate director of Johns Hopkins Center for Psychedelic and Consciousness Research, suggests that psychedelic scientists and clinicians should acquaint themselves with an eclectic collection of mystical traditions, Eastern religions, and Indigenous cultures to truly honor their role in holding this powerful yet delicate work. Clinicians commit to decolonizing psychedelic therapy by preparing themselves for the wide range of theological, cosmological, and ecstatic questions that may arise during psychedelic experiences. A primary undertaking here is attention to not privileging the dominant Judeo-Christian framework that underlies colonial society. A practical application involves commitment to self-exploration and embracing one's own metaphysical and theological questions and experiences. Again, Spirit first.

Lastly, a statement must be made here surrounding the therapist's awareness of their social location and the dominant identities they hold, including how these identities are positioned in relation to spiritual frameworks they introduce to clients. A commitment to decolonial practices in psychedelic therapy involves consistent attention to the ways we perpetuate harm through cultural appropriation by extracting sacred practices from non-dominant groups without reciprocity nor acknowledgment. When mystical or ineffable psychospiritual experiences occur, the mind seeks sense making, and otherwise unfamiliar rituals, ceremonies, and structures of non-dominant cultures' belief systems suddenly feel all too seductive. Dominant identities that hold positions of power have often maintained this seat through severance or disconnection from ancestral practices (for example, Pagan rituals, herbalism, and witchcraft), which, if sustained, would have resulted in more harm to their lineage. The result is what embodiment educator, Camille Barton, calls "the violence of the void:" the "sense of internal emptiness that many white people feel—a sense that there is no culture, no richness, no ancestral wisdom to connect to or lean upon." This void then becomes fertile ground for cultural appropriation or other harms associated with consumption and erasure. Barton's suggestion is a loving reminder to the body of us all, "Do not mistake the void for nothingness . . . we each come from rich histories, lineages filled with joy, loss, trials, tribulations and triumphs" (Barton, 2022). Each of us, gorgeously holding the capacity to fully honor the grief we embody and listen intimately and respond to the communications of the intuitive gut. Each of us, invited to return to a relationship with the seasons, with the unseen, with the ancestral. So abundant, there is no other direction but deeper.

Internalized Oppressions

Decolonizing psychedelic therapy is a commitment to examining the impact of colonialism, capitalism, and imperialism on the well-being of the clients we have the honor of working with. We observe and challenge attributes of these oppressive systems as they are communicated through our clients' embodied experience, and lovingly encourage narratives that embrace abundance, worthiness, and connection. We become intimate with the very structures we aim our arrow at. Intimate enough to name and recognize when internalized colonialism, capitalism, and imperialism are hiding beneath the masks of imposter syndrome, self-doubt, grief, shame, guilt, and fear. These masks are symptoms of a colonial mentality, and it is here that we become curious and compassionate. What is the origin story of these symptoms, and how do they feel familiar? When are these symptoms triggered, and under what circumstances are they quelled? How do these symptoms feel in the body, and what stories are they trying to tell?

Through time and trust with my clients, I will work with them to identify how these symptoms become embodied as internalized capitalism or supremacy.

Lovingly, I will remark at how perfect they were as students of systems, that there is and never will be anything wrong with them for the ways that they have adjusted to and survived these structures. Tenderly, I will get curious with them surrounding the definitions they hold of what "progress" looks like, of what it means to be "healed."

In this practice, we commit to healing that is in collaboration with our clients', our own, and our culture's past and future ancestors. We remember and honor lineage to encourage a sense of connection to an unseen, intangible world and invite space for the ancestral grief that surrounds disconnection, loss, and severance. Within this sorrow there is holy ground, and we build a foundation for the capacity to imagine generations that come after us. As we nourish this capacity for ourselves and our clients, we move toward a world that we know is possible.

Embracing Sacred Joy

As we commit to decolonizing the stories our clients have been told about who they are, we help them find the key that liberates their bodies from the cage of colonialism (Belcourt, 2015); the space around their bodies expands to become a vacancy for joy. Embodiment into the corners that once held self-doubt, grief, and fear allows for a truth of vastness and entitlement to the full sensory experience. Decolonization efforts must honor joy, pleasure, and play as much as they do grief and rage. To experience unapologetic joy as a medicine in and of itself is to open portals into new worlds that are sustained by love. Psychedelic therapists receive quite the responsibility here—many individuals of non-dominant identities may display subtle expressions of guilt, shame, regret, and even self-loathing when experiencing or even considering the experience of joy and pleasure. Can we encourage honoring and working within the paradox—the desire for healing and beauty alongside the experience of pain and suffering? Can we honor the difficulty of this coexistence in bodies that carry legacies positing that grace can be embodied by some, yet not all? Psychedelic therapists have the opportunity to attune to these inconspicuous forces, weaving in ancient worlds where joy and pleasure remain a birthright. Where there is intergenerational trauma, there is also intergenerational joy. We can be victors of play as the primary tool for becoming, much as we know as children. Psychedelic therapists must not forget the ways in which we are play therapists, our clients akin to the young in their intimacy with these medicines. Our spaces are portals. Our work is a practice of renewal, an offering, a way to shift stagnancy, and a connection to ancestral wisdom and to our most eternal self.

Conclusion

May you expand into every question and practice present here, inspiring or forgotten. Within a few years of this writing, the field of psychedelic therapy will be multiplied in its practice, its research, its efficacy, and with hope—its access. Stories of healing through this modality will be known from shorter distances between you and your extended community. Perhaps these stories of healing may be known as close to home as within your own body or those of your immediate kin. As the Spirit of this medicine work embodies and expands, our hands become wider in holding the responsibility of decolonizing the work; the task of protecting against neo-colonial practices that perpetuate when left unchecked; and the honor of bridging worlds we know, remember, and imagine. The practice of decolonization can feel almost ephemeral and perplexing, but I encourage your confidence in the work as an act of resistance. Show up. Stay attuned. Thank you for being here.

Note

1   For more information on the Sogorea Te' Land Trust, see: https://sogoreate-landtrust.org/

References

American Psychiatric Association. (n.d.). *Mental health disparities: American Indians and Alaskan natives fact sheet.* www.psychiatry.org/psychiatrists/cultural-competency/education/mental-health-facts

Anzaldúa, G. (2007). *Borderlands/La Frontera: The new mestiza.* Aunt Lute Books. Original work published 1987)

Barton, C. (2022, June 22). *The violence of the void.* https://xamillearton.medium.com/the-violence-of-the-void-f1f97c202043

Belcourt, B. R. (2015, September 22). Colonialism: A love story. *Billy-Ray Belcourt.* nakinisowin.wordpress.com/2015/09/22/colonialism-a-love-story/

Blackstock, C. (2011). The emergence of the breath of life theory. *Journal of Social Work Values and Ethics, 8.* White Hat Communications. https://jswve.org/download/2011-1/spr11-blackstock-Emergence-breath-of-life-theory.pdf

Butler, J. (2004). Precarious life: The powers of mourning and violence. *Verso.* www.wkv-stuttgart.de/uploads/media/butler-judith-precarious-life.pdf

Carlin, S. (2020). MDMA therapy training for communities of color. *MAPS Bulletin, 30*(Summer, 2). https://maps.org/news/bulletin/articles/444-bulletin-summer-2020/8308-mdma-therapy-training-for-communities-of-color

Comas-Díaz, L., & Rivera, E. (Eds.). (2020). *Liberation psychology: Theory, method, practice, and social justice.* American Psychological Association. Retrieved April 16, 2021, from www.jstor.org/stable/j.ctv1chs1sn

Corntassel, J., & Scow, M. (2017). Everyday acts of resurgence: Indigenous approaches to everydayness in fatherhood. *New Diversities, 19*(2), 55–68. https://newdiversities.mmg.mpg.de/?page_id=3194

Cross, T. (2007, September 20). *Through indigenous eyes: Rethinking theory and practice.* Paper presented at the 2007 Conference of the Secretariat of Aboriginal and Islander Child Care in Adelaide, Australia.

Duran, E. (2019). *Healing the soul wound: Trauma-informed counseling for Indigenous communities* (2nd ed.). Teachers College Press.

Fanon, F. (1963). *The wretched of the earth.* Grove Press.

Hart, C. (2021). *Drug use for grown-ups: Chasing liberty in the land of fear.* Penguin Press.

Herrera, J. (n.d.). https://medium.com/@muloka/this-quote-is-attributed-to-jonathan-her-rera-https-mcad-edu-faculty-jonathan-herrera-f25f0020faf6

Johnson, M. W. (2021). Consciousness, religion, and gurus: Pitfalls of psychedelic medi-cine. *ACS Pharmacology & Translational Science, 4*(2), 578–581. doi: 10.1021/acsptsci.0c00198

Kendi, I. X. (2019). *How to be an antiracist.* One World.

Laenui, P. (2006). *Processes of decolonization.* www.sjsu.edu/people/marcos.pizarro/maestros/Laenui.pdf

Love, S. (2021). Psychedelic therapy needs to confront the mystical. *Vice.* www.vice.com/en/article/xgz3wn/psychedelic-therapy-needs-to-confront-the-mystical

Marya, R. (2018). *Health and justice: The path of liberation through medicine.* Keynote Speech, 2018 National Bioneers Conference. www.youtube.com/watch?v=GyymzSE0VE8

Mitchell, S. (2018). *Sacred instructions: Indigenous wisdom for living spirit-based change.* North Atlantic Books.

Quijano, A., & Ennis, M. (2000). Coloniality of power, eurocentrism, and Latin America. *Nepantla: Views from South, 1*(3), 533–580. www.muse.jhu.edu/article/23906

Ritskes, E. (2012). What is decolonization and why does it matter? *Intercontinental Cry.* https://intercontinentalcry.org/what-is-decolonization-and-why-does-it-matter/

Tuck, E., & Yang, K. W. (2012). Decolonization is not a metaphor. *Decolonization: Indige-neity, Education, & Society, 1*(1).

Varanasi, A. (2021). Decolonizing therapy: Why an apolitical mental health system doesn't work. *Rewire.* www.rewire.org/decolonizing-therapy-mental-health/

Watkins, M. (2015). Psychosocial accompaniment. *Journal of Social and Political Psychol-ogy, 3*(1). http://jspp.psychopen.eu/article/view/103/html

Watkins, M., & Shulman, H. (2008). *Toward psychologies of liberation.* Palgrave Macmillan.

Chapter 4

Liberating Consent

A Kink-Informed Exploration of Consent in Psychedelic-Assisted Therapy

Emma Knighton

This chapter is dedicated to my switchy, witchy ancestors—living and transitioned, of blood and of community. For the right to ritual, for the modeling of liberated embodied expression, and for the reminder of co-constructed pleasure and healing in all consciousness bending forms. Thank you for reminding me who I am, thank you for never giving up, and thank you for showing me the way.

Much of the wisdom in this chapter comes from the queer, kink, and sex worker communities, some of which I am an active member of, and some of which I am not. I recognize the criminalized, violent, and traumatic histories of these communities, and I honor the living fight for queer, kink, and sex work liberation in our queer-phobic, sex-negative, and kink-shaming society. I recognize that it is the life, labor, and love of queer activists; the sex-positive movement; Black and Brown social justice activists; and their allies, as well as my embodied and passing privileges, that grant me the opportunity to write on this topic with some protection from retribution. I strive to represent my communities with honor and celebration, and to uplift and pay respect to those communities to which I do not share lived experience.

As psychedelic therapy transitions into mainstream health care, we must reckon with the reality of the lack of a unified standard around consent in our diverse community of practitioners. Psychedelic spaces are no strangers to reports of the spectrum of consent violations (Goldhill & Abbês, 2020). While we see many health-care workers taking it upon themselves to treat clients at a higher level of ethical care (American Counseling Association, 2014), the health-care field as a whole holds an archaic standard of consent (American Medical Association, 2016). So, how then does psychedelic practice integrate with health care without the promise of perpetuating consent violations? We look to the community with the most consent street cred: the kinksters—a community playing at the margins, where society has not given us rules of entry, so we came up with our own government, where safety is a necessary foundation to allow pleasure, healing, and transformation to reign free. While no one person, community, or way of being is perfect, it would do the field of psychedelic practitioners good to learn when to say that the way we have been doing consent is not working, and look to those who most commonly get it right.

In the pages that follow, we will look to one of the most robustly consent-oriented subcultures, the kink community, and explore how the consent practices embedded in

DOI: 10.4324/9781003167976-4

this community fluidly integrate with psychedelic-assisted therapy. My offering to you is a practice of liberation, packaged in protocols on how to build a trauma-informed, consensual container within which psychedelic-assisted therapy can intentionally occur. Let us liberate consent from the stale, standardized, and rushed exchange at the beginning of therapeutic, medical, and research interactions. Let us weave a tapestry of consensual connection, something that is alive, attuned, co-creative, dynamic, and engaging—revisioning consent as a co-constructed act that creates a sacred container for authentic human connection to self and other. Does that not sound more fun?

Definitions

Before we jump in, let us get on the same page. Some definitions for the purposes of this chapter:

Consent: a voluntary agreement, made without coercion, between persons with decision-making capacity, knowledge, understanding, and autonomy; it applies to *all forms* of interactions (Consent Academy, n.d.)

Negotiation: a conversation in which all people who wish to enter into the experience discuss their desires and interests, things they may be curious about but would prefer to explore once a prerequisite (such as trust) has been met, and finally the things they are not at all interested in or acts/actions that make them feel uncomfortable or unsafe (The Sex Ed, n.d.)

Kink play: childhood joyous play with adult sexual privilege, and cool toys

Power: the flame in each person (Boyer et al., 2010), which can be used with, for, and over; wielded individually, collectively, and systemically

Systemic oppression: the intentional disadvantaging of groups of people based on their identity while advantaging members of the dominant group (National Equity Project, n.d.) function to uphold the currently dominant, invented hierarchical systems of white supremacy, cis-heteronormativity, capitalism, colonization, patriarchy, and Christian hegemony

The Overlap of Kink and Psychedelics

Kink refers to socially unconventional sexual practice and is derived from the idea of a "bend" in someone's sexual desires and behavior, in contrast to "straight" or "vanilla" socially conventional sexual practices (The Sex Ed, n.d.). In a society dominated by heteronormativity and the engrained remnants of Puritan culture, being kinky is a radical, and historically dangerous, act. The kink community was born out of the radical queer movement and the fight to exist in authenticity outside of dominant oppressive norms.

Offering this kind of safe space for exploration is one of kink's great virtues, as it provides another option for relationship building and sexual expression that doesn't subscribe to traditional notions of how these structures should exist.

Kink includes rather than excludes, because it is built on the foundation of embracing what can otherwise be shunned and misunderstood.

(Glover, 2018)

Kink has been practiced largely underground due to curated stigma, fear of violence and punitive punishment, and the system's desire to suffocate liberated ways of being. Sound familiar? From a history of criminalization and freedom movements to practices that expand consciousness and challenge notions of normality, kink and psychedelic communities share many intersecting characteristics. A robust orientation toward intentional consensual engagement can be the next intersection solidifying these communities in comradery.

The consent protocols that follow are nonlinear and fluid. They are context, person, community, and moment dependent. Every protocol needs to be tailored to the practitioner(s) and client(s) present in the consent engagement, and every consent engagement is to be approached with the knowledge that they can and will adapt as the therapeutic relationship flows.

Power Dynamics

Kinky play often includes some level of consensual power differential and is most active in bondage and discipline, dominance and submission, sadism, and masochism (BDSM) scenes. Being with and feeling the flame of power are vulnerable, power is heavily sought after by organisms with developed brains, and the expression of power can flood our systems with feel-good chemicals (Engle, 2019). Playing with power is, well, powerful. There is nothing inherently wrong with power. Harm comes when power is abused and controlled, and when we are not accountable for our power. The kink community understands that to create safety around power play, robust consent practices and active accountability to negotiated power dynamics are non-negotiables. The right use of power is a delicate dance between all parties involved in an experience. Attending to the power dynamic dance floor and the bodies on it requires consistent verbal and non-verbal communication with the desire to be impeccable and the space for stumble and recovery.

There is an inherent power differential between a practitioner and a client in any therapeutic setting. As consent is impacted by power and the perception of power (The Consent Academy, n.d.), attending to power dynamics in the therapeutic relationship is of the utmost importance. The risk of saying no and the pressure to say yes is often amplified in the presence of a power differential. Practitioner self-disclosure is a necessary tool in the practice of flattening hierarchical structures (Brown, 2019). In addition to humanizing the practitioner, self-disclosure presents clients with increased opportunities to decide if they feel comfortable moving forward with the therapeutic relationship and treatment. This is particularly true at the beginning of the relationship, yet continues as the relationship deepens. Not only can practitioner self-disclosure enhance client autonomy, safety, and therapeutic rapport, but it also creates space for practitioners to own their potential for doing harm and increases accountability. By opening themselves to the vulnerability of being seen as human, imperfect, and capable of having blind spots and making mistakes, practitioners become more relatable while setting the stage for leaning into rupture rather than hiding behind shame and the projected perfection that often comes with the role of practitioner.

Specific to disclosure around privileged and marginalized identities, engaging in social location disclosures and subsequent processing of power differentials bring into dialogue that which is already in the room. An individual's social location is made up of a combination of identity markers, including gender, race, social class, age, visible and invisible disabilities, religion, sexual orientation, immigrant status, body size, and geographic location (Jamison, 2019). For example, clients with marginalized identities working with practitioners of related privileged identities (i.e., a Black or Brown client and a white practitioner) are given a better understanding of their practitioner's level of awareness and unlearning around internalized systems of oppression and associated potential for micro- or macro-aggressions. Should treatment continue, the therapeutic relationship is fortified through deeper consent due to the increased level of information, mutual sharing, and honest assessment of risk in the intensely vulnerable relational experience that occurs within psychedelic-assisted therapy. Here are some things for practitioners to consider and introduce into the therapeutic process to address these concerns.

Questions for Practitioners to Sit With

1. What is my social location, and how do systems of oppression apply to me?
2. How does my social location intersect with my client's social location, and how do these aspects of myself show up in my role as a psychedelic-assisted therapy practitioner?
3. What risk is my client with a different social location taking in working with me?
4. What work have I done/am I doing around my relationship to power as it relates to my social location and associated identities? How can I communicate that to my clients in a way that feels authentic, honest, and in alignment with my integrity and accountability?

Questions to Weave Into Preparation Sessions

1. How do our identities and experiences within society align? How do they differ? How might this alignment or difference come up in our relationship?
2. How do we check in about the power dynamics in our relationship?
3. How do we center accountability and liberation in our work together?

Embodied Consent

Someone in a kink class once said, "You can't say yes until you can say no." Knowing and expressing what we *do not* want is an essential part of knowing and expressing what we *do* want. Adrienne Marie Brown reminds us, "Your no makes the way for your yes. Being able to say no makes yes a choice" (Brown, 2019). Learning consent is an integral part of childhood development. (Anyone have a toddler in their family who runs around screaming "no" all day long?) The tragic reality is that many children (and adults) are taught to expect that their "no's" will be disrespected or they will be shamed for having a "no," and that a "yes" is not required for someone else to make an impactful decision on their behalf, especially related to touch. From family of origin to peer communities to colonization to Western culture as a whole, we are not good at setting and respecting boundaries . . . which means many of those accessing psychedelic-assisted therapy are going to have a hard time knowing and expressing their "no's" and "yes's."

When we have a history of trauma, it often takes years of dedicated work to truly own our needs and boundaries. With this in mind and the reality that most clients are not going to have a solid grasp on expressing needs and boundaries by the time medicine sessions start, psychedelic-assisted practitioners need to define what their baseline requirement is around their clients' ability to engage with consent practices. Kinky play partners must do the same; we need to be able to trust each others' "no" and "yes." Mine is: can this person have an embodied "no" and an embodied "yes"? Which means, do they know when they want to say no or yes, and can they express it to me? If they cannot, I will not proceed to consciousness-altered interactions and will work on this skill first. The following is a protocol to help clients cultivate their ability to find their authentic "no" and "yes."

A Protocol for Assessment and Practice of Embodied Consent[1]

1. Explain the following protocol in detail, demo it, ask the client what questions they have, and make it clear they can stop at any time. Ask if the client consents to engaging with this practice. ("Now that you have seen what this will look like, would you like to continue?") If yes, continue. If no, stop.
2. As they are able, have the client position themselves in a way that feels alert for their body.
3. Talk the client through three rounds of breathing.
4. Invite the client to think about a time when they were offered something and felt a strong "yes" in response. Have them hold this memory in their mind, and, as much as they are able, notice what arises in their body.
5. Invite the client to inhale deeply, exhale halfway, say "yes," and then exhale completely. Repeat this three times.
6. Process together: What did they notice? What did you notice? As before, pay specific attention to the tone, strength, and volume of their voice; the place that the "yes" resonates from in their body; and any images, memories, feelings, vibrations, dissociation, or other defenses that come up. Get curious about the spectrum of ways "yes" can be felt and expressed and what these feelings/ expressions mean.

7. Invite the client to think about a time when they were offered something and felt a "no" in response. Instruct them that this should be a 3–4 on a scale of 10 of how strong their "no" was. The intention here is to not have them bring up something triggering, and rather have them think of something with a mild emotional charge. Have them hold this memory in their mind, and, as much as they are able, notice what arises in their body.

8. Invite the client to inhale deeply, exhale halfway, say "no," and then exhale completely. Repeat this three times.

9. Process together: What did they notice? What did you notice? Pay specific attention to the tone, strength, and volume of their voice; the place that the "no" resonates from in their body; and any images, memories, feelings, vibrations, dissociation, or other defenses that come up. Get curious about the spectrum of ways "no" can be felt and expressed and what these feelings/expressions mean.

10. Repeat steps 4–9 and see what changes. Process together.

11. As they are able, do some somatic release, like rocking, exhaling loudly, humming, vibrating, shaking out the body, other forms of movement, or rubbing the bottom of the feet. This helps move lingering traumatic retention energy through the body and seeks to bring the nervous system into a grounded, present, and engaged state.

Embodied Trauma Assessment and Relational Trigger Mapping

When we look at therapeutic consent through the risk-aware consensual kink (RACK) lens, we see common tools for safety assessment and planning enhanced into consent protocols that can be applied to the consciousness-altered nature of psychedelic-assisted therapy. The RACK model is a way to approach a kink interaction, developed to address the reality that risk does exist and harm can happen. It posits that we can consensually engage in risky behavior, as long as all parties are informed of the risks ahead of time, and there is a mutually agreed upon plan for how to manage them. A RACK-oriented preparation includes answering three questions: Can you name the risks? Are you both able to affirm your consent to each other? Do you understand exactly what event/activity is about to take place? (Lords, 2018). Layer these questions onto the trauma-informed approach of assessing triggers that might arise during medicine sessions, and we have an informed consent protocol for moving into a vulnerable space that involves the potential for traumatic memories/retentions/reenactments, painful emotional and somatic experiences, and disorientation from consensus reality to arise.

When working with trauma survivors, it is imperative that the practitioner have an idea of what the client's trigger points are and how to move around and with them as they arise in the relationship and in the treatment room. For example, if a client is a sexual assault survivor, the practitioner needs to know what might activate this trauma and how to best interact with the client when they are in this state. Trigger points inform needs and boundaries, and needs and boundaries are foundational components of consent. Of course, most clients do not come into therapy with a list of their triggers, and most clients also could not sit down and rattle them off upon inquiry from their practitioner. A part of the natural unfolding of the trauma therapy process is building a trigger map—developing an understanding of where triggers exist, what they look like in action, and how to work with them. During this process, it is important to assess for individual, developmental, systemic, historical, and intergenerational traumas. If we are functioning within a time-bound psychedelic-assisted therapy model, it is important to have some sense of what triggers might arise and what they look like before we move into medicine sessions. This may require extending the preparation phase beyond the three preparatory sessions that are typical to many psychedelic-assisted therapy protocols.

I am oriented to the polyvagal theory, and I find it incredibly useful when doing initial and ongoing trigger mapping and trauma response assessments with clients. The polyvagal theory is a way of looking at how the nervous system functions in relation to emotional regulation, fear response, and social connection. For a more in-depth review of the polyvagal theory, see Chapters 6 and 7. Through this lens, we can look at the way trauma responses move through the nervous system of the client and start creating a map for how their basic trauma responses show up. The practitioner is able to start identifying which cues the client shows when their nervous system is activated into either of the sympathetic responses (fight or flight) or either of the dorsal vagal responses (freeze or fawn). For example, a cue might be the client tightening their hands into fists and raising their shoulders to their ears. Alternatively, cues could look like a client's eyes spacing out, or suddenly talking about something funny and off topic. This process also helps identify how the client shows up when they are in a healthy ventral vagal (social engagement) response. In creating this map together, the client increases their embodied awareness and ability to consent to working with a specific response, and the practitioner is armed with an amazing amount of non-verbal and verbal cues to attune to and utilize in present-moment processing and consent negotiations. People cannot give embodied consent when they are disassociated and cannot consensually change previously agreed upon boundaries when they are in an active fight, flight, freeze, or fawn response. It is therefore imperative that practitioners perceive when these responses are happening in their client's body so they can help hold previously agreed upon boundaries.

So, how long does this take? The classic therapist answer: it depends. It can look many ways and will evolve as the clients' nervous system responses are adapting throughout the course of therapy. For many trauma survivors, somatic awareness often takes years to develop, especially when dissociation was a part of how they survived the traumatic experience(s). Here, I am offering a basic tool, one that practitioners can use as the beginning of a road map to ensure there is some awareness of how trauma moves through the client's soma before inviting psychedelic molecules into the room.

The foundation of trigger mapping is the question, "Can you show me with your body what it looks like when you . . .?" Typically, people come to therapy with something they want to work on. We can use the client's reported symptoms to quickly get to a nervous system level understanding of what is happening, how it is likely going to show up in therapy, and what might activate it.

A Protocol for Embodied Trauma Assessment and Relational Trigger Mapping[2]

1. Explain the following protocol in detail, demo it, ask the client what questions they have, and make it clear they can stop at any time. Ask if the client consents to engaging with this practice. If yes, continue. If no, stop.
2. As they are able, have the client position themselves in a way that feels alert for their body.
3. Make a list of symptoms (i.e., what they want to work on and why they are participating in psychedelic-assisted therapy). Be attentive to potential overwhelm or need for titration as you are making this list.
4. As the client is able, do some somatic release, like rocking, exhaling loudly, humming, vibrating, shaking out the body, movement, or rubbing the bottom of the feet.
5. Ask the client to select a symptom to start with.
6. Ask, "Can you show me in your body what it looks like when you [insert symptom here]?"
7. Ask the client, "What do you notice right now?" and offer observations about non-verbal cues you witness in the client. Do not stay here for longer than a minute; watch for early cues of overwhelm.
8. Do a somatic release practice (examples in step 4).
9. Ask the client to name some examples of when this shows up in their life.
10. Ask, "Can you think of a situation where this might come up between us in an ordinary consciousness session or psychedelic-assisted session?"
11. Ask, "What could I do that might bring this up for you?" After they have provided a response, follow up with, "If that happens, what should we do?" Listen actively, engage with options for a plan of how to handle triggers, take notes, and process together. Know that clients might not always know the answer, and that is okay. The purpose of this is to explore together, start building an understanding of how their trauma shows up, explore how to respond in these moments, and build trust in the relational container.
12. Do a somatic release practice (examples in step 4).
13. When complete, ask the client if they would like to continue to the next item on the list. If yes, repeat steps 5–11. If no, stop and revisit in the next session.

Soft–Hard Boundaries Continuum

Queer theory, a foundation of the kink community, explores the oppressive power of dominant norms, particularly those relating to sexuality, and the suffering they cause to those who cannot, or do not wish to, live according to those norms. Queer theory invites us to get curious about and dismantle the forced binary and related hierarchies (i.e., man/woman, gay/straight) in the dominant norms that are projected into nearly every social structure in the modern world. With a foundational understanding of and ability to express the verbal binary "yes" or "no," we can open up the spectrum existing between and around these two statements, allowing for a greater acknowledgment and exploration of gray areas and soft boundaries (and by the way, "Yes." and "No." are full sentences). With an enthusiastic "FUCK YES" on one end and a strong "FUCK NO" on the other, we have a layered playground of ways to come to authentic and consensual connection.

The kink orientation to soft and hard limits provides a model for assessing boundaries and determining how to approach them in the therapeutic relationship. Every kink scene negotiation includes identifying hard and soft boundaries from all play partners; consent for play cannot exist without this discussion. Hard boundaries are unbreakable and must be respected by all parties *no matter what*; soft boundaries are open for negotiation in the moment of potential action (Criss, 2016). I often think about hard boundaries as the outermost fence that defines the area in which we can play. Soft boundaries are structures that exist within the fenced-off space where we have more room to explore, some requiring us to stop and go a different direction, some revealing a space of mystery and discovery we could have never imagined prior.

A hard boundary in psychedelic-assisted therapy might be that there will be no sexual touch, that there will be no touch of any kind, or that there will be no music of religious origin. A soft boundary could be that a client is okay with therapeutic touch but would like to have in-the-moment discussions about what kind of touch they are comfortable with at that time. Note: touch in psychedelic-assisted therapy is always *at least* a soft boundary, unless it is a hard boundary, meaning that there is never a "do whatever you want, it's all okay" rule around touch, but there could be a hard boundary of "touch is not an option," which must, in all circumstances, be respected. If it is a soft boundary, it is something to practice during preparation sessions—discussed in the section *Practicing Touch*. Another soft boundary might be the practitioner being open to self-disclosure, and they would need to decide in the moment what level of disclosure feels clinically and personally appropriate and comfortable, given the topic or type of inquiry from the client.

Both practitioner and client get to have hard and soft boundaries. Communicating and making a plan around how to respect and care for these boundaries throughout the therapeutic interaction build trust, show care, and prepare all parties for vulnerable connection that will ensue. Boundaries are about identifying the space within which we are comfortable experiencing relationship. They are not about keeping people out; they are how we consciously invite people in.

During preparation sessions, practitioners can engage clients in identifying hard and soft boundaries and making a plan around them for the relationship as a whole and the specific upcoming medicine sessions. This conversation will often be the most in-depth during initial preparation sessions, and it should be continually checked in on and updated as the therapeutic relationships progress.

By orienting toward a continuum of consent, the therapeutic relationship is grounded in the reality of the unknown. By acknowledging that we do not know what is to come and being intentional about asking what guidelines we want to take into the shared exploration, we do our best to prepare and enhance relational trust and accountability to the agreements made to guide the therapeutic dyad through ambiguous moments.

Safe Words

Safe words are an essential aspect of kink play. A safe word is a clear signal for the play to stop immediately or to shift in some way (Robyn, n.d.). Many approaches to container building outside of kink utilize this framework, and psychedelic-assisted therapy can too. Building a safe word into consent practices allows for quick, obvious communication between practitioner and client that something needs to change.

Safe words come in verbal and non-verbal varieties, and I recommend identifying both while developing the consent plan. If a client is in an altered state of consciousness where verbal ability is limited, there needs to be a way for them to clearly communicate "stop" or "no." A client may not want to answer a question the practitioner is asking or may not want to engage in supportive touch. A common example in the kink community is the traffic light system: "green" = keep going!; "yellow" = I'm nearing my limits/slow down; "red" = stop everything. Non-verbal safe words common in kinky play are holding up a hand, pushing away, dropping a ball held in the hand, or tapping in a specific way.

Practitioners and clients can get creative and come up with verbal and non-verbal safe words that work for them. They should be simple to express, something that will not be verbally said in the medicine session otherwise, and easy to remember. My usual non-verbal safe word? Tapping the thumb and pinky together, or dropping something. My usual verbal safe word? Pineapple.

Practicing Touch

In RACK, one of the guiding consent questions is, "Do you understand exactly what event/activity is about to take place?" It is commonplace in kink scene negotiation to engage with (look at, touch, and examine) toys, structures, and spaces prior to moving into active play. It is also common for partners to engage with lower-risk and lower-vulnerability play to assess safety and build trust before moving into higher-risk and higher-vulnerability play. While we cannot practice ingesting a psychedelic molecule and having an intense relational experience, we can practice vulnerable aspects of that experience ahead of time. If a client is consenting to having therapeutic touch incorporated into their therapy (reminder: this means it is a soft boundary), then practicing potential situations where touch might come up is a way to enhance safety, connection, and trust in the client and practitioner's ability to navigate negotiation around touch in the moment during medicine sessions. Practicing touch negotiation in an ordinary state of consciousness leaves room for exploring needs and boundaries that arise in the practice session and can be integrated into the consent plan, and processing whatever feelings come up around this process. Practicing ahead of time is a lower stakes way of figuring out what works and what does not. The goal is that practicing touch ahead of time increases the likelihood for successful use of touch during medicine sessions.

A Protocol for Practicing Touch[3]

Please note, only practitioners who are trained to use therapeutic touch should do this with their clients.

Please also note, this does not all need to be done at once. Take it slow and at a pace attuned to the client and the therapeutic relationship. Do somatic release throughout and at the end.

1. Explain the following protocol in detail, demo it, ask the client what questions they have, and make it clear they can stop at any time. Ask if the client consents to engaging with this practice. If yes, continue. If no, stop.
2. Practitioner and client position their bodies in the way they will likely be during the medicine session.
3. Agree on a form of touch to start with. I typically start with hand holding or a hand on the shoulder.
4. Practice client verbally requesting touch and practitioner verbally accepting and offering it. Process together.
5. Practice client non-verbally requesting touch and practitioner non-verbally accepting and offering it. Process together.
6. Practice practitioner verbally offering touch ("Would you like me to hold your hand?") and client checking in with self for a "yes" or "no" and any limits that show up alongside (for example, "yes, but only for a few moments" and "yes, but really light touch"), and then verbally accepting if there is a "yes" present and receiving it. If a "no" is present for the client, validate the no and do not touch the client. Process together.
7. Practice practitioner non-verbally offering touch (practitioner offers hand to client in a way the client can see) and client checking in with self, and then non-verbally accepting and receiving it. Process together.
8. Practice practitioner verbally offering touch and client verbally declining it. Process together.
9. Practice practitioner non-verbally offering touch and client non-verbally declining it. Process together.
10. Practice practitioner verbally offering touch and client verbally accepting it, then client changing mind and verbally declining it after physical contact has been made. Practitioner removes contact immediately upon change in consent. Process together.

11. Practice practitioner non-verbally offering touch and client non-verbally accepting it, then client changing mind and non-verbally declining it after physical contact has been made. Practitioner removes contact immediately upon change in consent. Process together.
12. Practice client verbally requesting touch and practitioner verbally declining and not offering it. Process together.

Revoke of Consent for Therapy Plan

In both kink play and typical health-care and research settings, consent can easily be revoked at any time. Someone says, "I'm done," and everything stops. The bondage comes off, the client leaves the therapy room, and the research protocol ends. Psychedelic-assisted therapy is different in that clients are under the influence of a significantly consciousness-altering substance that can last anywhere from 1 to 12+ hours. Psychedelic research informed consent documents require that participants not leave the facility until the morning after the medicine session (MAPS, n.d.). This is out of alignment with an integral aspect of consent: that it can be revoked at any time. It is true that someone cannot take the psychedelic substance out of their body once they have ingested it, but they can revoke consent for the accompanying therapy and the setting within which they started the therapy in. The psychedelic-assisted therapy field has not come up with a good answer for how this issue should be handled, and I have personally witnessed multiple experts respond to the question, "What if someone REALLY wants/needs to leave?" with "I don't know." We need to be prepared for this to happen, and we need to have a plan in place that does not involve calling the police. The answer will likely come from those who have been practicing underground and in traditional ceremonial settings. Those who stand to risk the most in these potential situations due to historical violence and oppression, namely, Black, Indigenous, and People of Color and LGBTQIA2S+ communities, need to be centered voices in the discussion.

In my practice, I always come up with a plan for how we would handle this should it arise. The plan looks different for each person and usually involves a support person coming quickly. My way is not *the* way; it is just what I have done out of necessity and the lack of a standard of care. My hope is that the field can come together to decide what the best course of action is to create a true consent-oriented container around the plan for total revocation of consent that is accessible, equitable, and safe for all who are participating.

Setting Up the Room

Psychedelic-assisted therapy settings have a wide range of aesthetics. From the "living room-like setting" in the research protocols to the nature-based settings of ceremonial spaces to hospice rooms, there is space to explore and co-create the setting of the psychedelic experience. While consent to the general setting of the therapy might be all or nothing, as the treatment space is generally determined by the practitioner or clinic, consent to the setup of the space and objects present is an important and often overlooked part of preparation. Asking clients how they would prefer the room to be set up, what objects they are or are not comfortable with being in the space, and if they would like to bring any items to personalize the space is a basic way of increasing client comfort, safety, and autonomy.

Particularly for clients with a history of religious and spiritual abuse, it is of the utmost importance to assess consent for the inclusion of any spiritual or religious objects or practices during preparation sessions. There is a common assumption that spiritual or religious artifacts or rituals should be integrated into psychedelic-assisted therapy. While this may be true for some people, there is a potential for triggering and re-traumatization within populations who have experienced similar artifacts, rituals, or belief systems in an abusive setting. Folks in the queer community who have experienced conversion therapy are one specific example. It is important to do an assessment with all clients around setting and be particularly attentive and consent oriented should someone disclose religious or spiritual trauma. More about cultivating client-centered ritual practices can be found in Chapter 10.

Aftercare Plan

Aftercare is a term in the kink community for what you do to make sure everyone is okay and taken care of after the play is over. It helps prevent complete crashing after experiencing the rush of oxytocin, dopamine, and prolactin that are typically released during sex or kink play. Aftercare helps to regulate the body's response as the chemicals dissipate (Garis, 2020).

The effects of psychedelic molecules can be similar to "subspace" in kink play, which is the often transcendental state people can enter when releasing control and power and in a submissive/dominant interaction. This correlation invites us to ask how we can mitigate the negative effects of "coming down" in psychedelic-assisted therapy through adopting the practice of aftercare. Planning for aftercare is as simple as practitioners being open, curious, and communicative with clients toward the end of psychedelic sessions about what they need and having options available. Agreeing on aftercare options (such as drawing, eating, sitting quietly together, going outside, or having a support person come in) ahead of time is a great way to prepare for what might come up. Once a practitioner and client have experienced a medicine session together, they can brainstorm for future sessions about what specific needs the client had when coming down from the medicine, what helped and what did not in the previous session, which aftercare options are accessible, and what plans can be in place to meet the client's needs going forward.

I remember being in a BDSM class when the facilitator started talking about aftercare and someone started a "tops need aftercare too!" chant. I would like to send my most heartfelt thank you to that person, because now I have a "practitioners need aftercare too!" chant that arises from my subconscious whenever planning medicine sessions. Tops and practitioners both hold the responsibility of maintaining the container and being accountable to the power dynamics present. Holding space with this level of responsibility can be exhausting and depleting. Practitioners need aftercare too. And, this needs to be done after the client leaves, so as not to put the client in a position of taking care of the practitioner. All practitioners should have a sense of what they need to care for themselves and decompress after medicine sessions, and they should have a plan in place to meet those needs after the session ends.

Building the Consent Plan

Following these protocols, there should be a clear, co-constructed, and communally understood plan for boundaries and consent written and signed prior to every medicine session. Check in during integration sessions about what went well, what did not, what was learned, and what should change in the consent plan. You can use this as a checklist, and I encourage personalizing it to suit the particular approach and dynamic of each unique therapeutic relationship.

Checklist for Building a Consent Plan

1. Assess client's relationship to "yes" and "no."
2. Discuss power dynamics present in the relationship and consenting to risk.
3. Do a trauma assessment and identify trigger points that could come up.
4. Identify hard and soft boundaries for the client.
5. Identify hard and soft boundaries for the practitioner.
6. Agree on a verbal safe word.
7. Agree on a non-verbal safe word.
8. (If a therapeutic touch is a soft boundary) Practice touch—accepting, declining, accepting then declining, declining then accepting, requesting, and negotiating.
9. Develop a plan for total revocation of consent for therapy after dosing. Review this plan with the client's support person.
10. Discuss the medicine room setup; consent to objects present.
11. Make an aftercare plan.

Conclusion

My hope for you, dear reader, is that this chapter has invited you to look at your own relationship to consent and how it flows in your life and practice. Consent is for each and every one of us, and it invites us into deeper connection with ourselves, others, and the world we live in. With a nod of reverence and gratitude to our kinky community members, may the psychedelic-assisted therapy field liberate consent and engage in an intentional restructuring and integration toward sustainable change and safer and more liberated experiences.

Notes

1   This practice is adapted from teachings I received from Betty Martin's "Like a Pro" training for touch practitioners who use the Wheel of Consent, and Christopher Hirsh, a radicalized and embodied facilitator and consultant of healing arts, justice activist, and storyteller. Christopher adapted these practices from voice, movement, and presence teachers Kristin Linklater and Stephen Buescher.
2   This practice is adapted from teachings I received from BDSM, EMDR, Cultural Somatics, Gestalt Therapy, and Psychosynthesis trainings and communities.
3   This practice is adapted from teachings I received from BDSM, Yoga, Psychosynthesis, and Psychedelic-Assisted Therapy trainings and communities. Betty Martin's Wheel of Consent and associated trainings are a great framework for understanding consensual exchange.

References

American Counseling Association. (2014). *ACA code of ethics*. https://www.counseling.org/resources/aca-code-of-ethics.pdf

American Medical Association. (2016). *AMA code of ethics*. https://www.ama-assn.org/system/files/2019-06/code-of-medical-ethics-chapter-2.pdf

Boyer, M. F., Johnson, G. R., Goodwin, L., Nieto, L., & Smith, L. C. (2010). *Beyond inclusion, beyond empowerment: A developmental strategy to liberate everyone*. Cuetzpalin.

Brown, A. M. (2019). *Pleasure activism: The politics of feeling good*. AK Press.

Consent Complexities: The Consent Academy. (n.d.). *The consent academy*. Retrieved January 18, 2022, from www.consent.academy/consent-complexities.html

Criss, C. (2016, September 9). Your BDSM essentials: Boundaries. *World Association of Sex Coaches*. https://worldassociationofsexcoaches.org/bdsm-essentials-boundaries/

Engle, G. (2019, 11–15). How "subspace" can help us better understand consent. *Dame*. https://dame.com/what-is-subspace/

Garis, M. G. (2020, October 20). Sexual aftercare isn't just a BDSM thing: Here's why everyone should try it. *Well and Good*. www.wellandgood.com/aftercare-after-sex/

Glover, C. (2018, 11–18). It's time to recenter kink and BDSM as part of radical queer history. *Slate*. https://slate.com/human-interest/2018/11/kink-bdsm-radical-queer-history.html

Goldhill, O., & Abbês, B. (2020, March 3). Psychedelic therapy has a sexual abuse problem. *Quartz*. https://qz.com/1809184/psychedelic-therapy-has-a-sexual-abuse-problem-3/

Jamison, T. (2019, April 4). Inclusion and diversity committee report: What's your social location? *National Council on Family Relations*. Retrieved January 18, 2022, from www.ncfr.org/ncfr-report/spring-2019/inclusion-and-diversity-social-location

Lords, K. (2018, May 2). Safety in BDSM: Understanding SSC, RACK, and PRICK. *Loving BDSM*. https://lovingbdsm.net/2018/05/02/ssc-rack-prick/

MAPS' FDA-approved MDMA/PTSD Protocol. (n.d.). *Multidisciplinary Association for Psychedelic Studies—MAPS*. Retrieved January 18, 2022, from https://maps.org/research-archive/mdma/protocol/ic_070705.html

National Equity Project. (n.d.). *Lens of systemic oppression*. www.nationalequityproject.org/frameworks/lens-of-systemic-oppression

Robyn, X. (n.d.). What is a safe word? Learn the basics of kink communication. *Lovense Blog*. www.lovense.com/sex-blog/kink-bdsm/what-is-a-safe-word

The Sex Ed. (n.d.). Sexpedia. *The Sex Ed*. www.thesexed.com/sexpedia#gloss_k

Chapter 5

The Heart of the Work

Relational Psychedelic-Assisted
Therapy

Genesee Herzberg and Jason A. Butler

Introduction

Relatedness as a Healing Agent

The psychological and physiological impact of trauma is notoriously slow and challenging to treat through standard psychotherapeutic and pharmacological interventions; it takes significant time to develop the safety and trust necessary to make contact with deeply dissociated aspects of the client's traumatic experience that lie at the root of their symptoms. Although psychedelic medicines are proving to be powerful tools for deepening and accelerating trauma recovery (Halstead et al., 2021; Krediet et al., 2020; Liriano et al., 2019; Mithoefer et al., 2011; Mithoefer et al., 2013; Ross et al., 2019), standard psychedelic therapy models often struggle to address ingrained remnants of traumatic wounding due to the short-term nature of the treatment, an inadequate foundation of safety and trust in the therapeutic relationship, the persistence of the client's protective defenses, or inattention to underlying relational dynamics.

Research corroborates what seasoned psychedelic therapists know from experience—trust and safety between client and therapist are foundational to a transformative psychedelic therapy treatment (Carhart-Harris & Nutt, 2017; Carhart-Harris, 2018; Grof, 1980; Herzberg, 2012; Johnson et al., 2008; Richards, 2015). In traditional psychotherapy, the degree of trust in the therapeutic relationship is the strongest predictor of an effective treatment (Safran & Muran, 2000; Wampold, 2015); this trust is even more critical in psychedelic therapy because psychedelic medicines are known to amplify emotional intensity, engender deeply vulnerable states, enhance sensitivity to physical and interpersonal environments, and compromise one's ability to give full-bodied consent.

Leading psychedelic therapist Stanislov Grof (1980) has famously described psychedelic medicines as "nonspecific amplifiers of consciousness" (p. 143), suggesting that these compounds are profound catalysts for facilitating the emergence and amplification of unconscious material into awareness. Psychedelics are known to temporarily relax the constrictive force of psychological defenses, bringing forward emotions, memories, and complexes that may otherwise be difficult to access

DOI: 10.4324/9781003167976-5

(Nutt & Carhart-Harris, 2020). MDMA,[1] for example, quiets activity in the amygdala—the "smoke detector" of the brain—calming the fear response and facilitating a temporary bypass of habitual defenses, such as protective self-states[2] and negative transference reactions (Mitchell et al., 2021).

Conversely, psychedelics can intensify transference feelings, in which the client experiences the therapist and the environment through the lens of internal working models formed in early attachment relationships. Grof, who supervised or guided over 4,500 LSD psychotherapy sessions, emphasized this point:

> Even an ideal interpersonal situation cannot completely prevent the occurrence of significant distortions under the influence of the drug. However, if there is a clear and solid relationship between the [patient] and the [therapist] outside of the session context, the drug-induced distortions become an important opportunity for learning and for corrective emotional experiences, rather than a danger to the psychedelic process. A good therapeutic relationship helps the patient to let go of psychological defenses, surrender to the experience, and endure the difficult periods of the session characterized by intense physical and emotional suffering or confusion. *The quality of the therapeutic relationship is essential for working through one of the most crucial situations in psychedelic therapy: the crisis of basic trust* [emphasis added].
>
> (Grof, 1980, p. 90)

Underlying relational processes are likely to surface and influence a psychedelic treatment, regardless of the therapist's approach, their capacity to perceive these dynamics, or their decision to bring them into the client's awareness. Given the potential for "drug-induced distortions" (i.e., transference-related projections) or a "crisis of basic trust" to surface in psychedelic sessions, it is incumbent upon the therapist to learn to recognize and work with relational dynamics as they arise within the treatment. When handled without skill and close attunement, intensified transference reactions have the potential to trigger therapeutic ruptures, cause significant adverse experiences during a psychedelic session, and have a lasting harmful impact on the client's well-being (Herzberg, 2012). Conversely, when there is a strong foundation of trust and safety and when transference–countertransference dynamics and ruptures in the therapeutic relationship are handled skillfully, psychedelic therapy can be a potent approach to treating a wide range of psychological concerns.

Introduction to Relational Psychedelic Therapy

Therapists can use a relational approach to cultivate an optimal context for maximizing psychedelic medicine's unique transformative capabilities and mitigating its harmful potential. Relational approaches in psychotherapy emphasize the collaborative process of building safety and trust, addressing therapeutic ruptures, and exploring the interpersonal client–therapist dynamics that spontaneously unfold. Throughout this chapter, we lay out a model for relational psychedelic therapy by weaving foundational elements from relational psychoanalysis with observations from our clinical experience with MDMA- and ketamine-assisted therapy, as well as scientific findings from psychedelic research and interpersonal neurobiology. We also integrate features of IFS to provide an accessible framework for working with the multiplicity of the psyche.

Relational psychedelic therapy aims to use the myriad therapeutic effects of psychedelics to catalyze a relational approach to psychotherapy. Synergistically, this model fosters opportune interpersonal conditions to maximize psychedelic medicines' healing potential through the central tenets described as follows.

A safe therapeutic relationship is a primary agent in psychological transformation and trauma recovery. The therapist uses attentive verbal and non-verbal body-centered interventions to facilitate right-brain to right-brain (Schore, 2012) co-regulation of nervous system hyper- and hypo-arousal to cultivate an overall atmosphere of safety and attunement. In building relational safety and trust, the therapist fosters an optimal context to explore the client's inner world, to work with relational dynamics as they surface in the therapy, and for the client to delve into the deeply vulnerable states evoked by psychedelics.

The emergent, here-and-now interpersonal dynamics between therapist and client—often amplified by psychedelics—become a microcosm of the client's relational world, unveiling interpersonal patterns formed in primary relationships that continue to play out in their current life. The therapist aims to cultivate an environment in which these unconscious interpersonal dynamics can safely surface and be known (e.g., through transference, countertransference, and enactment). The therapist endeavors to bring their full presence to interactions with the client, allowing themselves to be impacted while remaining mindful of how they are impacting the client. The client is encouraged to express any feelings that arise in response to the therapist. In turn, the therapist facilitates well-timed collaborative conversation about the dyad's moment-to-moment emotional exchanges.

The therapeutic process unfolds between the conscious and unconscious dimensions of both client and therapist, forming a co-created "relational field" that is fundamental to relational psychedelic therapy. The relational field is the intersubjective, shared unconscious space formed "at every encounter between bodies and minds" (Ferro & Civitarese, 2015, p. xv). In this co-created field, "neither member of the couple can be understood without the other" (Baranger & Baranger, 1961–1962/2009, pp. 795–796).

Emotion is considered more primary than cognition, and process and context are emphasized over content. The therapist consistently orients to the emotional tone of the relational field and attends to the underlying process of the dyad's interactions.

The therapist holds a lens of multiplicity and is prepared for the dynamic emergence of the client's diversity of parts, which are amplified by psychedelic states of consciousness. The therapist tracks and therapeutically engages with the full range of the client's parts, including protective and traumatized parts, and supports the client in cultivating their relationship with what IFS refers to as the "Self" (Schwartz, 2001), which carries deep wisdom, compassion, acceptance, curiosity, and unconditional love. This essential aspect of human nature exists in each of us and is frequently rendered more accessible by the effects of psychedelic medicines. The therapist helps each of the client's parts find full expression, acceptance, and reintegration within the client's psychic landscape.

In this chapter, we give specific attention to the treatment of developmental trauma. Although developmental trauma is generally associated with repeated adverse experiences in childhood, we extend this term to include more subtle experiences of attachment trauma, such as chronic misattunement, rejection, or denial of one's emotional experience by primary attachment figures, as well as relationally traumatic experiences that can occur throughout the life span, such as emotional or physical abuse, divorce, and betrayal. While developmental trauma is not a formal diagnosis in the *Diagnostic and Statistical Manual of Mental Disorders*, Fifth Edition, it has been widely regarded by clinicians as a primary diagnostic feature in many clients' histories (Van der Kolk, 2005).

The relational psychedelic approach can be applied in both long-term and time-limited therapies; however, it is most effective in ongoing treatment with a consistent therapist, where the client can glean the benefits of trust, safety, and attachment that are only built over time. The internalization of the therapist as a reparative attachment figure is a central component in healing developmental trauma, and this attachment process is significantly accelerated by psychedelic medicines; it is therefore incumbent upon the psychedelic therapist to recognize their role as an attachment figure and to hold that significant responsibility with intentionality and care. A long-term therapeutic relationship supports the client in firmly internalizing this reparative relationship and developing earned secure attachment.

What Is to Come

In the following pages, we introduce the challenges and opportunities of relational psychedelic therapy, illustrated through an example of an MDMA-assisted therapy treatment. Next, we describe key aspects of the therapist's stance in a relational psychedelic approach, providing a framework for tracking and tending the relational field, and facilitating co-regulation. We then describe our theory of change in relational psychedelic therapy, outlining the fundamental processes through which healing occurs and how these are facilitated by psychedelics. These processes include the cultivation of relational safety; engagement with dissociated self-states; the reparative and therapeutic uses of transference, countertransference, and enactments; and the facilitation of self-integration. We provide guidelines for transforming transference reactions and enactments from potential dead-end impasses, emotional ruptures, and retraumatizing experiences into generative opportunities for deep psychological transformation. We then discuss key relational considerations and frameworks for facilitating psychological and psychedelic integration. Finally, we close the chapter with an illustration of the final stages of trauma recovery through the relational psychedelic therapy lens.

Because MDMA's therapeutic qualities significantly support trauma work, we focus on this compound throughout this chapter, highlighting its subjective effects and mechanisms of action that potentiate transformation within relational psychedelic therapy. The mechanisms of action described throughout this chapter can be readily translated to therapeutic work with most other empathogenic[3] compounds; likewise, the relational psychedelic model detailed in this chapter provides a useful framework and effective set of interventions for psychedelic-assisted therapy with a wide range of medicines.

The Challenges and Opportunities of Relational Psychedelic Therapy

The dissolution of a client's ordinary internal and interpersonal boundaries induced by psychedelics inevitably softens the boundaries between therapist and client, and facilitates the deepening of the empathic connection. This "sympathetic resonance" naturally potentiates an amplification of significance in the relational field (Ferro & Civitarese, 2015, p. xv). When attending to this field, the therapist engages their embodied, imaginal, and emotional experience to indirectly "catch the drift" (Freud, 1923/1975, p. 239) of interpersonal dynamics through their symbolic and somatic manifestations. Attunement to the subtleties in the field helps draw out latent relational potentials of the therapist and client—where the palliatives of deep emotional holding and containment co-exist with the triggering irritants of trauma-based transference reactions and enactments.

Herein lies the challenging opportunity of the relational psychedelic therapy model: how to best make use of the surfacing unconscious interpersonal patterns evoked by psychedelics for the sake of working through the client's wounding while mitigating the harm they may cause under the wrong conditions. Through thoughtfully responding (and not responding) to what arises—and recognizing their own attunement and misattunement to the client's experience—the relational therapist may be able to facilitate reparative emotional experiences and a cohesive integration of previously dissociated parts of the client's self.

We propose that relational psychedelic therapy, when skillfully practiced, opens opportunities for the client to develop qualities essential to meaningful and fulfilling relationships, such as intersubjectivity,[4] interpersonal intimacy, emotional intelligence, greater freedom vis-à-vis defensive patterns of relating, and expanded compassion for the diverse parts of self. When the therapist remains unconscious of interpersonal dynamics or responds with defensiveness, however, the potential for a transformative experience is foreclosed; instead, the client's self-protective patterns are reinforced, which can lead to therapeutic impasse, re-traumatization, or even ongoing psychological harm. The following case example illustrates one such missed opportunity and the lasting harm it caused.

"She Wasn't Gonna Stick Around": Vera and the Vanishing Therapist

Vera,[5] a white, queer-identified graduate student in her early 30s, had a vibrant and fiery personality, with a hint of cynicism. Her charm, wit, and charisma made her easy to connect with, while a veil of sardonic sarcasm diligently shielded her vulnerability and subtly conveyed "don't get too close." Vera's family emigrated to New York City when she was an infant, and the stress of immigration weighed heavily on her parents, especially her mother. Unable to feel at home in this new environment, overwhelmed by the stress of parenthood and struggling with severe depression and untreated complex trauma, her mother suddenly and permanently left 2-year-old Vera and her father and returned to their home country. Vera's brokenhearted father did not know how to cope with his own grief, much less help his toddler process the confusing mix of intense emotions evoked by this abrupt abandonment. Her father turned to work and alcohol to manage his feelings, often leaving Vera home alone or with a family friend.

Vera sought psychotherapy as an adult to address the repercussions of her early trauma, including a lifelong struggle with depression, a series of unsuccessful relationships, and a general feeling of numbness. Vera described her first year of therapy by saying, "I had been super cerebral in all our sessions, packing things away, sometimes deliberately. Like, I know there are feelings there, but I don't want to deal with them now." She was able to recall several important details about her experience growing up—yet, each time she shared her story, it felt like she was detachedly talking about someone else, with a faraway look in her eyes. Vera and her therapist tried a number of somatic interventions to help her connect with her body and mitigate the dissociative pattern, but the process was slow going, and Vera became increasingly frustrated with it. She felt stuck: unable to work through her long-standing pattern of burying her trauma nor understand why she pursued relationships with people who "could never really show up."

After a particularly frustrating session the previous week, Vera's therapist mentioned that she was trained in MDMA-assisted psychotherapy and suggested that an MDMA session together might help Vera break through her pattern of dissociation and access her underlying emotions and trauma. Vera was intrigued by the idea and began to feel a renewed sense of hope: this approach could very well crack the vault in which she had sealed her feelings. Vera's therapist would be moving out of the country in four months, and Vera hoped that the session could offer closure and perhaps function as a ritual to mark the end of their work. Vera described feeling close to her therapist and trusting her as they took this significant step toward the difficult confrontation of past trauma.

Despite her hopefulness going into the MDMA session, Vera reflected, and the experience was a significant disappointment. Vera noted that her therapist prepared her for the MDMA session "a little too lackadaisically," leaving her with an inadequate understanding of what to expect in terms of the session setting, the type of guidance the therapist would provide, and the "rules of engagement." Most importantly, the therapist failed to prepare Vera for the significant impact that the therapist's pending move would have on her.

With a tone of sarcasm in her voice, Vera described her therapist's presence in the MDMA session as emotionally distant and disinterested, "Kinda just supervising, making sure I didn't hurt myself or whatever." She added, "I remember being pretty much left to my own devices." In reaction to the therapist's lack of engagement, Vera felt the need to self-contain and enacted her typical protective patterns. She noted, "There was a lot of the 'me' that normally controls 'me' present in the situation. My therapist didn't really relieve me of those duties." Vera was concerned about her therapist throughout much of the session; she worried that she was bored and felt like she should be entertaining her. Although motivated to make good use of the session, Vera felt distracted throughout, unable "to keep [her] attention on any one thought or idea for too long before the music would take [her] away again." Vera found herself fluctuating between "being a little girl again, trying to work through some of the early events" and "running away to do other things."

Vera described one poignant moment in which she was looking at black-and-white photos of herself as an infant with her mother and became filled with emotion. She had a vision in which she was a fetus in the womb having a conversation with her pregnant mother, who told her that "she wasn't gonna stick around and she was kinda sorry about all that." She had an image of her heart "shattering into tiny pieces" after her mother's half-hearted apology. Vera's fetus-self then turned her back on her mother, shielding herself from the profound pain of abandonment. Vera relayed this vision to her therapist during the session, but she felt that her therapist seemed preoccupied; she did not engage with her in a way that helped her deepen into the experience. She soon went back to dancing and frolicking around the room.

Vera and her therapist had four integration sessions prior to the therapist's departure. Although Vera was "filled with feelings that she was on the verge of really feeling," she was uncomfortable sharing them with her therapist and chose to "push them back down again." Concordantly, the therapist did not broach Vera's underlying disappointment, frustration, and the heart-shattering grief of her abandonment; instead, they stayed at the surface as they reviewed the events of the MDMA session and concluded their work together. Vera noted that the material that had emerged during the session "kinda just disappeared, or became stashed in places that I didn't revisit for a long, long time."

Vera's experience of her therapist's "lackadaisical" therapeutic holding, alongside their lack of attention to the impact of the termination, had a lasting harmful effect. For weeks after the session, Vera reported feeling "really sensitive," "flooded with a bunch of unspoken feelings," and "just wanting to be left alone." She noted that she did not feel comfortable in her home or able to access support from her partner, and thus she found herself turning her back to him, acting compulsively, and "checking out." She described a feeling of dismay that "peppered everything around" her and lasted for years after the session.

A Missed Opportunity

Vera's account speaks strongly to the dual potential of relational enactments. Her therapist failed to recognize or address the fact that the pending termination set up the conditions for Vera to reexperience the abandonment trauma she had come to therapy to treat. Rather than serving as an opportunity to work through this trauma, the treatment became a painful reenactment of her experience of abandonment by a trusted person. When unaddressed, enactments reinforce the client's protective defenses as well as their core beliefs about themselves and others. Additionally, as was true in Vera's experience, unresolved enactments can significantly amplify the intensity of the client's symptoms. For years after this session, Vera struggled in intimate relationships; she believed her emotional experience would be too much for others and returned to her lifelong pattern of self-containment.

Conversely, if the therapist had recognized the potential enactment and spoken to the here-and-now relational implications of Vera's imaginal conversation with her mother, the session could have evolved into a poignant opportunity to discuss the parallel separation happening in the therapeutic relationship. The therapist could have accompanied Vera in grieving both the heart-shattering loss of her mother and the loss of her therapist, gathering the fragmented pieces of Vera's heart through compassionate containment and empathic reflection, and giving Vera an opportunity to have her grief recognized and mutually felt. In acknowledging the effects of the therapist's unconsciousness and insensitivity, she could have wholeheartedly recognized the impact with far more care than Vera's imaginal mother, who was merely "kinda sorry" about leaving.

The Therapist's Stance

Tending the Relational Field

Drawing from Merleau-Ponty's *Phenomenology of Perception*, psychoanalysts Antonino Ferro and Giuseppe Civitarese (2015) describe the metaphor of the relational field as "the rigorously interdependent relationship that comes into being between subject and context, the reciprocal and constant influence of self and other, and the dynamic continuity arising between consciousness and the spatiotemporal parameters of experience of the world" (Ferro & Civitarese, 2015, p. 2). The relational field is the ambiance and atmosphere that permeates the therapeutic space and the subjective experience of client and therapist, as generated through the totality of conscious and unconscious interactions within the therapeutic dyad. The field shapes (and takes the shape of) the client and therapist's experience of each other, their experience of self, and their experience of the environment. As depicted in the following figure, the relational field is an emergent property born out of the client and therapist's somatic, emotional, imaginal, energetic, and relational modes of expression, explicit and implicit. The relational field is also influenced by the setting, the cultural and ecological context (the cultural field), as well as the transpersonal field, including intergenerational influences and archetypal energies constellated in the collective. As the amalgam of these powerful contextual influences, the relational field is considered the most influential factor of the psychedelic set and setting (e.g., MAPS, 2017).

The therapist's "tending" of the field is analogous to tending a garden. First, we attune to the condition and needs of each plant by taking in its aesthetic

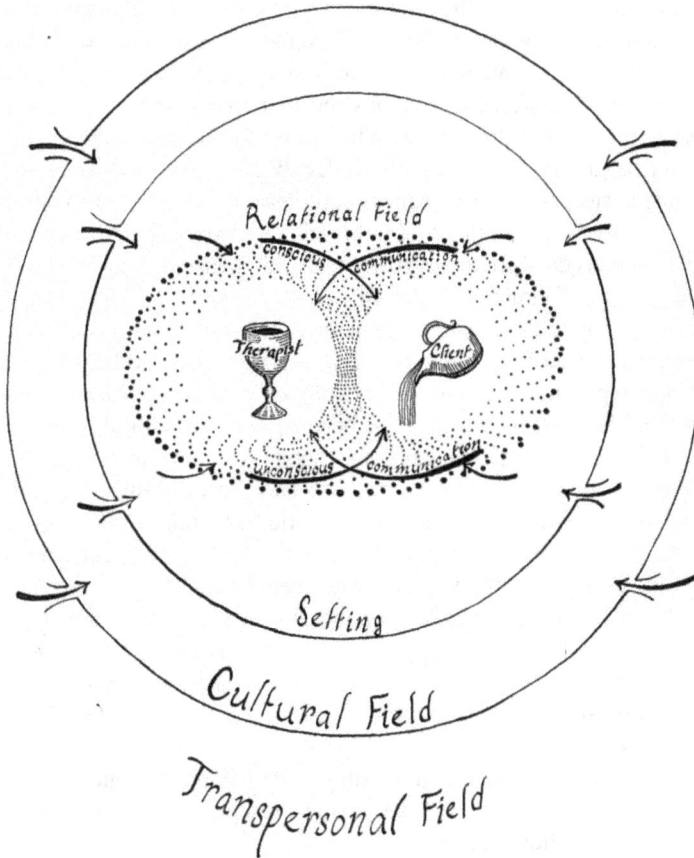

Figure 5.1 The relational field

Source: (Diagram illustrated by Inaê Cintra Mattiazzi)

presentation—the qualities present in the soil, stem, leaves, flowers, and fruit—by opening our heart to their displays of image, vibrancy, fragrant emanations, and any other communications. We might enter a state of embodied presence and notice how we feel as we take the plant in. We can then respond to the needs and communications we perceive by trimming away dead leaves, watering, offering nourishment, providing the appropriate environmental conditions, and harvesting the fruit.

Likewise, the therapist tends the relational field through receptivity and responsiveness to the aesthetics of the emergent expressions of the therapist–client encounter. The relational field is perceptible through mindful observation of the client and therapist's emotional experience and expression, somatic sensations, reverie, thought processes, flow of subtle energies, and non-verbal cues (i.e., facial expressions, gaze, skin tone, subtle movements, nervous tics, etc.). Sensitive attention to the aesthetics of the co-created field enables the therapist to cultivate empathic attunement, modulate affective exchanges and levels of arousal, support the containment and metabolization of trauma-related affect, and identify and attend to emergent transference reactions and enactments—processes we will elaborate upon in the sections that follow. When carefully cultivated, the relational field becomes fertile ground that gives life to deeply embodied emotional poignancy; vibrant images steeped in significance; and clear, generative, and vital thinking. When left unattended, the relational field—like a garden—begins to decay into a barren and vacuous dead space or grows wild with invasive unconscious dynamics that get in the way of intentional growth.

The key pathway to establishing a generative relational field, according to Ferro (2017), is through accessing moments of *at-one-ment* (unison) between client and therapist and repairing moments of breakdown in unison. When we notice the relational field has lost its aliveness or become charged with unformulated relational dynamics, we can take that as a cue that a breakdown or psychic retreat has occurred and needs tending. As we describe as follows, identifying and tending to moments of breakdown through co-regulation and relational negotiation is a direct route to reestablishing unison. At-one-ment in the therapeutic dyad is contingent on the therapist's ability to cultivate deep emotional interconnectedness, a "willingness to dare to open one's heart and soul to another human being" (Eshel, 2019, p. 3). By "feeling with" the client, the therapist helps "forge an emergent new entity of interconnectedness or 'withnessing' that goes beyond the confines of their separate subjectivities and the simple summation of the two—*a two-in-oneness*" (p. 1).

The experience of at-one-ment is similar to the phenomenon of resonance between musical instruments. Jungian analyst Joseph Cambray (2009) describes resonance with the following example:

> Consider a tuning fork used to tune a piano: striking the fork against a solid surface will set it vibrating at a specific frequency, producing a reference pitch; the relevant string on a piano can then be adjusted (tightened or loosened) so that the string resonates at the same frequency, so that the pitches match. In fact, if the vibrating fork is put in proximity with the tuned string, this will then begin to vibrate with the same frequency—the two are said to be in resonance.
>
> (p. 68)

Drawing a parallel to the psychotherapy process, Cambray adds that resonance is a form of "attunement among elements or agents in a field" (p. 68), which in turn amplifies the field's emergent properties. These properties include synchronicity, emotionally resonant countertransference, empathic reverie, concordant somatic experience, co-regulation, telepathic thoughts, and other subtle field phenomena.

The notions of resonance and emergence have important relevance for relational psychedelic therapy, where medicines act as profound amplifiers of emergent field phenomena. As psychedelic medicines generate an upwelling of the client's unconscious processes, the "vibrations" of these expressions saturate the shared space of the relational field with a broad range of empathic possibilities. The amplification of unformulated affect evoked by psychedelic medicines heightens the probability that these will affect the therapist's inner experience. When these frequencies are empathically met by the psychedelic therapist's open and receptive mind, a strong form of intersubjective resonance and attunement between client and therapist takes shape, and a highly dynamic relational field emerges.

In relational psychedelic therapy, the therapist aims to use their resonant countertransference feelings, somatic and energetic experiences, unbidden reveries, and intuitive perceptions to join the client in deep emotional connectedness. Carefully tending the relational field gives the therapist access to a multidimensional framework and approach for helping the client contain, metabolize, and understand the raw emotional intensity and meaningful implications embedded in their psychedelic visions, unformulated emotional and somatic experiences, unconscious interpersonal dynamics, and verbal expressions.

Co-Regulation

To cultivate states of resonance, enhance receptivity to the relational field, and identify moments of breakdown, the therapist opens their heart and reflective mind to the client's shifting states as well as their own embodied countertransference experience. Through meditative presence, the therapist brings awareness to the subtle emotional, somatic, and energetic qualities present in the field. As neuropsychologist Alan Schore (2012) describes,

> The empathic clinician's psycho-biologically attuned right brain tracks at a preconscious level, not only the arousal rhythms and flows of the patient's affective states but also [their] own somatic countertransferential, interoceptive, body-based affective responses to the patient's implicit facial, prosodic, and gestural communications.
>
> (p. 41)

By meeting the client at the affective and somatic levels of experience and attending to subtle unconscious processes, the therapist facilitates right-brain to right-brain communication and brain-activity alignment. This attunement occurs through non-verbal interactions, such as facial expressions, eye contact, subtle vocalizations, body gestures, and emotional resonance (Siegel, 1999).

The therapist's embodied attunement and empathic responsivity to the client's shifting states constitute what trauma researcher Stephen Porges (2017) and others call *co-regulation*. As "an interactive regulator of the patient's psychobiological states," the therapist

> is learning the nonverbal moment-to-moment rhythmic structures of the client's internal states, and is relatively flexibly and fluidly modifying [their] own

behavior to synchronize with that structure, thereby co-creating with the client a growth-facilitating context for the organization of the therapeutic alliance.

(Schore, 2012, p. 42)

Co-regulation facilitates states of resonance while also supporting the repair of moments of breakdown in unison through modulating hypo- and hyperarousal. Tracking the client's subtle non-verbal cues, nervous system arousal, and level of emotional engagement allows the therapist to discern whether resting in a state of resonance, implicitly engaging in co-regulation, or explicitly working toward interpersonal repair is indicated.

In moments of deep resonance, dissociated affective states become intensified; when mutual attunement is sustained within the relational field, the amplified affect may rise into conscious awareness. As the therapeutic dyad immerses in the felt sense of their subjective emotional experience, sensory and symbolic communications may emerge through subtle sensing, intuition, insight, or reverie. Instead of searching for meaning, the therapist remains open to whatever arises spontaneously such that verbal processing stays connected to the emergent process rather than moving away from it. As Bromberg (2006) explains,

When [a therapist] gives up their attempts to "understand" their patient and allows themself to know their patient through the ongoing intersubjective field they are sharing at the moment, an act of recognition (not understanding) takes place in which words and thoughts come to symbolize experience instead of substitute for it.

(p. 11)

By offering reflection and representation of the client's affective experience through symbolization, the therapist furthers the process of emotional metabolization by bringing previously unconscious affect into conscious awareness, thus facilitating integration between the limbic and prefrontal regions of the brain and supporting the organization of the client's mental processes (Siegel, 1999). Over time, as psychiatrist and researcher Dan Siegel (2013) posits, "dyadic regulation shapes self-regulation" as the client internalizes the therapist's regulating function (p. 103).

Co-regulation involves two or more nervous systems "talking" non-verbally with each other. Trauma, by definition, distorts the implicit "signals" sent from one body to another: hypervigilance, a hallmark of trauma, overinterprets signs of threat and under-interprets signs of safety. Conversely, MDMA quiets the brain's fear center, amplifying receptivity to indications of safety while diminishing perception of potential threats (Feduccia & Mithoefer, 2018). This prosocial effect is a significant boon for the use of co-regulation strategies in MDMA-assisted therapy because it increases client receptivity to experiences of resonance and co-regulation. Co-regulation can be particularly supportive during MDMA's onset, moments of intense trauma processing, and the medicine's comedown, when the client has greater potential for high levels of nervous system activation.

In the case described previously, Vera noted that throughout significant portions of the MDMA session she felt unsettled, distracted, and "left to her own devices," relying on typical patterns of hypervigilance and dissociation triggered by the therapist's lack of attunement. Imagine that her therapist, rather than "kinda just supervising," tunes into the relational field and notices Vera's difficulties settling into her experience. Turning toward her countertransference, the therapist senses an unformulated, bodily felt sense: a tight ball of energy in her solar plexus emitting palpable jolts at any unexpected sound or movement. As she tracks her somatic experience, she realizes that Vera just shared a childhood memory of being lost for several hours in a shopping center, terrified of the strangers around her, and unsure whether her father was still looking for her. The emotional resonance of the memory sends a strong wave through the therapist's body, leaving an affective impression of painful abandonment and emotional betrayal.

The therapist, working to contain and regulate her own body, first deepens her breath and aligns her subtle behavioral responses with the client's non-verbal cues, letting her heart open to fully experience the emotional resonance surfacing in the relational field. As the therapist gains a more grounded and embodied position within these unsettling feelings, she offers Vera a reflective comment about the terror of being left alone in an unfamiliar place as a child. Her voice is tuned to the frequency of Vera's expression, matching the emotional quality and adding resonant notes of empathic care. Her comments seem to have an impact on Vera, and the client responds by shifting her body into a more settled position. From that point forward, Vera drops more deeply into herself and is able to access embodied elaborations of her childhood experiences of emotional abandonment.

Trauma Recovery Through Relational Psychedelic Therapy

Developmental Trauma

According to leading trauma expert Bessel Van der Kolk (2005), developmental trauma stems from "multiple or chronic exposure to one or more forms of developmentally adverse interpersonal trauma (e.g., abandonment, betrayal, physical assaults, sexual assaults, threats to bodily integrity, coercive practices, emotional abuse, witnessing violence and death)" (p. 404). For our purposes, we will broaden this definition to include *relational trauma* caused by less severe, yet still highly impactful, repeated experiences of compromised emotional safety within primary attachment relationships due to chronic neglect, rejection, criticism, or attack of core aspects of the self.

This array of traumatic experiences can lead to self-regulatory impairments as well as fragmentation of the personality through disidentification and dissociation from the parts of the self that make one vulnerable to harm. These traumatized, dissociated parts carry overwhelming feelings, memories, and patterns of bodily tension associated with the trauma—while the traumatized psyche develops protective systems that work incessantly to keep those vulnerable and feeling-laden parts at bay. Despite the shielding offered by protective parts, dissociated self-states and the overwhelming emotions they hold can emerge suddenly in reaction to relational and environmental triggers reminiscent of the initial trauma. When triggered, these states hijack the body and mind, leading to emotional dysregulation and distorted perceptions of self and other. It is through this process that traumatic patterns of relating are imprinted and then continue to play out in intimate relationships throughout the life span.

Relational Theory of Change

In this and the subsequent section, we provide a summary of how the process of healing trauma unfolds through relational psychedelic therapy—a model we will elaborate upon in the sections that follow. We propose that the resolution of developmental trauma occurs through the cultivation of a therapeutic relationship that proves itself safe enough for protective parts, dissociated self-states, and dysfunctional patterns of relating to emerge and be met with witnessing, validation, curiosity, empathy, and care. We view relational psychedelic therapy as an ideal treatment modality to support the cultivation of this healing relationship and facilitate deep and lasting change. The therapist's sensitive attunement to the relational field, compassionate receptivity, and tactful opening of intersubjective dialogue fosters an atmosphere of deep safety, emotional honesty, and trust.

In this context, traumatically generated parts of the self and internalized interpersonal dynamics are afforded the opportunity to see and be seen, feel and be felt. To facilitate this process, the therapist sensitively engages the client's protective systems and invites them to share their experiences and perspectives, helping the client understand the role these parts play in stabilizing the psyche and protecting against re-traumatization. Over time, protective parts can be brought into negotiation with the client's diverse emotional needs, especially the need for vulnerable expression and intimate connection. As protective parts begin to feel seen and respected, they may sit back, or can be invited to step aside, such that the therapist and client can make contact with previously dissociated parts of the client. The therapist compassionately receives these traumatized parts, holding them with sensitive attunement and caring containment as they rise to the surface, find expression, and release through deeply embodied, emotional, imaginal, and energetic reexperiencing of previously intolerable affect. Interpersonal patterns rooted in traumatic relationships may manifest in the relational field through transference reactions or enactment; the skillful relational therapist brings these unconscious expressions into awareness and facilitates repair through carefully guided emotion-focused reflection, interpersonal negotiation, and the provision of unmet needs.

With time, the client gains greater self-understanding, disconfirms trauma-induced expectations and fantasies about self and other, and begins internalizing novel and reparative experiences of healthy relating. As the healing process unfolds, the client develops greater freedom and flexibility in how they respond to triggering situations, increased empathy toward their protective and traumatized self-states, and new pathways to meeting previously neglected core needs. Eventually, these self-states find a home in the client's conscious awareness, where they can be reclaimed as integral parts of the psyche without compromising the fundamental integrity of the self.

How Psychedelics Potentiate Relational Therapy

In standard psychotherapy, no matter the approach or modality, it can take many months or even years to gain access to the client's deeply dissociated, pain-ridden parts—much less to broach here-and-now dialogue about emergent transference dynamics and enactments in the therapeutic relationship—making trauma recovery an infamously slow process. Psychedelics, however, are powerful potentiators that can deepen and accelerate recovery from developmental trauma, leading to lasting characterological change. The potent neurochemical effects of psychedelic medicines can expediently bring traumatized self-states to the fore while heightening insight into interpersonal dynamics. These effects facilitate engagement and transformative work with self-states, transference reactions, and enactments that can otherwise be challenging to effectively access and engage. Symbiotically, the safety, trust, emotional honesty, and interpersonal negotiation cultivated through a skillful relational approach serve as an ideal container for the ritual of psychedelic healing.

While many psychedelics can potentiate a relational therapeutic process, we view MDMA and other empathogenic compounds as some of the most useful tools presently available to support recovery from developmental trauma. In the context of a well-held therapeutic container, MDMA reliably generates profound subjective experiences of interpersonal safety, trust, empathy, and self-acceptance. Simultaneously, MDMA tends to reduce interpersonal fear and expand the window of tolerance (Mitchell et al., 2021), which can soften habitual defense mechanisms and enhance capacity to tolerate previously overwhelming emotions. Supported by these complementary effects, dissociated self-states become more accessible, and the full-bodied experiencing, expression, symbolization, and meaning making of traumatic experience naturally unfold.

Additionally, MDMA increases self-awareness and access to the observing self, facilitating honest emotional dialogue. Transference dynamics may become magnified, while awareness and insight around these dynamics are more readily available. In the context of a safe, trusting, and interpersonally attuned therapeutic container, MDMA supports processing and working through transference reactions and enactment within the therapeutic relationship. Cumulatively, these effects profoundly expand opportunities for reparative emotional experience, memory reconsolidation, and greater self-awareness about one's interpersonal patterns.

In the following sections, we provide a detailed account of the trauma recovery process through relational psychedelic therapy. We weave relational and IFS theory together with clinical observations and scientific findings to illustrate how trauma recovery can unfold in an MDMA-assisted therapy treatment on a psychological and neurobiological level. We illustrate how the relational therapist can work in conjunction with psychedelic medicines to do the following:

1. Cultivate a solid foundation of safety and trust in the therapeutic relationship
2. Engage and work effectively with protective parts
3. Support the expression and integration of traumatized self-states
4. Work productively with transference reactions and enactments as they arise in the treatment

Cultivating Relational Safety

Grof (1980) argued that the most important element determining the efficacy of a psychedelic session "is the feeling of safety and trust on the part of the experient" (p. 87). He added, "This is, of course, critically dependent on . . . *the nature of the relationship between the subject and this person* [italics added]" (p. 87). To maximize the therapeutic benefit of psychedelic medicines, it is vital for the therapist to tend the therapeutic relationship by collaborating with the client in the process of building, maintaining, and repairing safety and trust throughout the course of treatment. The level of safety the client experiences in the therapeutic relationship is not static, particularly for those with marginalized identities living in unsafe worlds and those with significant histories of trauma. The client's sense of safety may fluctuate moment to moment throughout the treatment, based on their changing inner states and in response to cues from the therapist and the environment; therefore, the therapist must continuously track the client's experience of safety and threat throughout the treatment.

The interpersonal conditions necessary for healing developmental trauma are primarily expressed through repeated experiences of the therapist's warm and genuine care, humility, and dependability. *Relational safety* is cultivated through a therapeutic stance that includes unconditional positive regard (Rogers, 1951), openhearted curiosity, attuned receptivity, and compassionate understanding. Interpersonal trust is built through the therapist's consistency, competence, authenticity, and willingness to take responsibility for their mistakes and misattunements. Tactful dialogue about the client and therapist's intersectional identities, and any enactments of power and privilege that emerge, is fundamental to building and repairing safety and trust. The cultivation of a safe and trusting therapeutic environment is supported by the therapist's careful tending of the relational field—facilitating states of co-regulation, watching for instances of relational rupture, and skillfully working toward repair. This approach lays an optimal foundation for the client to relax into the therapeutic container and develop the comfort necessary to explore the depths of their inner world, the dynamics of the therapeutic relationship, and the dyad's intersectional identities. As these explorations unfold, the client's positive experiences of safety and intimacy in the therapeutic relationship are healing agents in and of themselves.

MDMA is known for expediently facilitating a deep sense of safety, trust, and emotional intimacy, which can be a novel experience for those with significant histories of developmental trauma. Perhaps the strongest mediator of MDMA's subjective effects is the flooding of the brain with serotonin, promoting feelings of well-being, relaxation, acceptance, and openness (Feduccia & Mithoefer, 2018). These effects are compounded by a surge of oxytocin, the "love hormone," which enhances emotional bonding, empathy, and interpersonal trust. The expanded openness, acceptance, and connection fostered by these "feel-good hormones" provide the client with templates for healthy relating that they can internalize over time. Although these profoundly openhearted states tend to fade with the medicine, the client may come away with a newfound awareness of their capacity for authentic relating, greater access to self-acceptance and compassion, and a renewed desire to cultivate intimacy in their relationships. Additionally, the enhanced level of trust and capacity to receive the therapist's care frequently endure well beyond the medicine session. This supports the cultivation of a strong therapeutic alliance and a deepening of the therapeutic process, whether or not psychedelic medicines continue to be part of the treatment.

While this neurochemically enhanced acceleration of safety and trust can be incredibly healing, some clients may perceive it as threatening. For clients with complex trauma, safety, trust, and warmth can be activating for several reasons: the unfamiliarity of intimate feeling states, prior coupling of positive relational experiences with harm, intense activation of unmet needs for emotional connection, the threat of overwhelm by previously dissociated affective states, and the grief that moments of safety and trust can evoke (i.e., mourning all the times these qualities were absent). The relational therapist can mitigate these threats by attuning to the client's tolerance for deepening positive experiences and titrating the level of intimacy to meet the client's particular needs (for contact as well as protection). The principles of non-direction and trusting the client's "inner healing intelligence," or their innate capacity to heal—core tenets of most psychedelic therapy models—encourage the therapist to follow the client's lead throughout the course of treatment, particularly during medicine sessions. This therapeutic stance allows the client to proceed at their own pace based on the level of risk they feel is manageable, giving them the freedom to trust the safety of the therapeutic container when they are ready and decide when to engage more intense, emotionally laden material.

In addition, an extended preparation phase may be appropriate to cultivate genuine safety and trust in the therapeutic relationship prior to introducing medicine into the picture, as well as to prepare the client for what may ensue. No matter the length of the preparation phase, the relational therapist can inform the client of the potential for the medicine to rapidly accelerate levels of trust and intimacy in the therapeutic relationship and to bring previously dissociated traumatic memories and self-states to the surface. They can then elicit and work with any parts of the client that have concerns about these possibilities (as detailed in the following section).

Working With Protective Self-States

Trauma-informed therapies recognize the paradoxical tension between the need to be witnessed in one's authentic self-expression and the need to protect one's vulnerability from harm. Navigating the razor's edge between these disparate needs requires the psychotherapist to hold the therapeutic process delicately: some risk is necessary, but too much risk is harmful. Guiding a client too quickly into deep trauma work can elicit fear and mistrust, trigger protective defenses, and threaten the client's sense of autonomy; conversely, too much avoidance, delay, or hesitation on the therapist's part can communicate to the client that the therapist is unwilling or afraid to feel, accompany the client in, or face some element of the trauma.

Despite the therapist's efforts to carefully negotiate this paradoxical tension, titrate levels of intimacy, adequately prepare clients for the medicine session, and follow the client's lead, the subjective effects of MDMA may still activate the client's instinct to protect themselves. As we have mentioned, psychedelics have a propensity to evoke previously dissociated traumatic memories and affective states. The MDMA-induced release of norepinephrine and cortisol enhances emotional engagement and recall of difficult memories, bringing self-states tied to traumatic memories to the surface and facilitating engagement with them (Feduccia & Mithoefer, 2018). This can be experienced as a threat to the client's protective parts, which intend to keep these dreaded experiences out of conscious awareness. Alternatively, protective parts can be triggered by underlying fears that the therapist will be overwhelmed, disbelieving, or indifferent to their trauma.

In reaction to these triggers, the client's protective parts may experience strong reactions to the therapist, to their exiled self-states or to the treatment; these feelings may manifest as sudden waves of constrictive emotions, like mistrust, agitation, avoidance, hopelessness, or hostility. Furthermore, many clients with developmental trauma navigate the world from a range of near-constant defensive strategies (e.g., hypervigilance or avoidance), led by protective parts who feel they must perpetually be on guard to protect themselves from an unsafe world or overwhelming inner turmoil. Fortunately, if the client is able to identify the presence of a protective self-state—or the therapist senses them through attunement to the client's experience and shifts in the relational field—an opportunity arises to work directly with the client's self-protective strategies. This work can lead to greater understanding of the protective parts, reparation of emotional safety in the therapeutic relationship, and ultimately transformation of these parts into healthier contributors to the client's internal system.

When a protective part surfaces, it is important for the therapist to first immerse themselves in the emotional content present in the relational field. The therapist can then invite the client into a collaborative exploration aimed at understanding what this part is communicating by non-defensively inquiring into their here-and-now feelings, including feelings about and perceptions of the therapist and the dynamics at play. The protective part is given the opportunity to share their experience with a curious, receptive person. As this part begins to feel understood and cared for, the reality of the current situation as distinct from the initially traumatizing environment may become evident, either implicitly or through the therapist's thoughtful use of self-disclosure, which may range from subtle hints to explicit articulation of their real-time experience. The protective part may thus come to see the therapist as an ally in tending to the client's emotional safety, rather than a threat.

In moments when relational safety is reestablished with the therapist through emotional expression, interpersonal negotiation, and the disconfirmation of traumatically generated expectations, the client's observing self becomes more accessible, and they can join the therapist in an exploration of their protective self-states. Clients often benefit from relating to their defenses as personified figures, "protectors" who contribute a specific function to the overall internal system (Kalsched, 1996; Schwartz, 2001). Open discussion about the protectors' function in the therapeutic process and in day-to-day life helps the client learn through direct experience the interpersonal and intrapsychic benefit and cost of the protection. Relational therapist and trauma expert Harvey Schwartz (2013) notes that over time, the aggressive energy of the protective self-state, deformed by trauma into the dynamics of too much or not enough, can be transformed into usable and creative forms of aggression through the therapist's open and compassionate engagement with the client's healthy self-protection, self-assertion, and discernment.

With practice, protective parts learn to negotiate their needs and become integrated as part of the "full democracy" of the client's psyche. As they begin to feel seen, understood, and valued—and recognize the safety of the therapeutic container—they relinquish their tight control over the more vulnerable and traumatized parts of the psyche; even the most tightly held protectors can learn to sit back and trust the capacity of the therapist to offer consistent holding of a wide variety of emotional states. In turn, the client is gradually able to experience, explore, and integrate traumatized self-states that were previously felt to threaten the integrity of the psyche.

MDMA stimulates several neurobiological shifts that support protective parts in sitting back and allowing trauma-related affect and self-states to surface. As we have alluded to previously, MDMA reduces blood flow to the amygdala and insula, attenuating amygdala activation in response to fear-inducing stimuli, thus quieting the fear response and generating a bodily based feeling of safety and ease (Feduccia & Mithoefer, 2018). The compound simultaneously increases activity in the ventromedial prefrontal cortex (Gamma et al., 2000), reinforcing the capacity for emotional regulation. As the nervous system settles into greater relaxation and the affective window of tolerance expands, the client gains an enhanced capacity to tolerate intense emotional states without succumbing to typical protective strategies associated with trauma (e.g., hypervigilance, flooding, avoidance, freezing, and numbing).

In addition, similar to many other psychedelic compounds, MDMA is correlated with a decrease in default-mode network activity (Müller et al., 2020), affording the client a reprieve from self-consciousness, rumination, and negative thought patterns that may dominate their day-to-day experience. Protective parts no longer need to stand guard within the context of a safe, relationally attuned therapeutic container, a regulated nervous system, an expanded window of tolerance, and the attenuation of negative thought patterns—presenting the client with an opportunity for reestablishing associative connections to deeply disavowed self-states and fragments of traumatic experience, making these available for therapeutic processing.

Working With Traumatized Self-States

IFS uses the term *exiles* (Schwartz, 2001) to refer to the young wounded parts of the self that carry dissociated fragments of traumatically induced memories and overwhelming affect, such as fear, shame, guilt, abandonment, betrayal, grief, and rage. To call into being these banished self-states that hold unmetabolized trauma, the therapist and client need to make genuine emotional contact. As psychoanalyst Clay Whitehead (2006) explains,

> Every time we make therapeutic contact with our patients we are engaging processes that tap into essential life forces in ourselves and in those we work with. . . . Emotions are deepened in intensity and sustained in time when they are intersubjectively shared. This occurs at moments of deep contact.
>
> (p. 624)

In such instances, each party is emotionally impacted by the here-and-now encounter of the therapeutic relationship. The therapist's role is to cultivate deep emotional attunement and to stay present, without agenda, with whatever emotions arise in the relational field. Through such "moments of deep contact," previously dissociated affect may intensify to the point that it becomes conscious.

MDMA and many other psychedelics have been shown to act as "re-associatives," supporting the process of integrating dissociated self-states (both protectors and exiles) by stimulating a significant discharge of energy from the medial temporal regions to the association cortices[6] (Carhart-Harris, 2007; Gamma et al., 2000). The enhanced communication between these two brain regions is a counterforce to the impact of traumatic dissociation, which inhibits integration between these brain regions, thus preventing integration of traumatic experience (Paulsen & Lanius, 2014). This feature of psychedelic medicines, as "re-associatives," has significant implications for trauma-focused psychotherapy. As trauma experts Sandra Paulsen and Ulrich Lanius noted, "The association of that which had previously been dissociated pathologically is the path to mental health for the trauma-related conditions" (Paulsen & Lanius, 2014, para. 20).

Simultaneously, MDMA quiets the fear response while enhancing emotional engagement and recall. This combination of effects gives the client greater access to what trauma experts call "dual awareness"—the simultaneous grounding in present-moment awareness (the observing self) alongside the reexperiencing of trauma-induced affective states (Fisher, 2017)—a state of mind seen as fundamental in trauma processing.

Through genuine emotional contact between therapist and client, combined with the enhanced intra-brain communication and dual awareness afforded by MDMA, the client is in an ideal state to engage long-sequestered traumatic memories and emotions and experience them in a full, embodied way. Multifaceted manifestations of these previously dissociated self-states emerge through a complex web of memory, emotion, image, sensation, energetic constriction, and narratives of self and other. Crystalized psychic shards of terror, shame, guilt, despair, grief, or rage dissolve into tears, sobbing, vocalization, movement, shaking, or other forms of emotional, physical, and energetic expression. The founder of IFS, Richard Schwartz (2008), noted, "This process of identifying and releasing the extreme emotion or belief that a part carries is called unburdening and, in IFS, is equivalent to healing the part" (p. 147).

When these traumatized self-states emerge in the therapeutic context, being witnessed and held with full acceptance and attuned care is central to their healing. As Schore (2012) describes,

> Re-experiencing the traumatic experience in therapy with the safety and security of an empathic, supportive therapist provides the person with a new experience. This new experience is specifically the clinician's interactive regulation of the patient's communicated dysregulated right brain hyper- and hypo-aroused affective states.
>
> (p. 103)

As dissociated self-states are brought into the light of consciousness and given the opportunity to express the trauma-laden affect they have long been holding, the way is paved for reparative emotional experience through the therapist's curious, compassionate, and caring receptivity to these tender and traumatized parts.

The release of dopamine and norepinephrine stimulated by MDMA enhances the acuity of mental focus, sharpens thought processes, strengthens self-reflective capacity, and supports the client's ability to track internal sensation and affect, thereby facilitating emotional (re)learning. Dopamine also plays a part in the "destabilization" of memories, helping the client to incorporate new information from present-day reality (Feduccia & Mithoefer, 2018).

Parts previously perceived as shameful and alienating can be lovingly seen and held, dissipating any associated charge and incorporating the present-moment sense of safety and the therapist's care into the reorganization of the client's relationship to these parts. Through repeated instances of the therapist's demonstrated trustworthiness, the client internalizes the image of a "good enough" parent (Winnicott, 1953), who can relate to all of their parts with care and compassion. The therapeutic dyad can together help the client's traumatized parts meet core unmet needs by, for example, validating the reality of their trauma; dispelling negative self-perceptions/self-blame; offering reassurance that they are safe, seen, and cared for; and exploring new ways to protect them from future harm.

The therapist's interest in and desire to understand the client's subjective reality provide a context in which dissociated self-states can be understood, affirmed, and integrated. Each point of non-traumatizing contact made with a dissociated part is a stitch in the fabric of the client's psyche, an opportunity to modify the deeply ingrained belief that these parts are destructive and must be kept locked away. Collaborative meaning making and reconstruction of the trauma narrative enable the client to develop new, conscious relationships to these parts of themselves. With an expanded window of tolerance and increased cognitive and emotional flexibility, built through their MDMA-assisted therapy sessions, the client develops greater capacity to safely feel and express intense affect, becoming available for deeper levels of emotional fulfillment in their relationships.

The client repairs their sense of dignity as they gain empathy for their wounded self-states and learn to see them as necessary adaptations to a traumatic environment, rather than proof of their being worthless, damaged, or a failure. The client cultivates compassion for their protective parts as well as their traumatized child parts, and gains greater choice around how to respond, inwardly and outwardly, as these self-states arise in their intimate relationships going forward—ultimately giving them greater freedom to express the full range of their personality. The IFS theory suggests that traumatized parts can be integrated by identifying new qualities they would like to adopt or roles they can play in the client's present-day reality and making agreements to ensure ongoing contact with these young parts. This process of reconnection and repair between the inner parts of the client's psyche facilitates a deepening of trust and safety among the client's parts and within the therapeutic relationship.

Occasionally, certain self-states (exiles and protective parts alike) remain dissociated and unnamed, existing outside the conscious awareness of both therapist and client, as they did in Vera's case. In these situations, they may instead be expressed as unconscious communication via transference reactions, received through the therapist's subtle sensing of the relational field and their countertransference reactions. When these signals go unrecognized, the mutually dependent transference and countertransference reactions are acted out by therapist and client in a process called "enactment."

Transference, Countertransference, and Enactments

Negative transference reactions typically begin when the client experiences an emotional trigger in response to a perceived rupture in the therapeutic relationship. Ruptures can range from subtle misattunements consciously imperceptible to both parties to a gross error on the therapist's part. They may occur in response to inadequate preparation for a medicine session, misattunement to the client's emotional experience or identity, or other triggering aspects of the therapist's behavior or the environment reminiscent of the client's original traumatic experience.

Vera's MDMA treatment contained many rupturing elements. Her therapist overlooked several important topics during preparation, including adequately orientating Vera to what she could expect from the MDMA session and emphasizing the importance of sharing negative feelings that arise toward the therapist. The therapist also appeared tired and disengaged during key moments of the session, and neither addressed the emotional distance that developed in response nor made space for Vera's feelings of frustration, disappointment, and anger. Cumulatively, these oversights put Vera in the position of taking care of her therapist, rather than the reverse, and reiterated Vera's lifelong experience of isolation and alienation. Notable transference dynamics thus emerged in the MDMA session: first in the form of Vera's impulse to self-contain, distract, and caretake, and later through mistrust, distancing, and disguised hostility toward the therapist.

Clients with a history of developmental trauma frequently avoid conscious awareness and discussion of ruptures because they are fearful of compromising relational safety (Bromberg, 2011); this may be especially true if the therapist and client embody any oppressor–oppressed identities. Direct communication about challenges in the therapeutic relationship can raise the threat of conflict or harmful power dynamics. When the client's sense of threat reaches a certain threshold, they may dissociate from the triggered state, creating distance from their emotional reaction and diminishing the threat. As psychoanalyst Wilma Bucci describes,

Dissociative defenses serve to regulate relatedness to others. . . . The dissociative patient is attempting to stay enough in a relationship with the human environment to survive the present while, at the same time, keeping the needs for more intimate relatedness sequestered but alive.

(Bucci, 2002, p. 149)

The client's dissociation impacts the relational field, frequently evoking a parallel experience of dissociation in the therapist—what Bromberg (2011) calls a "dead space" or "dissociative cocoon." When mutual dissociation is at play, a breakdown in unison has occurred in the relational field. The states that arise in both client and therapist are initially unsymbolized—wordless and imageless—such that neither client nor therapist can reflect upon or give expression to the dynamics playing out. These states are expressed through the mutual reliving of an emotionally charged dynamic, in which both client and therapist enter into an activated self-state that is isolated from more reflective parts of the psyche. For example, the therapist may lose their self-reflective capacity, begin to feel disdain toward the client, and make an unintentionally judgmental comment, thus falling into an enactment of a critical parental figure. Enactments can also be experienced as deadness—a mutual flattening of emotional responsiveness between therapist and client.

Navigating these emotionally complicated entanglements requires the therapist's committed attunement to shifts in the relational field and specifically to the transference–countertransference matrix—the "fluctuating, moment to moment experience of what it is like for them to be with their patient and for their patient to be with them during the course of the session" (Bromberg, 2011, p. xxvii). The therapist directs close attention and honest emotional reflection to their countertransference experience: the felt sense of the therapeutic relationship, including the somatic, emotional, and energetic qualities present in their bodies and in the therapist–client interchange. The therapist takes in the overall feel of the relational field, noting the extent to which there is a sense of resonance in the therapeutic dyad; the level of vitality vs. deadness; and any palpable feeling tone, charge, or nebulous quality. The therapist's attunement to these subtle shifts in the field, to their subjective state of mind and body, and to the client's presentation can serve as a primary means to better understand unconscious communications and relational dynamics at play before a full enactment takes shape.

Countertransference reactions may include strong experiences of disconnection and emotional deadness, which can manifest as boredom, restlessness, difficulty focusing, or exhaustion—or through the sudden experience of intense affect, such as distress, irritation, confusion, and rage. Relational psychoanalyst Donnel Stern (2010) referred to these important emotional signals as "chafing" (p. 52). The therapist's somatic experience may also be an indicator of an emergent but not yet symbolized relational dynamic; some notable somatic signals include a persistent tightness in the chest, nausea, sweating, temperature changes, strong currents of energy moving through the body, nervous system activation, feeling aroused, or an impulse to laugh at an inappropriate time. In addition, the therapist can listen for implicit communications within the client's spoken narrative and non-verbal cues that may function as symbolic representations of the client's here-and-now emotional state and their experience of the therapeutic relationship.

When mutual dissociation remains unrecognized, the therapist falls prey to unconsciously enacting their countertransference reaction. For example, when Vera's therapist failed to recognize and work with the maternal transference that she carried, she unconsciously stepped into an enactment of Vera's early abandonment by her mother. In relational psychoanalysis, enactments are understood as a form of interpersonally enacted sub-symbolic communication of unbearable and unspeakable affective states (Bromberg, 2011). In an enactment, the therapist and client find themselves playing out salient interpersonal dynamics that originated in the client's traumatic history and simultaneously tie into the therapist's own relational wounding. Enactments—if recognized and addressed—provide an en vivo opportunity to live through old relational patterns with the goal of creating a different outcome. As Davies explains,

> We assume—indeed, we rely upon—the hope that analyst and patient together will become enmeshed in complicated reenactments of early, unformulated experiences with significant others that can shed light upon the patient's current interpersonal and intrapsychic difficulties by reopening in the [therapeutic] relationship prematurely foreclosed areas of experience.
>
> (Davies, 1994, p. 156)

The therapist's position in working through an enactment is as a participant observer, drawn into the enactment through initially unconscious countertransference reactions while tasked with the responsibility of observing what is unfolding relationally. Enactments can be intense, challenging, and evocative for both therapist and client; if left unaddressed, they can lead to impasse and even abrupt termination of the treatment.

Enactments, paradoxically, are a primary source of iatrogenic harm as well as a powerful way in which the client can experience reparative processing and breakthrough insights that help them move toward healing. Central to the catalytic capacity of psychedelics is the increased potential for reparative enactments, particularly in attachment-related trauma, where witnessing, holding, containing, and reparative emotional experience can be deeply transformative.

Because psychedelics significantly modify the relational field, the therapist's responses—along with their conscious and unconscious thoughts and feelings—have greater potential to be deeply impacted and guided by the client's emerging material. These conditions require the therapist to abandon formulaic ways of relating to the client while fostering a "beginner's mind" and attunement to embodied emotional responses to prepare for the spontaneous emergence of enactments. The therapist must be willing to participate as a proxy for a source of the patient's previously unprocessed trauma, as well as their unrealized opportunities for repair and resilience. Taking up this proxy position in psychedelic therapy, where the range of projections is amplified, calls for even more empathy, patience, flexibility, and self-awareness than is typically needed to process unconscious interpersonal dynamics in traditional psychotherapy.

Interpersonal Negotiation

Working with these transference/countertransference reactions and enactments toward expression, repair, and mutual recognition is subtle and complex. The therapist's capacity to withstand moments of intense countertransference and maintain awareness of their internal experience amid a deeply dissociative process opens up the possibility of engaging directly with the relational dynamic at play. Here, the therapist engages in a process of inquiry, emotional honesty, and a willingness to take responsibility for mistakes. They consider the fluctuations and disturbances in the field within the context of the client's history, their own relational wounding, the sociocultural context, and the power dynamics embedded in the relationship. Repair becomes possible as the therapeutic dyad begins to put words to the dynamics playing out.

The therapist should help the client feel permission to express any and all negative feelings about the therapist or therapy process, beginning in preparation and throughout the full arc of the treatment. Remaining sensitive to right timing, the therapist starts by drawing attention to the breakdown of the reflective capacities of the dyad and engaging the client in an exploration of the dynamics present in the relationship. They invite the client to express their here-and-now emotional experience and reactions to the therapist. It is essential that the therapist maintain a non-defensive stance throughout this process.

Whether or not the client is able to name their internal experience, the therapist may opt to self-disclose through honest articulation of their countertransference and experience of the relationship—modeling emotional transparency as a path toward embodied expression, collaborative meaning making, and increased safety and intimacy. This relational intervention aims to bring the unconscious interpersonal dynamics into awareness and to create a more inviting atmosphere for the client to share feelings that previously felt threatening. Through this process, the therapist makes efforts to understand and sensitively develop language for the feelings and experiences being communicated by the client, deepening the client's experience of themselves by giving voice to aspects of their transference reactions that were previously not felt or represented.

Working through unconscious interpersonal dynamics is rarely straightforward; inviting the client to engage in direct conversation about their experience of the therapist has the propensity to trigger significant fear and protective defenses. In working with developmental trauma, the therapist needs to account for both the need to work through interpersonal dynamics as well as the fear these conversations can evoke. As Bromberg (2011) noted, the therapy needs to be "safe but not too safe" (p. 17). The therapist demonstrates their commitment to relational safety by staying emotionally engaged with the client throughout these challenging interactions. It is important for the therapist to show their concern for the client's emotional experience in the here and now, keeping in mind that putting words to these feared and shame-filled self-states is often a significant challenge to the client's sense of safety. It is essential to hold the client's experience with care during "not too safe" moments: specifically, the therapist should track the potentially provocative, even disorganizing, impact of this process; communicate concern about the impact of their self-disclosures and other relationally focused conversations; and maintain an ongoing attunement to the client's emotional experience, sense of safety, and level of nervous system arousal.

MDMA is a powerful mediator for working through unconscious interpersonal entanglements and can be a particular boon in situations where the client would otherwise experience direct interpersonal negotiation as threatening. Because MDMA can both intensify transference reactions and increase interpersonal and inner awareness, MDMA-assisted therapy can offer valuable opportunities to work effectively with relational dynamics as they show up in the therapy. Neurobiologically, MDMA increases central blood flow to the ventromedial prefrontal cortex (Feduccia & Mithoefer, 2018), enhancing the client's ability to access an observing self that can witness and reflect on (rather than act out) their interpersonal emotional experience. With this support, the client may find it easier to identify that a transference reaction has been triggered; differentiate it from their core sense of self; and express that part's perceptions, fears, and needs. Alongside enhanced insight, clarity, and discernment, MDMA fosters greater compassion and curiosity in the client around their transference reactions as they arise in the therapeutic relationship, supporting the development of intersubjective awareness and the capacity for interpersonal negotiation.

Through interpersonal negotiation, the client and the therapist explore their different versions of the relational dynamic taking place and carefully piece together their subjective realities to form a shared understanding of the underlying unconscious dynamics at play and each person's respective roles. By putting words to these dynamics, the therapist aims to help the client better understand their unconscious relational patterns formed in early development. This dialogue facilitates opportunities for authentic connection and "an environment of shared inquiry, shared authority, and eventually mutual recognition and influence" (Schwartz, 2013, p. 168). Concurrently, the therapist helps the client come to recognize their own resources for navigating interpersonal differences and emotional conflict. In identifying patterns of projection and outdated interpersonal schemas, new and more expansive emotional experiences become possible in the therapeutic relationship; over time, these possibilities can be transferred to the client's other relationships.

This process of negotiation hinges on the therapist's capacity to maintain an intersubjective stance through holding their own subjective experience while simultaneously developing an embodied understanding of the client's version of emotional truth. Repeated experiences of successful interpersonal negotiation strengthen the client's own capacity for intersubjectivity and demonstrate that authentic emotional relating can be generative rather than threatening. These shifts in perspective and expanded ways of relating support the client in decreasing their reliance on projection and maladaptive interpersonal patterns.

As unconscious interpersonal dynamics are gradually articulated and understood, the client is increasingly able to differentiate between the original traumatic relationship and their current relationship with their therapist, seeing the therapist for who they are rather than who the client imagined them to be. Simultaneously, the client sees themselves in a new light, no longer damaged, worthless, unlovable, or disgraced. As the process unfolds, the client cultivates more stable and realistic self-esteem as well as greater vitality and curiosity about themselves and others. Reparative emotional experiences become possible as the client accesses from the therapist what was needed but not available from their primary caregivers. Over time and through repeated instances of such reparative experiences, the client is able to adjust their habitual interpersonal dynamics and adopt healthier protective strategies.

Imagine, in Vera's case, that in the integration process the therapist had inquired into Vera's experience of the therapeutic relationship during the MDMA session. We can imagine Vera reacting by placating the therapist, saying that it felt fine and then quickly looking away. Rather than responding immediately, however, the therapist sits with Vera in the palpable feeling of emptiness that pervades the room, privately noting through her countertransference feelings of exhaustion and blankness that a dissociative process masking an underlying transference reaction is underway. Suspecting that feelings of abandonment and betrayal are likely being veiled by Vera's self-protective dissociation, the therapist calls to mind an image of young Vera, abandoned by her mother. After making empathic contact with this image, she sensitively expresses curiosity about parts of Vera's experience that may be under the surface and not yet articulated. The therapist discloses the countertransference impression that arose for her, mentioning that she felt some distance between the two of them at certain points during the session. She gently wonders aloud whether Vera experienced something similar.

In opening this relational dialogue, the therapist supports Vera in feeling empowered to acknowledge her concerns that her therapist was bored and disengaged, as well as her impulse to self-contain out of a fear of being a burden by imposing her needs on others. Appreciating the therapist's receptivity to her experience, Vera then feels safe enough to express her anger at her therapist for being distant. The therapist's care, non-defensiveness, and active engagement in the conversation demonstrate her desire for connection, her openness to feedback, and that she does not feel burdened by Vera's feelings. To amplify Vera's sense of safety, the therapist explicitly appreciates Vera's willingness to be vulnerable by bringing her feelings forward.

The therapist then discloses her actual experience of Vera, noting that she has felt touched by instances in which she expressed her needs, and shares her desire to support Vera in getting her needs met. The therapist also takes a risk by disclosing a bit about her own experience during the MDMA session, admitting to and apologizing for the fact that she was somewhat tired that day due to stresses in her own life, and taking responsibility for the impact this had on her ability to be as fully present as she would have liked. These disclosures concurrently validate Vera's emotional experience and serve as a counterpoint to Vera's deeply held beliefs that she is too much and her feelings will push people away.

The conversation unfolds into an exploration that helps Vera see through her projections and identify her habitual modes of self-blame, uncovering the historical context of her feelings toward her therapist and recognizing the deep wounding she experienced in her relationship to her mother. Vera thereby gains greater access to her grief around the loss of her mother as well as the impending loss of her therapist. This process of authentic relating about the therapeutic dynamic brings to consciousness Vera's underlying fear of being too much and being rejected as a result, alongside her tendency to self-contain and push others away in self-protection. The ongoing exploration of Vera's protective patterns in the medicine and integration sessions enables her to see both the value and the harmful impact of these patterns, and it creates an opportunity to learn new, more adaptive protective strategies.

Working in the Transference

For some clients with significant histories of trauma, the risk of compromising the safety of the therapeutic relationship through direct emotional engagement and here-and-now dialogue about challenging interactions feels too threatening. One client described the conversations we had about our mutual experience of each other as "walking into a field of landmines"—she felt like the relationship could blow up at any minute. These clients may be unable to engage as the therapist attempts to bring dissociated dynamics into conscious dialogue; instead, these forays evoke protective parts that lean on defenses, such as hypervigilance, hypercompliance, avoidance, angry withdrawal, or dissociation to avoid the terrifying prospect of relational rupture. As Schore (2012) describes, "In characterological dissociation an autoregulatory strategy of involuntary autonomic dis-engagement is initiated and maintained to prevent potentially dysregulating intersubjective contact" (p. 102). Working explicitly with transference reactions and enactments may be impossible with these clients, and negative feelings toward the therapist may remain dissociated for months or even years.

While MDMA can increase awareness of transference reactions and enactments, sometimes clients will step into a transference reaction during a medicine session with little awareness of what is happening. Even in these instances, a useful process can still unfold: the therapist has the opportunity to relate directly to the client's feelings, which may be amplified by the medicine and thus easier for the therapist to identify. This requires the therapist to develop a keen awareness of emergent transference reactions in the relational field and respond to them with respect, compassion, and curiosity.

The therapist can start by inquiring into the client's experience of the relational dynamic, and determine the extent to which direct relational work is possible by gauging the client's response. Careful attention to the client's micro-movements and subtle shifts in the relational field may reveal more than the verbal content. Clients with more severe trauma and deeply ingrained defenses against authentic emotional contact may deny, change the topic, become emotionally activated, slide deeper into dissociation, or otherwise avoid the therapist's attempts at relational dialogue. In these cases, relational work must occur implicitly. When explicit discussion *of* transference reactions is either untenable or would disturb the flow of the session, the therapist can instead work *in* the transference.

The therapist can implicitly support emotional metabolization by empathically attuning to and compassionately relating with the client's transference feelings. In this approach, the therapist takes in aspects of the client's inner world and experience, with attentive receptivity to the reverberation evoked within, such that the therapist is able to feel herself to actually be that unwanted part of the client's self or that unbearable inner figure (Mitrani, 2001). From this place of deep emotional resonance, the therapist can help contain and metabolize overwhelming, unformulated emotion and cultivate a compassionate connection to these unwanted and unbearable parts.

The integration of MDMA into the treatment can support and accelerate working in the transference by enhancing the client's capacity to drop deeply into their own emotional experience, meet the therapist in a state of resonance, and receive the therapist's compassionate response to the emotional distress held by these inner figures. Over time, "as the patient continues through the change process, he or she becomes more able to forgo autoregulation for interactive regulation when under interpersonal stress" (Schore, 2012, p. 102), making explicit relational work more possible.

In this section, we have provided a general map of the relational psychedelic approach to the process of trauma recovery. However, every client's recovery process is unique, and disruptions in the therapeutic relationship frequently occur.

When enactments and other transference reactions are triggered during a psychedelic session and not properly tended by the therapist (often through normal human fallibility), the self-states evoked may become a dominant influence in the client's experience in the following days or weeks. These reactions can play out with the therapist or in other close relationships, requiring sensitive and skilled therapeutic attention throughout the integration process. If the rupture is not properly addressed, an impasse in the therapeutic process may ensue, leading the client to experience heightened symptoms for some time thereafter, as we saw in Vera's case. For this and numerous other reasons, skillful integration is an essential element of any psychedelic treatment.

Relational Psychedelic Integration

Psychedelic integration is a complex and multilayered undertaking that involves a range of therapeutic practices. Although a comprehensive review is outside the scope of this chapter, in this section we demonstrate how a relational approach can be an invaluable resource for facilitating psychedelic integration and addressing some of the most pervasive and intractable challenges that arise during this essential phase of treatment. We discuss how to work with backlash from protectors, support the transformation of states into traits, utilize interpersonal negotiation to facilitate the integration process, and support the client in making sense of their trauma and developing a new narrative. For further discussion of the opportunities and challenges of psychedelic integration, see Chapter 14.

We feel it is important to highlight the intense and potentially destabilizing nature of psychedelic therapy. It can be profoundly vulnerable to be witnessed and supported through the expansive and contracted states evoked by psychedelics—the waves of exultant and agonizing experience, as well as the broad spectrum of deeply evocative trauma processing, emotional expression, and somatic release. In the days or even weeks following a psychedelic session, clients often find themselves in a highly sensitive state and may experience sudden, dysregulating waves of emotions, resurfacing of traumatic memories, heightened feelings of hopelessness and despair, amplification of debilitating symptoms, negative feelings toward the therapist or therapy, and even increased levels of suicidality.

An experienced psychedelic therapist understands that these challenges are a common part of the process, may be indicators of deep reorganization of the psyche instigated by this powerful modality, and can be worked with effectively with adequate skill and attunement, as we will illustrate in the pages that follow. The potentially destabilizing nature of the process and symptoms that may result should be conveyed to the client in the preparation phase and referenced as needed throughout integration. To safely support the client through this sensitive phase of the treatment and optimize the conditions for a transformative experience, it is essential for the therapy dyad to allocate adequate time for integration and for the therapist to offer consistent emotional attunement, reliability, and availability for contact (extra sessions, phone calls, etc.) during this period.

Backlash of the Protectors

As Harvey Schwartz and Jessica Katzman clearly articulate in Chapter 14, integration is not linear: clients frequently experience some gradation of doubt, conflict, or contraction around their medicine session experiences, leading to challenges, relapses, setbacks, and resistances in their healing process. The tension between vulnerability and protection is an archetypal human experience and one of the primary themes that shapes any psychedelic therapy treatment. The therapist's task is to help the client work with the archetypal paradox between their need to maintain protection and self-coherence by staying the same and the equally important, yet vulnerable, need for change (Bromberg, 1998). With the therapist's support, the client can learn to better navigate their protective impulses as well as manage the vulnerability of accessing traumatized self-states and unconscious interpersonal dynamics for the sake of transformation.

Clients often find that protective parts and their corresponding contracted states are activated in the days after an intense medicine session—particularly one in which they went to a notably vulnerable or expansive place or had a deeply intimate experience with the therapist. They may find themselves in a destabilized place in such instances, struggling with feelings of disappointment, distress, anger, doubt, fear, shame, or confusion. In seeking safety through stabilization, they may dissociatively distance themselves from the therapist, the treatment, the medicine session, or any vulnerable states that arose, and shift into protective self-states they have relied on for survival. The client thus regresses into "an insulated version of reality that protectively defines what is 'me' at a given moment and forcing other self-states that are inharmonious with its truth to become 'not-me' and unavailable to participate in the complex negotiation we call internal conflict" (Bromberg, 2011, p. 15). This dissociative hyper-compartmentalization—"me" from "not me"—is a protection against unbearable internal conflict: unbearable because the disjunctive self-states are so discrepant (i.e., open and vulnerable vs. distant and protected) that their coexistence in a single state of consciousness risks destabilizing self-continuity.

This "backlash" of protective self-states comes in many forms and may be experienced and expressed directly as anger or mistrust toward the therapist for guiding them to an unsafe place. As Bromberg (2011) articulates,

> When the fail-safe protective system is softened by a moment of genuine self-reflectiveness, the parts of the self that are the guardians of affective stability become outraged, and the part that holds the unprocessed affect of developmental trauma caused by attachment failure becomes fearful, depressed, or both, causing distress to all parts—for which the therapist's idea of "success" is then blamed.
>
> (p. 76)

Backlash feelings may also be directed toward the treatment and/or the medicine for suddenly ripping away the client's ability to protect themselves, leaving them hesitant to continue engaging with the process. Alternatively, protector parts may turn against themselves for having risked re-traumatization by letting down their guard and allowing access to previously sequestered traumatic memories and intolerable emotions. These parts may camouflage shame for failing to do their job behind anger, provocation, distancing, or minimization of the significance of what took place in the medicine session. Additionally, protective parts may feel threatened, fearing that they are no longer needed or valued. Protector backlash is frequently aimed at the more expansive or vulnerable child parts that surfaced with the support of the medicine; when hijacked by a protector, the client may find themselves feeling indifferent, inhospitable, and even hostile toward these parts. Backlash feelings may also be experienced as disorientation or confusion—a sense of being unsure whether the vulnerability was indeed safe and consensual.

Ongoing negotiation with these protective parts during the integration process is often necessary to address the feelings and dynamics evoked. Relational approaches to integration make use of the therapist's intuitive imagination and embodied sensing to track the relational field. The relational therapist listens for the emergence of dissociated self-states, especially nihilistic protectors that negate and undermine anything hopeful in the client's experience, thus pushing them to recoil into default patterns. Once the presence of these protectors is identified, there are moves the therapist can make to mitigate the enactment of parts that strip meaning from or inject existential despair into the client's experience.

For one, the therapist can counter the nihilism of the protectors by helping the client make meaningful links between their intention for the work and the experiences that spontaneously surfaced during and after a medicine session. For example, one client had a vision of building and deconstructing a tower throughout his journey; later, he dismissed the experience as "just like playing a video game at home, a complete waste of time." The therapist gently highlighted the tower's significance by connecting it to his intention of "not escaping my life anymore," and then invited the client to reflect on how his psychedelic vision seemed to point to the choice he had to either build towers of isolation or take them down. The client's discovery of a meaningful context for his experience evoked a release of emotional tension and an expanded sense of receptivity, allowing him to see that his process was purposeful and imbued with meaning.

Protector backlash calls for the therapist to hold in mind all parts of the client throughout the integration process. Relational theorists understand integration of the personality as a process of building connections of conscious awareness and collaboration between dissociated self-states. In his article on treating dissociative disorders, H. Schwartz (1994) describes psychological integration as occurring "when two or more previously separated aspects of self, in their own time and of their own volition, recognize each other's experience to the extent that there is a shared memory, grieving, and relinquishment of dissociative controls" (p. 201). When working with a client's traumatized self-states in a medicine session, integration may involve an extended process of building greater access to and communication between protective and traumatized self-states, as well as their essential

Self. This work entails attending to the needs of both the traumatized child parts and the adult parts, "addressing individual sub-narratives" of each part "in its own terms, and enabling negotiation to take place between them" (p. 194). To facilitate this process, the therapist may act as a mediator and translator between conflicting parts of the client, building empathic connection between them; the therapist's intermediary role is particularly important when fear and denigration have built up between different self-states (Bromberg, 1998).

Throughout this process, the therapist engages the protectors with a sense of appreciation for the responsibility they hold. Simultaneously, the therapist is tasked with shielding the client's vulnerable parts from the protectors' aggressive attacks by gently calling attention to moments when the protector is turning against other parts of the self. Clients can learn the "voice" of their protectors and cultivate the ability to recognize when they are activated. Further movements toward integration involve the client coming to see the purpose and value of their aggression as self-protective and empowering. Eventually, the protector parts relinquish their hyper-aggressive stance and begin to accommodate the overall needs of the client—especially their needs to function in the world, befriend dissociated self-states, experience and express their vulnerability, and maintain intimate relationships. Although initially conceptualized for the treatment of dissociative disorders, this model for integrating self-states is equally useful in guiding psychedelic integration when treating clients with developmental trauma.

Transforming States Into Traits

Psychedelic researcher Roger Walsh (2012) proposes that psychedelic integration aims to anchor exceptional states of consciousness—and the expanded emotional and relational capacities they facilitate—into enduring traits. How exactly to do this? It is one thing to have stood at the peak of the mountain, another to remember how it felt, and still another to be able to access that feeling in day-to-day life.

The temporary softening of the dissociative defenses induced by psychedelics paves the way for an accelerated leap into the uncharted territory of the personal and collective unconscious and boundless transpersonal realms. This bursting open of the doors of perception saturates the psyche with previously unfathomable experiences, unconscious parts of self, and otherworldly entities. One cannot do justice to the vast range of exceptional experiences psychedelics can engender through any attempt to summarize them. For our purposes, it is helpful to note common experiences reported in psychedelic therapy, which span the range from contact with young, previously dissociated self-states to the unleashing of hostile protectors to the embodiment of as yet undiscovered aspects of one's identity; to deep connection to one's essential Self; to new levels of emotional intimacy; to communion with ancestors, spirits, or extraterrestrial beings; to dissolving into unity with infinite loving presence.

In the integration process, the therapist is tasked with helping to protect these emergent experiences and nascent selves. The therapist does so by making space in their own mind and heart for these nascent parts to live, allowing the client's "seedlings of emergent self-experience" to be "held there for safe-keeping" (Davies, 2003, p. 23). The therapist may need to incubate these seedlings internally at first to create space for the client to grapple with any destabilizing reactions these profound states can evoke while ensuring the seedlings do not get lost entirely. This may require a balance of patience and persistence—making space for the range of reactions the client has to the session while staying connected to the deep personal significance and value the seedlings hold.

It is not only wounded or protective parts breaking through dissociative barriers that can feel threatening after a medicine session, and thus be hard to integrate. Blissful experiences of expansion, transcendence, unity, and connection to Self can later feel confusing, disorienting, unbelievable, or threatening to one's sense of self or worldview. Moreover, these states can be notoriously difficult to access once the medicine fades. Clients graced with such experiences may feel intense grief or despair upon the return of their familiar ruminative patterns or low moods, which can evoke a grasping desire to "get back" to the exultant state, or conversely trigger a minimizing dismissal of the transcendent experience.

We can support clients through this tumultuous ride by inviting them to share all their experiences of and reactions to their psychedelic session—transcendent and blissful, dismissive and distressing. A central tenet of psychedelic therapy— particularly essential for integration—is to hold both positive and challenging experiences, expansion and contraction, as equally valuable. Grounded in this equanimous stance, we are best equipped to help clients remain open to the full range of their experiences while drawing out their curiosity, spontaneous expression, and reflective meaning making.

A stance of equanimity supports the therapist in holding the client's disappointment, disbelief, or despair—as well as any protective impulses to shut down emotionally, or dismiss their experience—without holding tightly to an agenda of *making* the client recognize the value of their experience or succumbing to their own countertransference feelings of disappointment, doubt, or frustration. No matter the client's capacity or willingness to acknowledge and embrace their nascent parts, the therapist can continue to hold them in mind and heart, seek out opportunities to gently reintroduce them into the field, and watch for and reinforce moments when they spontaneously arise. With an eye for appropriate timing, the therapist can reflect these seedlings back to the client, working collaboratively to integrate the full spectrum of parts into the tapestry of the client's psychological world.

A significant goal of relational psychedelic integration is to foster ongoing recognition, internal empathy, and cooperation between the client's multiplicity of self-states. The relational therapist helps the client direct attention to the dialectic between expansive states and insights experienced in the medicine sessions and their more constricted and protective self-states, where the larger perspective prompted by expansive states can illuminate patterns of constriction. In this sense, integration should support the client in cultivating an increasingly intimate connection between the diverse parts of the psyche and the essential Self.

Expanded states may elicit experiences of gratitude at the macro level, a transcendent gratitude in which the client recognizes all parts of their life as purposeful and accesses appreciation for the diverse parts of themselves. These experiences of expansion and profound shifts in perspective are often supported by the client's access to the Self and its inherent acceptance and compassion. Within this expanded state, disparate parts of the client's psyche may achieve mutual recognition, empathy, understanding, and depolarization.

In a classical example of the perspective shifts frequently elicited by psychedelic medicines, one client came to recognize that she would not exist without the survival instinct of her protector parts. Her integration work focused on developing compassion, mutuality, and cooperation between the anxious, insecure, and hopeless self-states that she returned to after the medicine session and the part of her that remained connected to the sense of purpose, meaning, and acceptance she felt during the session. She came to understand her anxiety, insecurity, and hopelessness as "growing pains." Inspired by this new perspective, she began a practice in which she imagined the constrictive bodily sensations associated with these feelings as held in the intimate embrace of the transcendent gratitude she discovered during the medicine session. Through the integration process, the client strengthened her capacity to hold internal conflict between vulnerable and protective parts while maintaining self-continuity. The expansive states she accessed in the medicine session evolved into an internal space, like a dynamic theater stage that she could revisit and use as a resource to connect with the cast of characters that populate her psyche. This approach helped her regulate overwhelming emotional states, assess her needs, and ease negotiation between parts.

Interpersonal Negotiation in the Integration Process

Relational psychedelic therapy approaches integration as an intersubjective process. We come to know ourselves through others' reflections, particularly those we trust: a mirror made from the way we are "held in mind." The relational therapist uses this intersubjective framework to facilitate integration by giving careful attention to the client and therapist's experience of each other with an eye toward promoting mutuality, recognition, and intersubjective understanding. Approaches to support this aim include tending to residual vulnerability, integrating moments of connection as well as rupture and repair that occurred during the medicine session, and addressing unresolved ruptures.

Integrating Moments of Connection

As we have noted, the use of psychedelic medicines in psychotherapy amplifies relational risk. One of these risks, especially with empathogens, is ironically also one of its primary benefits—the deepening of interpersonal intimacy, supported by a neurochemically enhanced state of openness and trust. Some clients may also experience unitive-type experiences or what Thich Nhat Hanh (2003) calls "interbeing," in which their sense of separate self dissolves, and they feel merged or "one" with the therapist. These expanded affective states may fade as the medicine's effect wanes, leaving the client vulnerable to sudden contraction and dramatic shifts in their experience of the therapist and the therapeutic relationship. In fact, the deep relational safety and emotional intimacy present in the medicine session may later be experienced by the client as threatening; they may begin to doubt the authenticity of the therapist's care and trustworthiness, and question whether the feelings of intimacy were mutual. The client may feel they have done something inappropriate to the therapist or the other way around. They may feel shame for sharing feelings of love and affection, or generally expressing themselves in an unfiltered and openhearted way—what some call a "vulnerability hangover." As a result of this rapid shift from a state of openheartedness and trust to a state of contraction, the client may fear, devalue, or deem the therapist and/or the therapy as untrustworthy.

The risk of unexpected feelings of connection during the medicine session and sudden swings in the opposite direction thereafter are first and foremost mitigated by building a reliable environment of relational safety beforehand. This reliable environment is born out of the therapist's consistent emotional holding, in which they address and repair relational ruptures as needed. However, even when the therapy dyad has a solid foundation of trust prior to incorporating psychedelics, the deepened emotional intimacy of a medicine session may be experienced by the client as destabilizing afterward and elicit feelings of fear, mistrust, shame, or doubt, as well as contraction relative to the therapist.

The therapist can respond to the client's contraction and shifting levels of trust by making space for the client to express their concerns and inviting careful reflection of their felt experience of threatening moments. It is important for the therapist to reflect, normalize, and empathize with these often sensitive and vulnerable feelings, which may include significant guilt or shame. This exploration may indicate that more conversation is needed around consent to clarify whether there are certain forms of contact the client is not comfortable with, and to make new agreements that would increase the client's sense of safety. This set of interventions allows the client to experience the therapist's attunement, curiosity, and care for their safety, and feel that their concerns are being received and understood.

After mistrust and consent have been adequately explored and safety reestablished, the therapist may sense the client's need for an affirmation of the validity of their connection; through countertransference disclosure, the therapist can then share their authentic experience of genuine moments of shared intimacy. The therapist's disclosure of their own experiences of connection demonstrates to the client that the intimacy was not imagined; rather, it was a mutual and reciprocal encounter meaningful to both parties. A pathway is cleared for an honest exploration of these intimate moments, which can serve as points of reflection and reconnection. As the client feels more trusting of the tender feelings that arose, they may feel freer to describe the emotional intimacy they experienced during the session and how they were impacted.

This kind of deeply personal relational dialogue—involving mutual disclosure of feelings of warmth, affection, connectedness, and care—can generate levels of intimacy in the present moment similar to those experienced in the medicine session, reinforcing the authenticity and enduring nature of the strengthened connection that has been cultivated. Through this process, the client is able to integrate an embodied experience of deep, authentic relatedness, opening to new ways of being with the therapist and, by extension, their whole relational world. Repeated experiences of openhearted relatedness within the therapeutic relationship help the client expand their overall capacity for intimacy, intersubjectivity, and emotional fulfillment.

It is important to note here that moments of intimacy during a psychedelic session can elicit both erotic transference and countertransference. While elaborate discussion of this topic is beyond the scope of this chapter, we will touch on some key points related to erotic transference and countertransference here. First and foremost, erotic transference should be explored with care for the client's vulnerability, assuring them that the boundaries around sexual contact are clear, and their erotic feelings can be safely felt and expressed. These feelings can then be explored in the same way we would open up any relational dialogue—inviting the client to express their experience, helping them find words for their feelings, normalizing them, and working together to understand these feelings in the context of the client's early relational experiences.

The therapist needs to hold a delicate balance between welcoming the expression of erotic feelings, desires, and fantasies, on the one hand, and holding clear energetic, emotional, and physical boundaries on the other. When done with skill, this process can help the client connect to a sense of being lovable, and learn that their desire is safe and can be expressed without triggering feelings of rejection and shame. Erotic transference can be a vehicle for working through deep wounding around sexuality as well as childhood love and grief at what was not possible in relation to primary attachment figures. In instances of erotic countertransference, the therapist should first make their feelings as conscious as possible and work to understand the feelings in the context of any relational enactments that are present as well as their own early attachment experiences. The therapist needs to look out for instances in which erotic transference/countertransference dynamics are serving to meet the therapists own needs for emotional and sexual fulfillment, work to attend to these needs outside of the therapeutic relationship, and take care around how their needs may be sending inappropriate or mixed messages to the client around the boundaries of the therapeutic relationship. It is essential to assess whether consultation is needed and to tread carefully around self-disclosure.

Integrating Rupture and Repair

During a medicine session, the enhanced sense of safety and openness sometimes give clients the courage to name challenging feelings and transference reactions (e.g., idealization, devaluation, paranoia, erotic feelings, parental love, abandonment, intrusion, or sadistic hostility) during medicine sessions. These reactions may be responses to ruptures that occurred during the medicine session or in prior therapy sessions. Ruptures can result from an experience in the medicine session of misattunement, inadequate holding, a sudden shift in the amount of contact leading to feelings of abandonment or overstimulation, or intrusion (e.g., too much directiveness, interpretation that does not resonate or feels hurtful, or over-disclosure from the therapist). Ruptures may also result from broaching topics or traumas before trust is established, unwanted or inadequate consent for touch, or cultural enactments such as microaggressions and invalidations.

While ruptures can and should be processed during the medicine session when possible, it is important to return to these conversations during the integration phase. By revisiting the client's expressed feelings, the interpersonal dialogue that followed, and any resultant reparative emotional experience, the therapist demonstrates that they value these interchanges and take seriously the client's concerns; additionally, this conversation can reinforce the trust built through the initial encounter. This process might involve the following relational interventions:

- Appreciating the client's willingness to share their challenging feelings
- Developing clear agreements about any requested adjustments
- Joining with the client in mutual appreciation for the expanded trust and emotional intimacy they built together
- Helping the client make links to their experiences of relational trauma and resulting interpersonal patterns

These activities strengthen the client's capacity to speak authentically to their experience and engage in generative interpersonal dialogue, opening the client and the treatment to new levels of relational work.

Addressing Unresolved Ruptures

There are also instances in which relational ruptures occur during a medicine session but are not processed in the moment. In these cases, a rupture may remain a part of the client's experience thereafter, manifesting as feelings, such as hurt, anger, disappointment, abandonment, or betrayal. As we have noted, the client may not be able to identify the challenging feelings they are experiencing in relation to the therapist, much less bring them forward or articulate them. Clients may experience these feelings as overwhelming or threatening to the connection with the therapist, and avoid or dissociate from them altogether, as we witnessed with Vera. This could lead to avoidant or dissociative behavior in integration sessions, emotional distancing from the therapist, or even withdrawal from the treatment. It is essential that the therapist find a way to identify and work with these feelings during the integration process, either explicitly or in the transference, to avoid future enactments and premature termination and also because these feelings are central to the therapeutic process, and repair has the potential to be healing on multiple levels.

In some instances, it is clear to the therapist that a rupture occurred during a medicine session that needs tending. In other instances, the therapist senses that something feels off but may not have a clear notion of what caused the rupture; and in still others, they may be completely oblivious. Whether or not there are clear indications of a rupture or transference feelings post-medicine session, it is important for the therapist to closely track the relational field and attune to the client's feeling states and their own countertransference to listen for protective defenses and signs of dissociation in the days following a medicine session.

If the therapist picks up on something that needs tending, they can gently inquire about the feelings they perceive or the rupture they witnessed in the medicine session. When the therapist is uncertain whether something needs tending, it never hurts to ask—the client can always say no and is likely to appreciate the therapist's thoughtfulness and concern. When the client is not able to explicitly name or actively engage in dialogue around a relational dynamic that appears to be present, the therapist can listen to the client's narrative, affective exchanges, and non-verbal cues for what the protective defenses are communicating, paying particular attention to what these defenses signify about the client's experience of the therapist and the pacing of the therapeutic process.

The therapist can help the client navigate challenging feelings that arise by receiving negative transference reactions and feedback non-defensively, whether they are named explicitly or inferred through the client's implicit communications. The therapist demonstrates that feedback and exploration of challenging interpersonal dynamics are welcome and can lead to repair by:

- Maintaining an open, receptive, non-defensive, and empathic stance to the client's feelings and experiences
- Helping the client put words to any unconscious or unformulated feelings toward the therapist
- Acknowledging and taking responsibility for ways they negatively impacted the client
- Exploring what is needed in order to achieve repair
- Demonstrating their commitment to learning from the experience and making necessary adjustments to address the client's concerns

Through this process of rupture and repair, the client develops their capacity to understand and accept their inner experience and hold this alongside an empathic understanding of others' subjective experience (intersubjectivity), helping them build stability, security, and emotional fulfillment in attachment relationships.

Case Example

Let us take Vera's case as an example. Due to her significant experience of early abandonment by her mother, Vera unconsciously took control of her childhood situation by transforming her overwhelming feelings of hurt, powerlessness, and loss into self-criticism and self-blame, seeing herself as not good enough to keep her mother around. Throughout her life, Vera held impossibly high expectations for herself, which forced her to repeatedly confront the discrepancy between who she was and who she expected herself to be, leading to a deep sense of shame and worthlessness. Naturally, she brought these high expectations of herself into her medicine session, experiencing a pervasive sense that she needed to perform in a certain way, entertain her therapist, and make the experience meaningful for them both. She also projected her high standards for herself onto the therapist and the session, leading to a specific idea of how the session would go and how the therapist would show up. When the session did not go as she had hoped, Vera felt a deep sense of disappointment in herself, the therapist, and the treatment as a whole.

Imagine that prior to the MDMA session, Vera's therapist engages her in an exploration of her expectations for the treatment, painting a realistic picture of what is possible in the one MDMA session they have planned prior to termination. Vera's therapist discusses the potential for disappointment to arise during and after the medicine session. The dyad also touches on the significance of the impending end of their work together. The therapist encourages Vera to speak to any challenging feelings about the therapy and the therapeutic relationship as a whole, highlighting the importance of these feelings as well as the valuable potential for repair through interpersonal dialogue. In this imagined scenario, the therapist's thorough preparation provides Vera with a framework that helps her understand and relate to the challenging feelings triggered in her MDMA session.

During the integration sessions, let us say that the therapist identifies and draws out Vera's feelings of disappointment, opening space to explore these feelings. The therapist then normalizes and empathizes with Vera's feelings and takes responsibility for the ways in which she did not adequately show up during the session, thereby modeling how to take ownership for one's mistakes and work toward repair without collapsing into shame or guilt. The therapist also shows a desire to learn from her mistakes and shift her behavior accordingly. Together, they explore Vera's desire to feel her therapist's engagement and care; in the process, the therapist expresses the authentic care she feels for Vera in that moment, as well as her commitment to showing up with clear presence, attunement, and active participation. Through this interchange, Vera and her therapist experience a deep sense of connection and mutual appreciation for the trust they have cultivated.

Afterward, the dyad begins exploring Vera's disappointment in herself, relativizing it as a wishful part that seeks to avoid loss by being perfect, "If only she had done it just right, the session would have been so profound and meaningful that the bond between Vera and her therapist would endure forever." Highlighting the split between who Vera thinks she should be (perfect and therefore lovable) and who she fears she is (deeply flawed and therefore bound to be rejected) allows Vera to find acceptance for who she actually is—human, flawed, *and* completely lovable. She also comes to accept her powerlessness to control her environment through an all-star performance. The naming of Vera's hopes for a meaningful and lasting bond with her therapist inspires the dyad to explore and honor the connection that does exist between them and investigate ways they can continue carrying each other in their hearts and minds without a need for Vera to be perfect.

As the dyad engages with Vera's disappointment in the treatment itself, the therapist skillfully holds the reality of the meaningful work that did unfold alongside Vera's disappointment about what did not, helping Vera access embodied awareness and emotionally congruent expression of her disappointed expectations. Together, they grieve the work they were unable to achieve in the medicine session. Vera is then able to contact her grief about the experiences she desperately wanted but did not get to have with her therapist—and at a deeper level, with her mother—before they each left her in a state of need. As the grief moves through and Vera experiences the depths of her helplessness in each situation, she realizes that the intense losses she endured were, in fact, beyond her control. This relational process provides Vera with relief from long-held pain, an expanded capacity for relational intimacy, and deeper integration between her child and adult selves.

This example highlights the true nature of psychedelic-assisted trauma therapy, revealing it for the potent treatment that it is—not a cure but a deep and meaningful process of self-discovery, affective expression and reembodiment, personality reintegration, and rupture and resolution that leads to reparative emotional experiences and deep interpersonal healing.

Collaborative Meaning Making and the Creation of a New Narrative

A key aspect of psychedelic integration involves helping the client weave the threads of their original trauma and its impact on their life into a coherent narrative, a tapestry illustrating their unique healing journey. As the client gains greater self-acceptance, they can move more freely into creative play and collaborative meaning making. Previously unconscious self-states become imbued with significance and find a more integrated home within the client's narrative and sense of self. The trauma narrative and the figures involved (e.g., the perpetrator, disappointing parent, or rejecting partner) may be viewed through a lens of compassion and acceptance. Forgiveness of both self and others may enter the realm of possibility when it had previously been inconceivable.

In this stage of the healing journey, the scope of the treatment expands to include a multiplicity of archetypal potentials as the client develops experiential insight into the mythopoetic trajectory of healing and transformation. For example, the client's process may be meaningfully understood through the archetypal image of death and rebirth: the initial trauma becomes a forced descent into the underworld—the dark night of the soul, marked by experiences of "corrupted innocence, struggle, failure, suffering, hopelessness" (Schwartz, 2013, p. 196). This journey through the shadowy realms of the underworld is undertaken for the sake of recovering lost parts of self and grieving loss associated with the trauma. The "sacred return" from the underworld and subsequent rebirth of self, of disintegration and reintegration, is like the phoenix "rising in flight from the ashes, after all hope has been destroyed by an all-consuming fire" (Schwartz, 2013, p. 196).

After careful trauma processing, including significant periods of grieving the pain and outrageous unfairness of the trauma, the client may eventually come to see their past experience as a valuable source of wisdom, resilience, and pathway into meaningful service. Tedeschi and Calhoun (2004) describe this stage of trauma recovery as the generative process of post-traumatic growth. Much like the Japanese art of *kintsugi*, in which broken pottery is repaired with a lacquer of powdered gold, silver, or platinum to create something more beautiful than the original and celebrate the object's history—including its breakage and repair (Kemske, 2021)—the client can come to appreciate and revere their whole self, not in spite of their traumas but because of them.

With time, the client's courageous confrontation with their trauma gives way to "unexpected opportunities, hope, awakening, and redemption" (Schwartz, 2013, p. 196). Like the image of the spiral labyrinth, clients begin to understand their journey as the cyclical path toward the integrative wholeness of self. Subsequent reflections on their direct experience of these mythic themes diminish the influence of "self-defeating narratives which pre-empt the potentials for hope and recovery," embracing a narrative of strength, resilience, and empowerment in which each step in their recovery reveals itself as a reenactment of "the universal process of maturation and liberation" (p. 197).

The Heart of the Work

Psychedelic medicines foster experiences of expansive play between the diverse parts that collectively shape the client's psyche and the emergence of a more expansive identity and experience of the world. In joining with the client in this dynamic play, the psychedelic therapist has an opportunity to hold them through a profoundly transformative process. The therapist witnesses and reflects back who the client becomes when they have relief from the constricting force of trauma defenses. The therapist nurtures the client's blossoming selves through carefully tending the relational field, emotionally attuned mirroring, and an intersubjective (I-Thou) style of relating, helping the client to nourish the garden in which these selves can thrive.

Relational psychedelic therapy ushers in expanded possibilities for effectively accessing and reworking traumatic relational and attachment dynamics; we have found this approach to be effective for mitigating the pervasive impact of developmental trauma and its myriad enduring symptoms that make trauma recovery a notoriously slow, challenging process. In emphasizing careful, heart-centered attunement to the relational field, we aim to create a therapeutic context that amplifies the transformative potential of psychedelic medicines by supporting the client's regulatory capacity through co-regulation, engaging relationally in the client's healing process, tracking and responding to the emotional vicissitudes of the interpersonal encounter, and thoughtfully working through ruptures and enactments as they arise, promoting collaborative repair and mutual understanding. We aim to provide a space for the ghosts of trauma to safely emerge, for the exiled parts of self to be felt and reclaimed, and for the gradual expansion of the client's relational and emotional capacities. Joy and resilience bloom from the bridges built that connect back to the heart.

Notes

1 MDMA is the abbreviation for 3,4-methylenedioxymethamphetamine, the pure form of the street drug known as "ecstasy" or "molly." Although MDMA is considered an empathogenic compound and not a classical psychedelic, our use of the term *psychedelic* throughout this chapter includes classical psychedelics and empathogens, as well as dissociative anesthetics like ketamine.
2 We will use the terms *self-states*, *parts of self*, and *parts* interchangeably throughout this chapter. When using any of these terms, we are referring to the multiple parts of self that exist in all of us, initially developed through the dynamics of our formative relationships. These parts are then activated throughout our lives in response to changing interpersonal, environmental, and emotional cues.
3 *Empathogen* is a term coined by Ralph Metzner and David E. Nichols that means "empathy generating." A related term that is used for this same class of psychedelic medicines is *entactogen*, meaning "to touch within." Empathogenic compounds include MDMA, MDA, 3-MMC, MDEA, MDOH, MBDB, 6-APB, methylone, mephedrone, GHB, and low-dose ketamine, among others.
4 *Intersubjectivity* is understood as the ability to recognize "another mind who can be 'felt with,' yet has a distinct, separate center of feeling and perception" (Benjamin, 2004, p. 6), an orientation to the other that philosopher Martin Buber (2000) described as an I-Thou relationship.
5 This vignette is a summary of an interview of a participant's experience of MDMA-assisted psychotherapy. Excerpts from the interview were initially published in a qualitative study conducted by Dr. Genesee Herzberg entitled "The phenomenology and sequelae of MDMA-assisted psychotherapy." "Vera" is a pseudonym, and some details of the story have been changed to protect the identity of the participant.
6 The medial temporal regions are responsible for encoding memory and processing emotion, and the association cortices are responsible for "the ability to attend to external stimuli or internal motivation, to identify the significance of such stimuli, and to plan meaningful responses to them" (Purves et al., 2001, p. 238).

References

Baranger, M., & Baranger, W. (2009). The analytic situation as a dynamic field. *International Journal of Psychoanalysis*, 89, 795–826. (Original work published 1961–1962)

Benjamin, J. (2004). *Beyond doer and done to: Recognition theory, intersubjectivity and the third*. Routledge.

Bromberg, P. (1998). Staying the same while changing: Reflections on clinical judgment. In *Standing in the spaces: Essays on clinical process, trauma and dissociation* (pp. 291–307). The Analytic Press.

Bromberg, P. (2006). *Awakening the dreamer: Clinical journeys*. Routledge.

Bromberg, P. (2011). *The shadow of the tsunami and the growth of the relational mind*. Routledge.

Buber, M. (2000). *I and thou.* Scribner.

Bucci, W. (2002). The referential process, consciousness, and the sense of self. *Psychoanalytic Inquiry, 22*(5), 766–793. https://doi.org/10.1080/07351692209349017

Cambray, J. (2009). *Synchronicity: Nature and psyche in an interconnected universe.* Texas A&M University Press.

Carhart-Harris, R. L. (2007). Waves of the unconscious: The neurophysiology of dreamlike phenomena and its implications for the psychodynamic model of the mind. *Neuropsychoanalysis, 9*(2), 183–211. https://doi.org/10.1080/15294145.2007.10773557

Carhart-Harris, R. L. (2018). Serotonin, psychedelics and psychiatry. *World Psychiatry, 17*(3), 358–359. https://doi.org/10.1002/wps.20555

Carhart-Harris, R. L., & Nutt, D. J. (2017). Serotonin and brain function: A tale of two receptors. *Journal of Psychopharmacology, 9*(31), 1091–1120. https://doi.org/10.1177/0269881117725915

Davies, J. M. (1994). Love in the afternoon: A relational reconsideration of desire and dread in the countertransference. *Psychoanalytic Dialogues, 4*(2), 153–170. https://doi.org/10.1080/10481889409539011

Davies, J. M. (2003). Falling in love with love: Oedipal and post-Oedipal manifestations of idealization, mourning and erotic masochism. *Psychoanalytic Dialogues, 13*(1), 1–27. https://doi.org/10.1080/10481881309348718

Eshel, O. (2019). *The emergence of analytic oneness: Into the heart of psychoanalysis.* Routledge.

Feduccia, A. A., & Mithoefer, M. C. (2018). MDMA-assisted psychotherapy for PTSD: Are memory reconsolidation and fear extinction underlying mechanisms? *Progress in Neuro-Psychopharmacology and Biological Psychiatry, 84*(Part A), 221–228. https://doi.org/10.1016/j.pnpbp.2018.03.003

Ferro, A. (2017). Dream model of the mind. In A. Ferro (Ed.), *Contemporary Bionian theory and technique in psychoanalysis* (pp. 114–148). Routledge.

Ferro, A., & Civitarese, G. (2015). *The analytic field and its transformations.* Karnac Books.

Fisher, J. (2017). *Healing the fragmented selves of trauma survivors: Overcoming internal self-alienation.* Routledge.

Freud, S. (1975). Two encyclopedia articles. In J. Strachey (Trans. & Ed.), *The standard edition of the complete psychological works of Sigmund Freud, Volume 22 (1932–1936): New introductory lectures on psycho-analysis and other works* (pp. 235–259). Hogarth Press & The Institute of Psycho-Analysis. (Original work published 1923)

Gamma, A., Buck, A., Berthold, T., Hell, D., & Vollenweider, F. X. (2000). 3,4-Methylenedioxymethamphetamine (MDMA) modulates cortical and limbic brain activity as measured by $[H_2{}^{15}O]$-PET in healthy humans. *Neuropsychopharmacology, 23*(4), 388–395. https://doi.org/10.1016/S0893-133X(00)00130-5

Grof, S. (1980). *LSD psychotherapy.* Hunter House.

Halstead, M., Reed, S., Krause, R., & Williams, M. (2021). Ketamine-assisted psychotherapy for PTSD related to racial discrimination. *Clinical Case Studies, 20*(4), 310–330. https://doi.org/10.1177/1534650121990894

Hanh, T. N. (2003). *Interbeing: Fourteen guidelines for engaged Buddhism* (New ed.). Full Circle Publishing.

Herzberg, G. (2012). *The phenomenology and sequelae of MDMA-assisted psychotherapy* (Dissertation No. 3545616) (Doctoral dissertation). California Institute of Integral Studies. ProQuest Dissertations and Theses Global.

Johnson, M., Richards, B., & Griffiths, R. (2008). Human hallucinogen research: Guidelines for safety. *Journal of Psychopharmacology, 22*(6), 603–620. https://doi.org/10.1177/0269881108093587

Kalsched, D. (1996). *The inner world of trauma: Archetypal defenses of the personal spirit.* Routledge.

Kemske, B. (2021). *Kintsugi: The poetic mend.* Herbert Press.

Krediet, E., Bostoen, T., Breeksema, J., van Schagen, A., Passie, T., & Vermetten, E. (2020). Reviewing the potential of psychedelics for the treatment of PTSD. *International Journal of Neuropsychopharmacology, 23*(6), 385–400. https://doi.org/10.1093/ijnp/pyaa018

Liriano, F., Hatten, C., & Schwartz, T. L. (2019). Ketamine as treatment for post-traumatic stress disorder: A review. *Drugs in Context, 8,* 212305. doi: 10.7573/dic.212305. www.ncbi.nlm.nih.gov/pmc/articles/PMC6457782/

MAPS. (2017, May 10). Elizabeth Nielson & Jeffrey Guss: Therapeutic process in psilocybin-assisted therapy. [Video]. *YouTube.* www.youtube.com/watch?v=R71mfgfPBkw&ab_channel=MAPS

Mitchell, J. M., Bogenschutz, M., Lilienstein, A., et al. (2021). MDMA-assisted therapy for severe PTSD: A randomized, double-blind, placebo-controlled phase 3 study. *Nature Medicine, 27,* 1025–1033. https://doi.org/10.1038/s41591-021-01336-3

Mithoefer, M. C., Wagner, M. T., & Mithoefer, A. T. (2011). The safety and efficacy of ±3,4-methylenedioxymethamphetamine-assisted psychotherapy in subjects with chronic, treatment-resistant posttraumatic stress disorder: The first randomized controlled pilot study. *Journal of Psychopharmacology, 25,* 439–452.

Mithoefer, M. C., Wagner, M. T., Mithoefer, A. T., Jerome, L., Martin, S. F., Yazar-Klosinski, B., Michel, Y., Brewerton, T. D., & Doblin, R. (2013). Durability of improvement in post-traumatic stress disorder symptoms and absence of harmful effects or drug dependency after 3,4-methylenedioxymethamphetamine-assisted psychotherapy: A prospective long-term follow-up study. *Journal of Psychopharmacology (Oxford, England), 27*(1), 28–39. https://doi.org/10.1177/0269881112456611

Mitrani, J. L. (2001). 'Taking the transference': Some technical implications in three papers by Bion. *The International Journal of Psychoanalysis, 82*(6), 1085–1104. https://doi.org/10.1516/JECN-FBNV-TUUE-NUHX

Müller, F., Holze, F., Dolder, P., Ley, L., Vizeli, P., Soltermann, A., Liechti, E., & Borgwardt, S. (2020). MDMA-induced changes in within-network connectivity contradict the specificity of these alterations for the effects of serotonergic hallucinogens. *Neuropsychopharmacology, 46,* 545–553. https://doi.org/10.1038/s41386-020-00906-2

Nutt, D., & Carhart-Harris, R. (2020). The current status of psychedelics in psychiatry. *JAMA Psychiatry.* doi: 10.1001/jamapsychiatry.2020.2171

Paulsen, S. L., & Lanius, U. F. (2014). Introduction: The ubiquity of dissociation. In U. Lanius, S. Paulsen, & F. M. Corrigan (Eds.), *Neurobiology and treatment of traumatic dissociation: Toward and embodied self.* Springer.

Porges, S. W. (2017). *The pocket guide to the polyvagal theory: The transformative power of feeling safe.* W. W. Norton & Company.

Purves, D., Augustine, G. J., Fitzpatrick, D., et al. (Eds.). (2001). *Neuroscience* (2nd ed.). Sinauer Associates. Chapter 26, The Association Cortices. www.ncbi.nlm.nih.gov/books/NBK11109/

Richards, B. (2015). *Sacred knowledge: Psychedelics and religious experiences.* Columbia University Press.

Rogers, C. (1951). *Client-centered therapy: Its current practice, implications and theory.* Constable.

Ross, C., Jain, R., Bonnett, C. J., & Wolfson, P. (2019). High-dose ketamine infusion for the treatment of posttraumatic stress disorder in combat veterans. *Annals of Clinical Psychiatry*, *31*(4), 271–279. www.ncbi.nlm.nih.gov/pubmed/31675388

Safran, J. D., & Muran, J. C. (2000). *Negotiating the therapeutic alliance: A relational treatment guide.* Guilford Press.

Schore, A. (2012). *The science of the art of psychotherapy.* W.W. Norton and Company.

Schwartz, H. L. (1994). From dissociation to negotiation: A relational psychoanalytic perspective on multiple personality disorder. *Psychoanalytic Psychology*, *11*(2), 189–231. https://doi.org/10.1037/h0079545

Schwartz, H. L. (2013). *The alchemy of wolves and sheep: A relational approach to internalized perpetration in complex trauma survivors.* Routledge.

Schwartz, R. C. (2001). *Introduction to the internal family systems model.* Trailheads Publications.

Schwartz, R. C. (2008). *You are the one you've been waiting for: Bringing courageous love to intimate relationships.* Trailheads Publications.

Siegel, D. J. (1999). *The developing mind: Toward a neurobiology of interpersonal experience.* Guilford Press.

Siegel, D. J. (2013). *Parenting from the inside out: How a deeper self-understanding can help you raise children who thrive.* TarcherPerigee.

Stern, D. (2010). *Partners in thought: Working with unformulated experience, dissociation, and enactment.* Routledge.

Tedeschi, R. G., & Calhoun, L. (2004). Posttraumatic growth: A new perspective on psychotraumatology. *Psychiatric Times*, *21*(4).

Van der Kolk, B. A. (2005). Developmental trauma disorder: Toward a rational diagnosis for children with complex trauma histories. *Psychiatric Annals*, *35*(5), 401–408. doi: 10.3928/00485713-20050501-06

Walsh, R. (2012). From state to trait: The challenge of transforming transient insights into enduring change. In T. B. Roberts (Ed.), *Spiritual growth with entheogens: Psychoactive sacramentals and human transformation* (pp. 24–30). Park Street Press.

Wampold, B. E. (2015). How important are the common factors in psychotherapy? An update. *World Psychiatry*, *14*(3), 270–277. doi: 10.1002/wps.20238

Whitehead, C. C. (2006). Neo-psychoanalysis: A paradigm for the 21st century. *Journal of the American Academy of Psychoanalysis & Dynamic Psychiatry*, *34*(4), 603–627. https://doi.org/10.1521/jaap.2006.34.4.603

Winnicott, D. W. (1953). Transitional objects and transitional phenomena: A study of the first not-me possession. *International Journal of Psycho-Analysis*, *34*(2), 89–97.

Chapter 6

A Somatic Approach to Psychedelic-Assisted Therapy

Veronika Gold

Context and Acknowledgment[1]

Early in my career as a psychotherapist, I began seeing clients with histories of sexual abuse. As I worked with them, I became aware of their need to do more than just talk about their trauma. It was clear they needed more from me than empathy, psychoeducation, distress regulation, and cognitive reframing. Their protracted suffering, alongside the limited efficacy of my current therapeutic toolbox, indicated that I should expand my range of interventions. I sought out training in Eye Movement Desensitization and Reprocessing therapy, which significantly enhanced my ability to work with clients with trauma histories. Yet, even after integrating this modality, I continued to observe trauma-related patterns held in the body that my existing therapeutic tools could not adequately address.

Over the next decade, I pursued further training in Hakomi, Somatic Experiencing, Organic Intelligence, and embodiment practices taught as a part of the realization process (Blackstone, 2018). These models brought me a deeper understanding of my clients' somatic experiences, expressions, and processing. Working with MDMA in the MAPS[2]-sponsored clinical trials for the treatment of PTSD, and with ketamine at Polaris Insight Center, opened an even wider lens that expanded my understanding of trauma recovery. My clinical work has also been informed by my personal experiences growing up under the oppressive communist regime in Czechoslovakia, as well as by the therapists who supported me in healing my own trauma. However, far beyond my academic training, it has been my clients who entrusted me with their pain and suffering that taught me the most about the depths of the human condition and the process of integrating and healing of trauma.

Introduction

Physical touch and other somatic practices have been used in healing traditions for thousands of years. Its roots reach back to the earliest shamanic and religious rituals using touch alongside prayer, dance, connecting with spirit, physical and spiritual healing, and energetic clearing (Levitan & Johnson, 1986; Smith et al., 1998). In the West, however, the body had not been acknowledged as an important part of

DOI: 10.4324/9781003167976-6

psychological healing until the 1920s when German psychoanalyst Wilhelm Reich began advocating for including the body in psychoanalysis. Since Reich, many approaches to somatic therapy have been developed. Presently, the United States Association for Body Psychotherapy is dedicated to developing and advancing practices of somatic therapy that affirm the inseparability of mind, body, and spirit.

It has become more widely acknowledged over the past 50 years that traumatic experiences are held in the body, to the point that somatic work[3] is now considered by many trauma experts to be an essential component of trauma recovery. In the contemporary field of trauma therapy, healing trauma happens not only through the release of fear-based beliefs, thoughts, emotions, and cognitive schemas associated with the trauma but also through a process of somatic releasing and reinhabiting the body in a new and vital way (Van der Kolk, 2015; Kain, & Terrell, 2018; Levine, & Frederick, 1997).

Nevertheless, little has been written about somatic work in the context of psychedelic therapy. Pauline McCririck and Joyce Martin developed "fusion therapy" in 1965 that involved using a moderate dose of LSD paired with consensual touch, "like a good mother would do with her child" (Grof, 2019, vol. 1). Dr. Stanislav Grof, one of the founders of transpersonal psychology and leading LSD-assisted therapy researcher, was inspired by McCririck's work. Subsequently, Grof and his wife Christina incorporated physical components (what they called "focused energy release bodywork") into their Holotropic Breathwork method.[4] Dr. Michael and Annie Mithoefer used Grof's theory and techniques as a foundation for their pioneering work with the MAPS and its MDMA-Assisted Therapy Manual (Mithoefer et al., 2014).

Building on these foundational contributions, I have found that in the context of therapy, the use of psychedelic medicines presents an opportunity to place the body at the center of the mind, body, and spirit continuum—with somatic approaches/ interventions as the most immediately available tools when encountering and processing trauma. In the pages that follow, I will redefine trauma through a non-pathologizing lens, present an overview of how the body and nervous system are impacted by trauma, and describe a somatic approach to treating trauma through psychedelic-assisted therapy (PAT). In the second half of this chapter, I will discuss considerations for the use of therapeutic touch in psychedelic therapy and then share case examples from my practice to illustrate opportunities for incorporating touch and somatic work in the treatment of trauma.

De-Pathologizing Trauma

All therapists work with trauma regardless of whether or not it is their specialty. Varying degrees of trauma are present in most clients' histories. In the broadest sense, we can think of trauma as any event that had a lasting negative effect on us emotionally, cognitively, relationally, somatically, or spiritually. Unfortunately, trauma is too-often seen as just a set of distressing symptoms that meet the criteria for the diagnosis of PTSD in the *Diagnostic and Statistical Manual of Mental*

Disorders, Fifth Edition. While the acronym PTSD is widely accepted in denoting the sequelae of trauma, I support the use of the less pathologizing term post-traumatic stress syndrome (PTSS) coined by Peter Levine (1997). Most trauma experts, including Bessel Van Der Kolk, Richard Schwartz, Peter Levine, Harvey Schwartz, Michael and Annie Mithoefer, and Marcela Ot'Alora, emphasize trauma symptoms as natural lifesaving responses to a situation in which adequate resources for processing a traumatic experience were not available.

Seeing trauma symptoms as an adaptive response, rather than as indications of a disorder, changes how clinicians relate to their clients—in particular how they contextualize their clients' symptoms and what strategies they employ for healing. The label PTSD indicates a medicalized treatment of a pathology. The PTSS model identifies the residual trauma stress response as the result of short-term self-protective responses, becoming debilitating when extended into the long-term.

Although a therapist/client relationship is inherently hierarchical, psychedelic therapists can give authority back to the client by stepping away from the role of all-knowing figure and following the client's lead. PTSS moves beyond imposing a medicalized "outside observer/expert" paradigm and instead puts the client's own observations of their inner experiences at the center of therapeutic relationship, inviting new understanding of the client and the unfolding therapeutic process. Depathologizing trauma opens the way for a more client-centered approach.

Trauma and the Body

Trauma and the Nervous System

The nervous system starts to develop four weeks after conception, eventually acquiring both sensory and motor functions. It consists of two components: the central nervous system (brain and spinal cord) and the peripheral nervous system (nerves across the body and appendages). The peripheral nervous system is further divided into the somatic (or voluntary) nervous system and the autonomic (or vegetative) nervous system, which we will focus on here. The autonomic nervous system is broken up into the sympathetic, parasympathetic, and enteric nervous systems. The sympathetic division, regulated by the amygdala, is responsible for the "fight or flight" response and the parasympathetic for the so-called rest-and-digest and freeze or submit responses, as well as the "social engagement" system (S. Hoskinson, personal communication, May 2, 2016).

Steven Porges's groundbreaking polyvagal theory explains the mechanics of nervous system regulation and dysregulation. In his book, *The Polyvagal Theory* (Porges, 2011), Porges describes the neurological architecture and two branches of the vagus nerve within the parasympathetic nervous system: dorsal and ventral. The ventral (or "facing forward") vagal branch is activated during social engagement. When a person is distressed or in danger, they generally first attempt to regulate through engagement with another person—through connection, negotiation, or submission (Kain & Terrel, 2018). If this approach is unsuccessful, the sympathetic nervous system kicks in and fight/flight behaviors occur. If this strategy fails, the dorsal vagal nerve is activated, triggering the freeze or submit/ collapse response.

States in which the nervous system is well regulated are known as the "optimal arousal zone" or the "window of tolerance" (Siegel, 2012). When within the window of tolerance, neither part (sympathetic nor parasympathetic) of the autonomic nervous system is overactivated. In this state, one feels calm, engaged with life, and safe to seek connection with others. One can receive, process, and integrate information and respond to the everyday demands of life with ease (Siegel, 2012).

Nervous system dysregulation can occur when an individual feels unexpectedly overwhelmed, is unable to process and integrate the distressing experience, and cannot return to feeling safe. Suppose someone encounters a physical or emotional threat, which activates the sympathetic nervous system and the fight or flight response. Their heart beats faster, their eyes widen, breathing becomes more rapid and shallow, perspiration increases, and their muscles tense. If the person cannot move away from or through the situation, they might "remain stuck" in this sympathetic response, as the dorsal branch of the vagus nerve (within the parasympathetic nervous system) takes over and the freeze mechanism becomes engaged. During the freeze response, both the sympathetic and parasympathetic systems are activated; the muscles are tense and full of energy but are unable to release this tension.

The submit/collapse response (also known as hypo-arousal) is triggered when the threat is sustained or is perceived as inescapable. The breath slows down, and the person starts to feel numb, disconnected, dissociated, and without energy. Some people report a feeling of becoming small and invisible. The submit/collapse response serves the person during severe emotionally or physically traumatic events by decreasing sensitivity to external stimuli or essentially "removing" the person psychologically from a situation where they feel hopelessly trapped. During the submit/collapse response, there is less blood flow in the arms and legs, and the individual experiences diminished sensations in the body and greater immobility. Evolutionarily, this response could save an animal's life (by "playing dead," as predators do not like to eat dead bodies) or at least minimize the pain of the attack. PTSS develops when trauma cannot be processed after the event due to a lack of support, skill, space, acknowledgment, or the continuation of an ongoing traumatic situation (Levine & Frederick, 1997; Levine, 2017).

Dysregulation of the nervous system can also happen gradually through repeated exposure to situations that evoke fear, powerlessness, hopelessness, terror, anger, loneliness, or abandonment. This could result, for example, from an emotionally neglectful parent or an accumulation of microaggressions. Whether due to an acute or ongoing trauma, long-term dysregulation and an overactive fight/flight/freeze/ submit response can lead to chronic symptoms, including insomnia, hypervigilance, anxiety, depression, and feelings of disconnection. In many ways, PTSS is a chronic condition with recurring fight/flight/freeze/submit patterns that completely take over the individual's life, throwing them into a confusing survivalist mode of existence (H. Schwartz, personal communication, December 5, 2020).

Stephen Terrell talks about the "faux window of tolerance," a condition in which an individual is chronically operating outside the "window of tolerance" and has developed mechanisms for emotional coping that make them appear as if they are within the "window of tolerance" when instead they are constantly moving between freeze and flight/fight states (Kain & Terrell, 2018). Therapists can help their clients recognize this pattern by providing psychoeducation and, with the help of somatic practices, facilitate processing needed for nervous system deregulation and gradual return to "window of tolerance."

The Impact of Preverbal and Developmental Trauma

Developmental trauma can profoundly impact all aspects of one's develop-ment—neurological, psychological, and social—and compromise one's overall sense of self and safety in the world. The first six months of life are crucial to the development of the capacity to self-regulate and co-regulate. The myelina-tion of the ventral vagus nerve (which begins in the third trimester in utero and continues through adolescence) has its strongest phase of development in the first six months of life. Babies learn to make meaning of the sensations they are experiencing through interaction with their caregivers. With "good enough" parenting, babies are supported in developing 1) *interoception*: the capacity to assess and understand feelings and sensations inside one's body; 2) *exterocep-tion*: the capacity to evaluate information coming in from the outside world; and 3) *neuroception*: a process through which our nervous system senses whether another person is safe, dangerous, or life-threatening (Porges, 2011, 2016). Traumatic social and environmental conditions during early development can significantly disrupt this process and impair the development of these faculties (Kain & Terrell, 2018).

Arousal in the sympathetic nervous system changes our physiology, particu-larly during early development. These changes include, among others, protective alterations in visual and auditory perception, increasing attunement to sounds and sights of danger and threat. For example, the middle-ear muscle changes under stress such that we can better hear lower-frequency sounds (sometimes described as "predator" sounds). Those raised in chaotic early environments lack-ing accurate feedback regarding safety vs. threat often become compromised in their ability to differentiate between safety and danger. These individuals habitu-ally orient toward signs of danger (hypervigilance) and are limited in their ability to recognize safety (Kain & Terrell, 2018, p. 25). When someone is in a chronic hypervigilant state, they keep looking for the "predator sound" and simultane-ously become disconnected from other cues in the environment. They therefore cannot recognize and regulate through indicators of safety. For example, a client does not hear their therapist because they are focusing on steps they hear outside the room.

Psychedelic-Assisted Trauma Therapy

Creating Optimal Conditions for the Natural Resolution of Trauma

The human fight/flight/freeze/submit responses and the experiences that trigger these patterns of behavior often get "stuck" in the body, as if frozen in time. In spite of the challenges trauma causes to nervous systems and human lives, we have an organismic intelligence that includes an innate tendency toward self-healing and the completion of what remains incomplete (S. Hoskinson, personal communication, May 2, 2016; Levine, 1997, 2017; Grof et al., 2008). Many psychedelic therapy modalities often refer to the "inner healer" or "inner healing intelligence" to describe the intuitive wisdom and innately driven movement toward healing that can lead us to restoration and wholeness.

The role of the therapist is to co-create the optimal "set and setting"—inner and outer conditions for the inner healing process to unfold—so that previously intractable mental, emotional, and somatic processes can move toward completion. Optimal conditions are oriented toward cultivating safety and support. These include a therapeutic relationship, where the therapist communicates respect, curiosity, and openness, and attends to the client's "set"—their current state of mind, mood, attitude, somatic experience, interpersonal concerns, feelings about the therapist, beliefs about psychedelic medicines, and expectations for the treatment. The therapist also brings awareness to their own somatic process, current frame of mind, mood, outside concerns, and hopes for the session and the treatment as a whole. In addition, the therapist and client should consider the context of broader sociocultural values and perceptions about psychedelic therapy (such as political or religious perspectives) within the client's community and how these may influence the treatment. Optimal conditions for healing are also co-created by paying close attention to the "setting"—the physical space where the psychedelic session takes place, including the room's aesthetics, lighting, and decor, and the music used in the session (Gold & Sienknecht, 2020).

The goal of trauma therapy is to create these optimal conditions to allow the natural impulse toward healing and completion to be accessed and followed to reach its natural resolution, that is, to process what needs to be processed, to see what needs to be seen, to hear what needs to be heard, to feel what needs to be felt, to express what needs to be expressed, and to move what needs to be moved. In effective trauma therapy, resolution that did not happen during and after the traumatic event(s) finally has the opportunity to occur in a safe and supportive environment. When this processing of past traumatic events happens—now with the inclusion of previously unexpressed emotions and the completion of unfinished motor movements within the safety of the therapeutic relationship—the unmetabolized and inadequately processed past experience(s) can be integrated, and symptoms can begin to resolve.

Capacities Necessary for Healing Trauma

To help a client therapeutically process and integrate traumatic events successfully, three capacities need to be strengthened (Hartman & Zimberoff, 2006):

1. Containment: the sense of being resourced, such that one is able to feel, stay with, and process challenging sensations while increasing self-awareness. This requires developing the ability to observe and regulate nervous system responses and move through what feels overwhelming.
2. Positive body awareness: positive memories and resourcing states need to be uncovered, developed, and strengthened in the body. It is essential to support clients in connecting to these positive states and expanding their capacity to experience pleasure.
3. Dual awareness: increasing the ability to stay connected to the therapist in the present moment and simultaneously connect with the feelings and memories associated with past traumatic material, without dissociating. Increasing this ability becomes possible when the therapist stays attuned to the client's process and remains present even when the client dissociates.

In the following section, the sensation, image, behavior, affect, and meaning (SIBAM) model is presented as a helpful tool for cultivating greater somatic awareness and strengthening capacity across each of these three areas.

The SIBAM Model

The SIBAM model, developed in the 1970s by Peter Levine (2010), is a "bottom-up" model[5] used to help both client and therapist track, understand, and process multiple layers of the totality of a client's experience. It maps one's experience from physical sensations to feelings, perceptions, and meaning making. Levine uses the acronym of SIBAM to describe what he calls the five channels:

1. Sensation: the internal experience of physical sensations
2. Image: the internal representation of external stimuli, such as taste, smell, sight, tactical perception, and hearing
3. Behavior: observable movements and gestures
4. Affect: emotions and the "felt sense"
5. Meaning: beliefs about one's situation and oneself

Using this model, therapists can help a client notice, track, and connect with their experience by placing attention on each channel. Practicing these somatic exercises will enhance a client's capacity to slow down and more mindfully connect with their "full" experience. This, in turn, will strengthen their ability to connect with positive experience, expand capacity for dual awareness, and support their ability to stay with and process challenging experiences.

Processing Trauma With the SIBAM Model

When we experience trauma, our relationship to these channels becomes fragmented, and some parts of our experience become overemphasized (for example, smelling a significant odor or seeing a specific object) and others underemphasized (for example, distressing feelings or sensations). This can lead to narrowed behavioral patterns. Beginning to mindfully notice these fixed patterns of association/dissociation (also known as over-coupling and under-coupling) within the SIBAM channels can be illuminating for the therapeutic process. For example, if the sound of a car horn has been associated with fear due to a past car accident (over-coupling of image and affect), hearing a car horn can incite fear and panic, and the person might avoid being in traffic or driving altogether. Using the SIBAM model, a therapist can help the client slow down this sequence by tracking what is happening in each channel and noticing impulses toward a particular behavior pattern (e.g., traffic sounds that lead them to avoid driving). Slowing down and tracking these subtle aspects of experience can allow the client to access the unfinished fight/flight response, leading to the discharge of trapped energy. The therapist can also support this client by helping them bring attention to the "here and now" therapy space and invite them to pay attention to other channels, such as the color of the couch (image) or the texture of a decorative pillow (sensation).

Psychedelics and the Trauma Response

Expanded states of consciousness can support the client's ability to stay with difficult feelings by expanding the "window of tolerance," thereby facilitating greater opportunities for trauma processing. The client's defense mechanisms, which ordinarily keep them safe from threatening feelings, memories, and sensations that might otherwise be overwhelming, are mediated by the effects of many psychedelic medicines. This effect can allow previously dissociated information to surface without the usual sense of being alarmed, panicked, frightened, or shut down. This dissociated material can then be directly experienced and reparatively processed by the client.

Certain psychedelic medicines, such as MDMA, directly target and decrease activity in the amygdala, the part of the brain that controls the fight/flight/freeze/submit response (Mithoefer et al., 2014). Other psychedelic medicines, such as psilocybin, have been shown to decrease activity in the default mode network (DMN), which has been described as the "seat of the ego." The DMN is our self-conscious overseer that drives rumination and self-judgment. The dampening of the DMN softens our default habits of reactivity and trauma defenses while increasing overall brain connectivity, engaging parts of the brain that are not typically in communication with one another (Nutt & Carhart-Harris, 2020). Ketamine, classified as a dissociative anesthetic that often has a psychedelic effect, has been shown to have an antidepressant effect. The psychedelic dissociative effects of ketamine can enhance self-awareness; facilitate connection to positive feeling states; create distance from traumatic material and negative self-view; and facilitate feelings of peace, joy, sacredness, and transcending time and space (Wolfson, 2016).

A Somatic Approach to Psychedelic-Assisted Trauma Therapy

Unresolved trauma may surface more readily in expanded states of consciousness. As mentioned earlier, MDMA and other psychedelics can decrease the activation in the amygdala and the DMN and soften defensive structures, allowing the client to access unprocessed trauma memories without the usual sense of being overwhelmed, alarmed, panicked, or shut down. The trauma memories that then arise often manifest as—or are accompanied by—somatic symptoms, such as tightness in the chest, difficulty breathing, pain, tiredness, or restlessness in the body.

Some somatic interventions that can support working with these symptoms during a psychedelic-assisted session include noticing, tracking, allowing, breathing into, accentuating, expressing (vocalizing, verbalizing, moving, pushing, and kicking), focusing on the somatic manifestations of imagery and reparative fantasy, and using tools like weighted pillows or blankets. The use of touch is also an important means of supporting the client to feel safe and cared for and to connect deeply with their own tracking, experiencing, processing, and integrating traumatic material stored in the body.

When working with memories and current manifestations of trauma during psychedelic therapy sessions, the therapist should encourage the client to connect with whatever the process brings up; welcome and track sensations, emotions, and thoughts; and express any sensorial or emotional content through movement, sound, and/or language. At times, the therapist may ask the client to *accentuate* bodily sensations and associated emotions or to let the sensations *build up* for a moment to support their release. The therapist needs to find a balance between helping the client stay with their experience without intruding while at the same time helping the client feel supported when moving through the often uncomfortable process.

When to Use Somatic Interventions

For the therapist to best determine which type of somatic intervention would be most useful in any given moment, they should consider certain variables: the medicine that they are working with, the client's history, as well as the here-and-now somatic and psychodynamic process. Every client's journey is unique to them. The therapist must learn to attune to the client and their process and follow the client's lead. It is important for the client and therapist to work collaboratively, both trusting the client's inner healing intelligence rather than following a preconceived approach. Following the inner healing intelligence can look like listening to a client's felt sense, being led by and responsive to impulses, sensations, feelings, images, and memories that arise moment to moment, and supporting the client's process of releasing and moving toward wholeness.

It is important to recognize the various types of experiences that a client might have during a psychedelic session: from the perinatal and the biographical (personal) to the collective, archetypal, or mystical (transpersonal). The type of experience they are having should inform how to engage. For example, when the client is in a perinatal state, going through a birth memory, it might be appropriate to offer pressure or resistance, or hold their head. If the client is in a young, regressed state, the therapist might hold them with a lot of tenderness; use fewer words; and offer touch that is gentle, supportive, and nurturing. Alternatively, when someone is in a state of ego dissolution, the therapist might do best to stay present yet sit back and allow the process to unfold without offering somatic intervention.

Grof (2019, vol. 2) highlights the importance of the use of—and the risk of the underuse of—somatic work, especially in the later parts of PAT sessions. If a somatic process remains incomplete by the end of a medicine session, the client might end up feeling unwell or have physical pain in the days following the session. More importantly, the client can remain stuck in a deep emotional process for quite some time after the session. Grof suggests that during the active phase of the session, the therapist's use of somatic interventions should follow the lead of the client and their process. Toward the end of the session, Grof contends that the therapist should inquire more actively about the body. It is essential that the therapist be comfortable with bodywork and the potential intensity of the emotional and somatic releasing and expressions. The therapist should at times actively encourage and support these focused somatic, emotional, and energetic releases so that the client has the opportunity to arrive at a state of completion by the end of the session, characterized by a calm and a more relaxed state.

Somatic interventions used in the integration phase should be customized for each individual client and their own processing. For example, a client who has started reconnecting with their body might benefit from embodiment practices, such as gentle massage or exploration of slow movement practices. Alternatively, a client who has connected with their suppressed rage might benefit from unstructured dance or physical exercise (in moderation and with care to not exhaust the newly available energy).

Therapeutic Touch in Psychedelic-Assisted Therapy

Types of Therapeutic Touch

Touch in PAT can be differentiated into safety touch, supportive touch, and active touch. Safety touch is employed to ensure a client's safety. Although it might not seem to have psychotherapeutic value, safety touch can actually be a useful therapeutic intervention. For example, safety touch can be reparative for patients whose trauma involved not being physically protected. To illustrate the essential practice of safety touch, imagine a situation where the client is in a deep transpersonal state, possibly not even aware they are in an office. They unexpectedly get up onto their feet, and it appears they may fall and injure themselves. Or the client starts to fall off the couch to the floor. In such instances, the therapist must use their best judgment to protect the safety of the client.

Supportive touch is often a simple gesture, such as holding a client's hand, shoulder, or feet. This can provide a sense of connection, support, and companionship during challenging and emotional moments in the session. It can be used for invoking calm and reassociation or to facilitate a reparative experience. Supportive touch can also involve placing a hand at the back of the client's head, upper back, or kidney area. This method of touch can help with deregulation, reducing a client's anxiety and increasing a capacity for processing trauma. Supportive touch can foster reparative experiences when a client has been harmed by a previous lack of support. This form of touch is particularly useful when a client is experiencing states of regression, fear, or horror. It can give them the needed support to more effectively "stay in the process" with those challenging feelings. This might lead to energetic/emotional discharge, which could look like shaking, sweating, and/or crying, and such a release might then shift the client into states of relaxation, calm, or joy (Levine, 2017). For a more elaborate description of supportive touch, see Chapter 7 on relational touch.

Active touch can help a client process and release somatic tension and blocked emotions or energy, complete unfinished motor movements, and connect with sensations that arise during the process. This could look like pushing against a client's body, for example their hands or feet while they connect with an impulse to push or kick, or offering pressure to a place on their body where they are experiencing tension or discomfort.

Grof (2019, vol. 1) describes two ways of releasing unprocessed somatic and emotional material with the help of active touch: catharsis and abreaction. Catharsis involves release through crying, screaming, and vocalizations. Abreaction involves the client holding bodily tension in their awareness for an extended period of time, leading to an eventual release and redistribution of psychic and somatic energy. Somatic releases by way of touching areas of tension, adding pressure, or pushing against the client's body may then be expressed in many forms, including tremors, twitches, coughing, and vomiting. After these forms of release, the client might shift into states of relaxation, rest, or joy.

Informed Consent for Touch

Informed consent is an indispensable component of both therapeutic touch and PAT. To facilitate a supportive therapeutic container, the psychedelic therapist must provide consistent attention to the client's sense of safety and ongoing consent to the therapeutic process. During the informed consent process, the therapist and client discuss how they will and will not physically interact during sessions, and come to a mutual agreement that can be renegotiated in the future. Rather than being seen as a single conversation during the preparatory session, informed consent should be viewed as an ongoing process that happens across the entire course of treatment. The components of the agreement should be reviewed regularly prior to each medicine session.

In the initial conversation regarding consent for therapeutic touch, the therapist might start by detailing the different types of therapeutic touch that are available and why and when these might be offered, as articulated previously. The initial conversation with a client about touch options should lead to a mutual and explicit agreement outlining the client's level of comfort with different types of touch. During this conversation, the therapist should identify hypothetical situations when the unexpected use of touch is required for the patient's safety even if it cannot be obtained in the moment, so it becomes part of the client and the therapist's shared understanding and agreement.

Importantly, the clear boundary of no sexual touch must be clearly verbalized and expressly agreed upon by the therapist and the client, even though it may seem obvious (and so tacitly agreed upon).

Therapists must be aware of cultural factors related to consent and therapeutic touch; preferences regarding touch vary greatly across cultures. It is important to make efforts to understand each client's background, comfort level, and preferred methods of expression in relation to touch (Tseng, 2001). For example, a client might greet their therapist with a kiss on a cheek, a custom in some cultures, but may feel uncomfortable with touch by their clinician during a session. Thus, inquiry, flexibility, and open conversation are essential at the beginning of a therapeutic relationship that may involve touch.

Part of the consent negotiations for incorporating touch into the work should include a discussion of when the therapist can offer touch unsolicited and when the therapist should wait for the client to request touch. The therapist should ask if there are any specific areas of the body where the client is not comfortable being touched, and discuss whether the client has any areas with physical sensitivity and/ or injuries. The client's relationship to and feelings about their body should be explored and understood. Vulnerable areas that evoke feelings of shame or self-judgment should be noted. A verbal and non-verbal method for signaling a request for contact should be established.

During the consent process, the therapist should discuss how touch will be initiated when checking in with the client during the session. During MDMA-AT sessions, clients are encouraged to have alternating periods of inner and outer focus. It is helpful to make an agreement that if the client does not connect with the therapist(s) for an extended period of time, the therapist will check in with them. If the client prefers touch as a way of checking in, it should be expressly agreed that permission for touch will not be requested before the checking-in touch/prompt. The therapist should ask the client how they would like to be physically prompted; some prefer a light touch on the arm, shoulder, or hand. This agreement will prepare the client for the prompt and help avoid startling them in the middle of a deep process.

Sometimes, clients indicate in the preparatory phase that they do not want to include touch but later ask for touch during the medicine session. This potential scenario points to a challenge, for both client and therapist, that needs to be recognized, explored, and agreed upon before a medicine session. There are two divergent clinical perspectives on this issue. One perspective encourages the therapist to let the client know that they can always decline pre-approved touch during the medicine session, but the therapist will not offer touch that was expressly declined during the consent process, with the intention of respecting the boundary expressed in a non-altered state of consciousness.

Another perspective, as identified by McLane et al. (2021), brings attention to the potential downfall of this first approach. What if the client under the influence of the medicine is more attuned to their present-moment needs, and therefore, denying their spontaneous request for touch in the session might stand in the way of the healing process? From this perspective, the therapist's denial of touch may fail to respect the client's autonomy and agency during the session or trigger feelings of abandonment. This begs the question: is it possible that a client has the capacity for embodied consent when in an altered state of consciousness? Working from this perspective, if a client declines the use of touch during preparation, the therapist can let them know that at times people who initially state they do not want touch feel differently during the medicine session and find themselves wanting physical contact. The client and the therapist can then discuss how to navigate this situation and clarify how the client would want to proceed in such an instance.

It is also important to determine a safe word and non-verbal gesture that can be used by both therapist and client as a signal to stop any therapeutic touch work. It is best to use a neutral word like "stop" or "enough." When negotiating this safe word, it is important to take into consideration that words or phrases, like "no," "fuck off," or "get away from me" may be expressed as a part of the reparative processing of a past abuse trauma. For this reason, identifying a *neutral* safe word is important. Additionally, a physical gesture, like presenting the raised palm of the hand, can be useful when a client is unable to easily verbalize from within their expanded state of consciousness. See Chapter 4 for an in-depth discussion of clarifying client boundaries around touch, as well as specific protocols for practicing requesting, denying, and discontinuing therapeutic touch.

Case Example: Annie

Annie, a 45-year-old woman, sought treatment for chronic depression. As a child, Annie had been emotionally and physically abused by her father. Her father laid out a system of rules she had to follow daily. When she failed to obey or made a mistake, she was punished by having to sit with her hands under her thighs while he shook and slapped her. A memory of one of these events came up during a ketamine-assisted therapy session.

Annie reported feeling tension in her hands and a desire to move them but also feeling frozen. Making use of a technique to help facilitate connection with the material arising, I encouraged her to breathe into the sensation to make more space for what was coming up for her. (This request is not the same as asking someone to breathe deeply to calm an unpleasant feeling.) As she connected with the sensations in her hands, Annie started to feel anger and a desire to push her father away. I encouraged her to imagine doing that. Her hands moved out from underneath her and forward in a pushing motion. I offered to provide physical resistance. She liked the idea, and she started to push against my hands while focusing on her inner experience.

Annie began to add her voice, expressing anger and saying, "Go away! Get your fucking hands away from me!" The words were clearly meant for her father and did not indicate that she wanted me to go away or stop. Because we had the agreement to use the specific safe word "enough" if she wanted me to stop the touch, there was no confusion in my mind about how to proceed. Over the course of the next several minutes, she pushed my hands with increasing vigor and force. The process continued, and she yelled, "Now he is gone! I have my strength back, and he has no chance of coming back." She laid down and sought connection with her younger self, expressing compassion and empathy for what she had been through as a little girl. She imagined giving herself a teddy bear (which she was not allowed to have as a child), tearing her father's list of rules into pieces, and taking the little girl with her away from the childhood home. In the integration sessions, Annie was able to share more of her childhood memories. In the past, shame kept her from being able to connect with herself and others. After processing this trauma—through the lens of restorative and reparative fantasy, somatic processing, and reconnecting with her younger self—she was able to develop and sustain more compassion for herself and started to engage in her life more fully.

When to Incorporate Touch

When to use and when not to use touch are not always clear. For example, for a client who is expressing their internal process by moving around and crying, touch could be counterproductive, interrupting their deep internal process. Conversely, with another client who is presenting similarly, yet has a history of developmental trauma, a therapist who opts not to use touch might miss an opportunity to provide support for their healing. In this case, not offering physical contact could counterproductively increase dysregulation or may even be retraumatizing for the client. It is therefore vital for the therapist to remain aware of the larger context of the client's history as well as their longitudinal process when determining whether touch is a potential benefit or hindrance in each unfolding moment. Simultaneously, it is important to keep in mind that there is no one perfect intervention. When mistakes or missed opportunities occur, therapists should approach them as possibilities for learning with and about the client, with the understanding that processing misattunement holds the potential for reparative experience. See Chapter 5 for an extensive discussion of relational repair.

The MAPS MDMA-Assisted Therapy Manual recommends offering supportive touch early in a session as a way to help clients regulate anxiety that sometimes arises as the effects of the medicine begin to take hold (Mithoefer et al., 2014).

Therapeutic touch can then be used at various points throughout a psychedelic session, following the lead of the client and their process. Whether earlier or later in the session, Mithoefer et al. (2014) and Grof (2019, vol. 1) suggest first inviting the patient to connect with their body through mindful intention and breath before offering touch. If appropriate, the client might be invited to place their hands on their body before the therapist joins with physical contact or engages in further therapeutic touch. This approach honors the inner healing intelligence and allows internal exploration before additional intervention is offered.

From Grof's (2019, vol. 1) perspective, "focused energy release" bodywork is best suited for the later part of a medicine session. In the later part of a session, when the effects of the medicine are subsiding, the client might need additional help through the therapist's use of touch-based interventions. More active touch work, such as Grof's bodywork, can facilitate the release of pent-up energy by applying pressure to stuck areas or holding the energy for a period of time. As mentioned earlier, this helps avoid the potential for somatic symptoms or challenging emotions to remain "stuck" in the system following the session.

If touch is used in a medicine session, it is essential to revisit the experience during the integration. The therapist and client should explore how the touch work felt, whether the client expected or hoped for something different, what worked, what did not work, and what could have been more useful. The therapist and client can then use this information to guide future sessions. In integration sessions, self-touch and/or bodywork can continue somatic processing—particularly if the client continues to experience somatic symptoms after the medicine session—by completing unfinished motor movements, working with stagnant energy, grounding in a sense of calm, or reconnecting with one's body.

"Why Am I Touching?"

Psychedelic therapists have a heightened responsibility to get to know their own limits, boundaries, and sensitivities, as well as the various ways they respond to challenging clinical situations. If a therapist is not well attuned to their internal processes, they run a higher risk of counterproductively intruding on the client's process by trying to control or overdirect it. Or, with a lack of self-awareness, they might inappropriately withhold, withdraw, or abandon the client.

Many clients seek out PAT after enormous challenges, traumatic events, and the failure of traditional therapy or medical treatments. A PAT therapist therefore needs to remain continually mindful of how they can be vicariously impacted by the tremendous amount of suffering they encounter in a psychedelic session. This can then influence when and how a therapist engages with therapeutic touch.

A valuable way to cultivate self-awareness practices can be found in the acronym WAIT? (Why Am I Talking?), introduced by Richard Schwartz in Internal Family Systems Training (M. Mithofer, personal communication, September 12, 2016). I suggest a slight modification for somatic work, "Why Am I Touching?" Before we, as therapists, initiate any touch work, we should ask ourselves: Where is the impulse to touch coming from? Am I touching because the client's process or content is too overwhelming for me? Do I feel the need to intervene to help regulate my own nervous system rather than doing what is best for the client? Although there are many times when intervention, somatic support, or bodywork is appropriate, "Why Am I Touching?" is most always a good self-check across all aspects of PAT.

Opportunities for Therapeutic Touch in Psychedelic-Assisted Therapy

Supportive Touch at the Beginning of a Medicine Session

Supportive touch, such as holding the client's hand or placing a hand on the shoulder, can be helpful in the early part of a psychedelic session to mitigate anxiety that sometimes arises as clients enter the medicine space. This gentle form of touch can help the client become comfortable with the transition into expanded states of consciousness and establish safety and trust in the process.

Case Example: Lucas

Lucas, an older male client in an MDMA-AT treatment for complex PTSD, was feeling very anxious at the beginning of a medicine session. He could not remain still and kept taking his eyeshades off and initiating conversation with the therapists. He was invited to talk about how he was feeling and use a breathing technique to help calm his anxiety while waiting for the medicine to take effect. Despite previous practice with the breathing technique in our earlier preparation sessions, it did not seem to reduce his anxiety. We offered supportive somatic touch, and the client consented, asking for touch from both therapists. The male therapist held his hand and I placed my hands on his feet. Within a couple of minutes, he started to report a decrease in anxiety. Several minutes later, he put his eyeshades on and relaxed into the session's initial stage. Soon after that, he expressed appreciation for the touch and indirectly let us know he no longer wanted touch by saying, "I am okay to just be with myself with the music and wait for the medicine."

Touch and Perinatal and Birth Trauma

Sometimes, expanded states of consciousness can facilitate unique insights into perinatal and birth experiences that continue to impact a client's life. Stanislav Grof et al. (2008) introduced the concept of Birth Perinatal Matrices (BPM), which outlines the birth process from the vantage point of the fetus's experiential patterns across four stages of birth. BPM I refers to the perinatal experience (before the onset of labor), which may be characterized by oceanic bliss; tranquility and cosmic unity; or, in the case of a challenging pregnancy, by malaise, disgust, paranoia, or anxiety. BPM II refers to the phase after contractions have started, yet before the fetus has moved into the birth canal, which may be experienced as stuckness, helplessness, hopelessness, or guilt. BPM III refers to the movement through the birth canal, which often involves struggle, life/death crisis, rage, anxiety, and discharge of energy. BPM IV refers to the final physical separation from the mother, which often comes with a sense of relief, liberation, love, and divine oneness. While it is possible to experience challenges in each of these stages, they most often show up in BPM II and III.

Grof identifies these very early experiences—both challenging and positive—as potential templates for later life patterns. For example, an adult client may present with symptoms of severe depression, hopelessness, and "feeling stuck" that correspond with the second perinatal matrix (BPM II) challenges. Those born via Cesarean section will have only experienced the initial phases of the birth process, which might manifest later in life as a strong capacity to start projects alongside intense struggles carrying them to completion. Grof believes experiences within the perinatal matrices impact all human beings. He contends that the nature and quality of one's early developmental experiences—specifically early instances of abandonment, abuse, oppression, and/or recurring feelings of guilt, shame, powerlessness, anxiety, and depression—influence how one's prenatal and birth challenges show up later in life. For example, good-enough care by early attachment figures and a predominance of positive childhood experiences can help mitigate BPM I though BPM IV challenges. On the other hand, adverse childhood experiences can lead to future "echoing" of challenges from BPM I through BPM IV.

Ray Castellino was another pioneer in the field of prenatal and perinatal therapy, and he was an early advocate of using somatic approaches to facilitate attachment and bonding for infants and their caregivers, as well as for clients in later stages of life. His work focused on resolving prenatal, birth, and early childhood trauma. Castellino viewed the use of touch and co-regulation with the therapist as indispensable for a successful resolution of the residual influences of prenatal and perinatal challenges for adult clients, as words and mental understanding are not available in these developmental stages. PAT frequently brings forth somatic and imaginal memories of perinatal experiences, providing the opportunity to access, engage, and process challenging birth experiences. In the context of psychedelic therapy, therapeutic touch in service of processing and integrating preverbal and birth trauma may prove to be a powerful tool for resolving current-day symptomatology of early trauma. Touch used in these scenarios can provide a sense of safety through co-regulation with the therapist, support the completion of unfinished motor movements initiated during and after birth, provide missing experience of nurturance and care, and support reconnection with dissociated sensations and emotions. Therapeutic touch might entail placing a hand on the client's shoulder or hand, or under their head or kidney area to support regulation. Some approaches to therapeutic touch, such as Grof's focused energy release bodywork, include the therapist providing resistance to movements arising organically from the client's body. This is illustrated in the following example, in which I place my hands on the client's head and shoulders to simulate the birth experience.

Case Example: Simone

Simone came to KAP treatment due to her increasingly unmanageable symptoms of depression and because she felt hopelessly stuck in her relationship. She described her inability to leave her partner of three years, even though it was clear they had grown apart. She told me that despite their multiple efforts to reconnect, she continued to feel alone in the relationship, yet was unable to find the energy to leave. Simone recognized this immobility as a pattern in her intimate relationships. She said that when she feels hopeless, her depression increases, and this makes it challenging to mobilize into action.

In her first and second KAP sessions, she reported feeling calm and relaxed in a way she had not remembered feeling in a long time. She reported sensations of floating, being "in the universe," and feeling connected to everyone and everything. These pleasurable experiences provided a new distance from familiar feelings of hopelessness.

Simone's intention for her third KAP session was to understand more about the roots of her depression. In her initial intake, Simone had reported that her birth process was rather long and that her mother told her she had been "stuck" for a while, and a C-section was considered, although ultimately determined unnecessary. In the KAP session, soon after the medicine was administered, Simone curled up into a fetal position and started to push her head into the pillow. I kept my mind open to the many different interpretations of what she may have been experiencing. Based on her movements, I started to wonder if she was reexperiencing her birth, so I asked Simone for permission to apply touch. With her consent, I began to touch her head and shoulders to simulate pressures during the birth process. She responded positively to the touch by pushing against my hands and using her feet to push herself forward. As the intensity peaked, she said, "I feel stuck," "It's hard to breathe," and "I want to get out." I verbally encouraged her to follow her somatic impulses and express any sounds or words that came up. After some time, she moved forward, let out an extended sigh, and then took a deep breath. She relaxed, curled up, and looked like she might fall asleep. After a few minutes, she put her thumb in her mouth and rested peacefully. As the medicine wore off, Simone shared her experience. She said, "I think I relived my own birth. . . . I'm not sure what that means, but it felt important." She expressed feeling calm and connected." In the weeks following, Simone began to feel more hopeful and was better able to ask for what she needed in her relationships—both at work and at home. She no longer felt completely defeated and hopeless. She decided to give couples counseling another try. Simone reported that she felt more capable of leaving her partner if the relationship did not change for the better.

Touch and Early Developmental Trauma

Psychedelic-assisted therapy sessions that include touch can provide unique opportunities for reparative relational healing of developmental trauma, especially trauma experienced in the preverbal phase of development. In psychedelic sessions, clients may experience the manifestations of early trauma in their body without a specific visual memory or story attached to it. With the support of the medicine, the client can gain insight into their hypervigilance, or they might find that this response is suspended during the session, providing a novel experience of feeling safe. The use of supportive, nourishing touch can be very effective in healing early trauma as the therapist can temporarily step into the role of caregiver and provide the missing experience of safety through care and co-regulation.

Case Example: Tom

Tom, a 55-year-old male patient, sought out PAT for help with treatment-resistant depression. Tom was a twin, and due to a dangerously low birth weight, he was placed in an incubator for a month, where he likely was not receiving adequate human touch. He described himself as always feeling hopeless and disconnected from himself and his life energy. His treatment included 10 KAP sessions over three months. During his second KAP session, he started to make infant-like sounds of distress, exhibiting movements centered in the spine, which looked separate from other disjointed movements in his arms and legs. This type of somatic response has been described as "larval swimming movement," often a sign of a very early life defense response to threat or overwhelm (Levine, 2017). Tom's head was shaking, so with his permission, I gently placed a hand on the top of his head. The distress movements slowed down, and Tom began expressing softer, calmer sounds and eventually settled into peaceful silence. Later in the session, Tom described feeling safe and protected by the gentle touch of my hand, such that he could let the move-ments happen without feeling overwhelmed. In subsequent sessions, his larval movement returned but became less pronounced and over time not as overwhelm-ing and eventually stopped. I continued to use somatic support, and Tom eventually started engaging with me by touching my hand with his fingers—demonstrating the exploratory touch infants use when they feel safe.

As our work progressed, Tom reported being able to internalize my touch along-side a sense of safety that felt like "being held comfortably as a baby." He expressed feeling supported and connected. Over the next few weeks, Tom reported feeling more energetic and engaged in his daily activities, including an impulse to reach out to others and a renewed ability to make friends. Four months later, Tom weaned off antidepressant medications. A year later, he continued to be depression free and reported being better able to maintain meaningful relationships.

Working With the Freeze and Submit/Collapse Response

As mentioned previously, when one is "stuck" in a freeze response, they are expe-riencing both sympathetic and parasympathetic arousal. It is as if they are stand-ing on the gas and brake pedals simultaneously. The fight/flight activation that the nervous system has not been able to discharge lies underneath the immobility of the freeze response. This high activation state can lead to chronic lack of energy, depression, and eventually the submit/collapse response (also known as hypo-arousal). Catatonia, sometimes diagnosed as a motor disorder, is an example of an extreme state of unresolved collapse response (Moskowitz, 2004).

The therapeutic process of working with the submit/collapse response involves first helping the client move out of collapse into freeze and then out of freeze. The client will reconnect with sensations, feelings, and/or memories (reassociation of the under-coupled aspects of their experience), which may be connected with releases of energy and accompanied by movements, sounds, verbalization, sweating, crying, shaking, or purging. This can be painful, intense, or frightening. The release and deactivation of the stuck energy of a freeze response and reconnecting with all aspects of experience facilitate a shift into regulation. During and after medicine sessions that involve working through a freeze state, the client may experience increased anxiety, distress, rage, or grief. The process might continue in the hours, days, or weeks after the session. For many clients, the return from the freeze state can be exhausting but can ultimately lead to feeling powerful and energized "like coming alive again." However, without adequate preparation and support, this process can lead to further overwhelm and a return to the freeze or collapse state.

In preparation for PAT with a client in a freeze or submit/collapse response, the therapist should help them expand their capacity to track and "be with" sensations in their body and support their development of self-care practices and self-soothing strategies. Additionally, it is important to discuss and normalize the possible discomfort that may arise in the medicine session and subsequent integration process. As therapists, we can facilitate successful completion of the client's process by attentively stewarding them through their emerging sensations, emotions, physical movements, and memories, and support their unfolding meaning making. After sessions involving processing trauma with aspects of freeze or submit/collapse states, therapists should make themselves available for additional follow-up check-ins or integration sessions, if needed.

Case Example: Carla

Carla, a 50-year-old female, was referred to KAP after a severe episode of suicidal ideation and brief hospitalization resulting from the sudden death of her partner. In her intake session, Carla found it challenging to talk about her experience and share her history. It was difficult for her to speak, and she exhibited slow, rigid movements, a blank stare, and emotionless facial expressions. Her primary therapist shared details of her trauma history with me. She was a survivor of multiple traumatic events since her early childhood, and the recent death of her long-term partner had triggered her current severe depressive episode. It was clear she was stuck in a state of hypo-arousal/collapse.

Carla's treatment took place over five months. During the initial four weeks, I saw Carla for KAP medicine sessions twice a week, with integration sessions once or twice a week. With the support of ketamine, she experienced relief from the collapse response. She started to verbally process her recent loss. She was able to track sensations and feelings in her body and express significant grief. Despite the process that occurred in the office during these medicine sessions, in between sessions, she felt stuck in the freeze response. She began to experience high levels of sympathetic activation, which presented as anxiety, fear, and anger, which she was not able to move through alone.

During the next series of KAP sessions, Carla expressed these feelings by kicking into the mattress, screaming, and pushing against my hands. She then described "witnessing" (in utero) her mother's experiences of being pregnant with her while in a volatile relationship with her father. She reported feeling consumed with fears about the future. As she got in touch with these prenatal memories (Grof, 2000) while I provided verbal and somatic support, her body began to tremble, shake, and vibrate, discharging pent-up energy. In the integration sessions, Carla began to tolerate her system's activation without needing to move away or getting stuck in a freeze response; she started to move through cycles of activation and deactivation with greater ease. She was able to process memories of her traumatic life events, as well as the vicarious experience of her mother's trauma while Carla was in utero. By the end of our work together, she reported feeling more alive, began reconnecting with friends, and even expressed openness to dating in the future. She began finding enjoyment in exploring new activities and felt more optimistic about her life.

Anchoring Positive Resource States

Anchoring is a technique that helps the client internalize a positive feeling state and carry it with them going forward, such that they can call on it at a later time. Anchoring supports the cultivation of resilience and is a useful tool for the integration process. When a client resolves past trauma and develops an increased capacity to self-regulate (increased coherence) or when they access a positive internal space, we can invite them to stay connected with this physiological and emotional feeling state in that moment to create "an anchor." Michael Vancura asks clients at the end of sessions, "Where in your body do you feel the most relaxed, the most at home right now?" and then uses that information for anchoring (personal communication, June, 9, 2022). Similar to how paying attention to the multiple channels identified by the SIBAM model can deepen a client's awareness of their internal experience, Vancura recommends prompting a client to provide detailed descriptions of feelings, sensations, and internal images to support effective anchoring. Anchoring grounds a feeling state as a somatic memory anchored in the body that can help make that feeling state more accessible. Anchoring can be further enhanced by self-touch or the therapist's touch. The client is then invited to continue to reconnect with the anchored state in the days and weeks after the session.

In the following example, I use anchoring to support a naturally occurring resourced state by inviting the client to connect with her body, sensations, and emotions to help her gain access to this positive state after the session.

Case Example: Sarah

Sarah, a 30-year-old female, was in treatment for post-traumatic stress. Symptoms stemmed from when a fire broke out in her house while she was asleep. In the process of fleeing the fire, she handed her daughter to the firefighter and then lost track of her. Even though they both survived, Sarah continued to experience a pervasive and dysregulated hypervigilance response. She had significant difficulty falling and staying asleep; during the daytime, she would have flashbacks of the smell of smoke. She was not able to feel relaxed around her daughter, even when she cognitively knew they both were safe.

After two KAP sessions in which we processed the memories of the event, she reported a decrease in flashbacks; yet, she continued to struggle with hypervigilance. In her third ketamine session, she connected with the fact that she had saved her daughter's life and came to see her hypervigilance as a strength. She began to feel a sense of peace and connected that feeling with how she used to feel prior to the fire trauma. Sarah reported that not only did she feel calmer, but she also felt appreciation for her hypervigilant self. I asked Sarah if she was aware of a specific place in her body that connected to her strength while in a relaxed physical state. She said she felt especially good in her solar plexus, so I invited her to place her hands on that area and further connect with the sensation. Sarah reported a vision of white soothing vibrations radiating out from her solar plexus and across her whole body. She described a vision of an ethereal being providing support to that area. I encouraged her to use her hand to set an anchor to the powerful sensations, emotions, transpersonal vision, and state of mind. I offered to place my hands on top of hers to further reinforce the anchor, which she gladly accepted. She later successfully used this anchor in the mornings and evenings while she was in bed. Over the next month, she reported a continued decrease in hypervigilance and sleep disturbances, an increased connection with herself, appreciation for her strength during the fire event, and confidence that she could successfully navigate the hypothetical instance of a future event.

Using Somatic Work at the End of a Session

Somatic work can be valuable at the end of a medicine session to assist clients in releasing whatever tensions surfaced in their body; help them move to a calmer, more grounded state (Grof, 2019, vol. 1); and incorporate new insights and ways of being. Therapeutic touch can help a client reinhabit their body and reconnect with the therapist as a medicine session nears its conclusion—particularly when using dissociative psychedelics, like ketamine. This type of grounding and reorienting touch might involve holding the feet, hands, head, or neck, or may include more vigorous bodywork. Clients can also be invited to use self-touch and physical movement.

The Importance of Self-Care With PAT

The importance of self-care for the psychedelic therapist cannot be overemphasized. With PAT, a large amount of psychic, emotional, and somatic material is processed in a relatively short time frame compared to traditional therapy. Furthermore, psychedelic therapy induces greater porosity, along with heightened suggestibility and boundary diffusion for both therapist and client, all of which infuses the shared relational field. Even with adequate training, therapists will take some of the processed material into their own bodies. In addition to regular consultation or supervision, PAT therapists should cultivate a strong practice of discharging, clearing, and rebalancing following medicine sessions. It is essential for therapists using somatic interventions to be fully present and feel grounded in their bodies, as their internal state and sensations will impact the client. By working with a somatic therapist, a therapist can continue to process their experiences and increase their somatic awareness, resilience, and internal coherence, allowing them to be more present, attuned, and effective therapists.

Other regular self-care practices might include salt baths, ocean soaks, aromatherapy, sound healing, flotation tank sessions, nature walks, or dance. Additionally, regular bodywork, acupuncture, massage, exercise, or movement practice can help offset or mitigate the potential internalizing of a client's trauma.

Conclusion

Physical touch is indispensable to healthy human development—without it, infants fail to thrive. Touch is a powerful vehicle for interpersonal connection for human beings of all ages, as well as an underappreciated component of physical and emotional healing. Physical touch carries enormous potential as a tool in PAT. Beyond the many somatic approaches that use touch, there are also non-touch techniques (used in conjunction with verbal processing) that can foster greater somatic awareness and positive outcomes in trauma processing. Whether using touch or non-touch methods, somatic work should be an integral part of PAT.

As Western culture and its professional practices continue to recognize the value of somatic therapy techniques, PAT—with its unique opportunities to effectively employ therapeutic touch—may help move the traditional psychotherapy field forward by its example. The inclusion of the physical body is an essential component of a fully integrated healing journey toward wholeness.

Notes

1 I am deeply grateful to my dear friends and colleagues who have helped me with the editing of this chapter, especially Leonard Cetrangolo, Sharon Bandy, Eric Sienknecht, and Harvey Schwartz.
2 MAPS is the Multidisciplinary Association for Psychedelic Studies.
3 I will use the term "somatic work" as a broader term to encompass somatic theory, use of touch by a therapist, as well as attunement to and working with the body's subtle processes, which can look like paying attention to and connecting with the body, breathing into sensations, or working with non-sexual self-touch.
4 Grof describes "Holotropic," meaning moving toward wholeness, as the goal of psychedelic-assisted therapy (Grof, 2006). Following the rescheduling of LSD as a controlled substance, when it was no longer legally available for clinicians to use in psychotherapy,

Stan and Christina Grof developed Holotropic Breathwork—a therapeutic modality that combines deep breathing, inner focus, bodywork, and music in a comfortable setting to elicit expanded states of consciousness (Grof, 2019).
5   Addressing trauma starting with the limbic system, in contrast to starting with the prefrontal cortex in "bottom-down" models.

References

Blackstone, J. (2018). *Trauma and the unbound body: The healing power of fundamental consciousness*. Sounds True.

Gold, V., & Sienknecht, E. (2020, July 31). Ambassadors to hidden territories: Set and setting in psychedelic-assisted psychotherapy. *Chacruna*. https://chacruna.net/ambassadors-to-hidden-territories-set-and-setting-in-psychedelic-assisted-psychotherapy/

Grof, S. (2000). *Psychology of the future: Lessons from modern consciousness research*. State University of New York Press.

Grof, S. (2019). *The way of the psychonaut* (Vol. 1, 2 vols.). Multidisciplinary Association for Psychedelic Studies (MAPS).

Grof, S., & Bennett, H. Z. (2006). *The holotropic mind: The three levels of human consciousness and how they shape our lives*. Harper San Francisco.

Grof, S., Hofmann, A., & Weil, A. (2008). *LSD psychotherapy*. Multidisciplinary Association for Psychedelic Studies.

Hartman, D., & Zimberoff, D. (2006). Healing the body-mind in heart-centered therapies. *Journal of Heart-Centered Therapies, 9*(2), 75–137.

Kain, K. L., & Terrell, S. J. (2018). *Nurturing resilience: Helping clients move forward from developmental trauma an integrative somatic approach*. North Atlantic Books.

Levine, P. A. (2010). *In an unspoken voice: How the body releases trauma and restores goodness*. North Atlantic Books.

Levine, P. A. (2017). *Somatic experiencing* [Healing Trauma Training Manual]. Foundation for Human Enrichment.

Levine, P. A., & Frederick, A. (1997). *Waking the tiger: Healing trauma: The innate capacity to transform overwhelming experiences*. North Atlantic Books.

Levitan, A. A., & Johnson, J. M. (1986). The role of touch in healing and hypnotherapy. *American Journal of Clinical Hypnosis 28*(4), 218–223. doi: 10.1080/00029157.1986.10402657

McLane, H., Hutchison, C., Wikler, D., Howell, T., & Knighton, E. (2021). https://blogs.bmj.com/medical-ethics/2021/12/22/respecting-autonomy-in-altered-states-navigating-ethical-quandaries-in-psychedelic-therapy/

Mithoefer, M., Doblin, R., Sola, E., Mithoefer, M. G., Gibson, E., Ruse, J., . . . Mithoefer, A. (2014). *A manual for MDMA-assisted psychotherapy in the treatment* . . . Retrieved January 5, 2021, from https://maps.org/research-archive/mdma/MDMA-Psychotherapy_Treatment_Manual_Version_6_FINAL.pdf

Moskowitz, A. K. (2004). "Scared stiff": Catatonia as an evolutionary-based fear response. *Psychological Review, 111*(4), 984–1002. doi: 10.1037/0033-295x.111.4.984

Nutt, D., & Carhart-Harris, R. (2020). The current status of psychedelics in psychiatry. *JAMA Psychiatry*. doi: 10.1001/jamapsychiatry.2020.2171

Porges, S. W. (2011). *The polyvagal theory: Neurophysiological foundations of emotions, attachment, communication, and self-regulation*. W.W. Norton.

Porges, S. W. (2016). Trauma and the polyvagal theory: A commentary. *International Journal of Multidisciplinary Trauma Studies, 1*, 24–30. doi: 10.3280/ijm2016-001003

Siegel, D. J., & Siegel, D. J. (2012). *The developing mind: Toward a neurobiology of interpersonal experience*. Guilford Press.

Smith, E. W., Clance, P. R., & Imes, S. (1998). *Touch in psychotherapy: Theory, research, and practice*. Guilford Press.

Tseng, W. (2001). Culture-relevant psychotherapy. *Handbook of Cultural Psychiatry*, 595–610. doi: 10.1016/b978-012701632-0/50112-1

Van der Kolk, B. (2015). *The body keeps the score: Brain, mind, and body in the healing of trauma*. IDreamBooks.

Wolfson, P. (2016). *Ketamine papers: Science, therapy, and transformation*. Multidisciplinary Association for Psychedelic Studies (MAPS).

Chapter 7

Relational Touch in Psychedelic-Assisted Therapy

Shirley Dvir and Jacki Hull

Introduction[1]

Touch, our very first language, is foundational for human development and has been used for healing around the world for centuries. However, the field of psychotherapy is conflicted about touch, with many practitioners holding fears of violating ethical boundaries. Here, our intention is first to raise awareness about professional touch in psychotherapy, which is safe and ethical when used with care, skill, consent, and good boundaries, and then to discuss the potential benefits of combining professional touch with ketamine-assisted therapy. This chapter is written from the perspective of Relational Somatic Healing—a method of working with relational touch in psychotherapy to heal developmental trauma.

Pej (Shirley as the Therapist)

Pej, a 45-year-old cisgender Caucasian man, was a stay-at-home dad for two school-age kids. He had recently fallen into a deep depression with little insight into its cause. From the outside, his life seemed good—he had a loving wife, two wonderful kids he used to enjoy taking care of, and many friends and family to support him. Despite my best efforts as an experienced somatic psychotherapist to guide him into a deeper relationship with his inner experiences, Pej told me he was tired of talk therapy. I sensed that he had given up on his hope to heal, and I watched him progressively decline into greater depression and shutdown. By that time, I had studied craniosacral touch therapy and was willing to try anything that would help, so I invited him to rest his body on my table and obtained consent to place my hands gently under his left shoulder and left knee. Pej was able to rest and feel held without the need to explain or do anything. Slowly with my hands holding him, his body started to relax and become less rigid, his breath expanded, and his thoughts quieted. I followed his body's progression from rest to release of tension and energy. I held him lovingly and welcomed his experience without judgment or the need to attach a story to it. Right there on the table, slowly, session after session, by feeling accepted and held, Pej started to loosen his rigidity and soften his frozen body. As he softened, memories and images started to surface, and we were able to

DOI: 10.4324/9781003167976-7

process them together while I held him. In less than three months of twice a week touch-oriented psychotherapy sessions, Pej was back to himself; he regained his aliveness, found renewed energy to be with his family, and was able to find a job. When I inquired about what had helped Pej, he told me that my touch supported him in feeling accepted such that he began to find acceptance toward himself.

An Introduction to Touch

Touch is one of the most essential senses in the mammalian kingdom; it is instinctual, organic, intuitive, and inherited. Touch plays a crucial role in development throughout the spectrum of the human life span: embryonic, infancy, childhood, adolescence, adulthood, aging, and dying (Field, 2014). The skin is the envelope of the body and the sensory system. Our skin is the first organ to develop and the largest, most important organ of the body, without which humans would not survive (Field, 2014; Montague, 1986). The skin has been called "the social organ" (Linden, 2015; Montague, 1986), the organ through which humans interact and communicate with each other.

Touch is the earliest and most profound medium of communication between caregiver and infant. Ashley Montague (1986) called touch the "mother of the senses" (p. 3). Unlike other senses, humans cannot survive without touch; as Montague (1986) wrote, "When the need for touch remains unsatisfied, abnormal behavior will result" (p. 46). In a research study investigating the role of a mother's touch in infant development, Polan and Ward (1994) found that infants who demonstrated a failure to thrive received less maternal touch, in the form of physical interaction and physical attention, compared to other infants. Other research on maternal touch in early development has shown that maternal touch not only promotes growth, but it significantly affects the infant's regulatory behaviors, reduces stress, and builds stress tolerance (Feldman et al., 2010; Jean et al., 2004).

Touch has been an ancient method of healing since before recorded time—at least as far back as 1800 BCE—and was considered a central component of medicine until the pharmaceutical revolution in the 1940s (Field, 1998). The practice of healing touch has its roots in many ancient cultures and traditions, such as entheogenic shamanism, Ayurveda, and traditional Chinese medicine, in which it is considered a sacred system of natural healing passed down through generations (Field, 2014).

Tiffany Field (2014), a leading researcher on the benefits of touch, noted that touch is an efficient method for reducing anxiety and creating a sense of ease and trust. From a biochemical perspective, touch stimulates complex chemical reactions in the body, including a decrease in stress hormones, such as cortisol, catecholamines, norepinephrine, and epinephrine, and an increase in prosocial hormones, such as serotonin and dopamine. Touch also stimulates the production of oxytocin, a pituitary hormone regarded as the "love hormone." Dopamine, serotonin, and oxytocin—also known as the "feel-good hormones"—each play a significant role in creating a sense of calm and safety and correlate with pleasant mood, emotional stability, focus, and stronger functioning of the immune system (Marcher et al., 2015).

Biases Around Touch in Psychotherapy

Despite the many benefits of touch, most psychotherapists express a high degree of caution regarding physical contact with clients. In a research survey of a national sample of 470 psychologists, close to 90% responded that they never or rarely offer touch to their clients (Stenzel & Rupert, 2004). The reasons psychotherapists do not use touch include a desire to avoid crossing ethical or legal boundaries and fears that touch may cause harm, lead to sexual exploitation, or be perceived by the client as harmful or abusive. While these are important concerns—particularly in the sensitive states evoked by psychedelic medicines—they overlook the healing potential of touch when held in a safe and ethical manner. Additionally, Milakovich (1998) found that therapists who do not use touch simply have no professional or personal experience with it.

Ethics of Touch

The United States Association for Body Psychotherapy (USABP, 2018) has a well-defined code of ethics in regard to the use of touch. It makes it clear that touch in psychotherapy is a legitimate and valuable modality when used skillfully with clear boundaries, sensitive application, and good clinical judgment. The USABP code of ethics articulates guidelines for therapists when incorporating touch into their practice. The guidelines state that therapists should have training and supervision in the use of touch, that touch is never utilized to gratify the personal needs of the therapist, and that sexual touch is never part of therapy. Additionally, the guidelines suggest using a signed informed consent regarding touch and obtaining consent not only in written or verbal form but also through ongoing non-verbal cues by listening to the client's body language.

In our opinion, the most important guideline is expressed in the statement, "The application of touch techniques requires a high degree of internal clarity and integration on the part of the therapist" (USABP, 2018). This statement speaks to the significance of the internal state of the therapist and the importance of cultivating a high level of self-awareness, mindfulness, and embodiment. Such qualities are essential to developing clear, safe boundaries within the therapeutic relationship—a foundational element of ethical touch in psychotherapy. Emphasizing the internal state of the therapist invites practitioners to become aware of their intention for offering touch as well as the quality of their touch.

Consent to Touch

Consent and re-consent are the most important elements of touch-based psychotherapy and differentiate it from other touch healing modalities, such as bodywork. Consent is not only an ethical guideline but a core clinical consideration and intervention. True consent goes beyond words or writing; because touch is a non-verbal communication, it needs to be met with non-verbal consent as well. The art of non-verbal consent involves somatic tracking, listening, and receiving the client in the moment: their body language, somatic positioning, movement, and energy. For example, notice the position of the client's body, especially their head—is it directed away from or toward the therapist? Is their body relaxed or tense? Does the client feel present or dissociated? What is their facial expression? Are their eyes closed or open, looking at the therapist or away? Is there tension in the mouth? What is their facial tone, color, and change of color—is it pale, pink, or red?

Therapists need to collect all these non-verbal cues and ask themselves, "Does the client's body consent to touch?" If their body is showing signs of pulling away, shutting down, closing, tensing, and so on, there needs to be a discussion about what is happening somatically, as the client may not be aware that their body is saying "no" or "not yet." Therapists also need to sense into their own non-verbal consent. Does the therapist's body feel open and receptive to touching the client, or does it feel hesitant, closed, or cautious? Listening for the therapist's own full consent is crucial when conducting safe and ethical touch-based psychotherapy. When the therapist does not have consent from their own body to touch, it is an indicator to listen to their "no" and discuss this important clinical issue with the client.

Beyond non-verbal cues, therapists need to consider a variety of additional elements in the process of consent, including the client's past experience of touch; their ability to truly feel safe saying "yes" or "no;" and their racial and cultural background, age, gender, sexuality, trauma history, and relationship to oppression, power, and privilege. Therapists need to ask themselves the following: Can this client truly consent, or will they comply on the outside and resist on the inside? Is it safe for them to say no? What does consent look like, say, between a female client of African descent working with a white male therapist? And finally, what would consent look like between an adult therapist and a child client, considering that adults rarely ask for a child's permission before they touch them.

Because many clients were violated with touch in their past, how can we ensure they feel safe to say "no" or "stop"? Sometimes, the process of consent takes several sessions, months, or even years to unfold. It is essential that therapists empower clients to feel their true "no" and only move into safe touch when they are ready to express their true "yes." Re-consent addresses the fact that what feels right in the current moment may not feel right in the next moment. It is therefore important to practice asking and reasking for consent each time there is a change in the position of the hands. This allows clients to feel in their body what is right for them in each moment and feel the power of owning their body and setting right boundaries for themselves. See Chapter 4 for an elaborate discussion of embodied consent and cultivating the capacity to feel and express one's true "yes" and "no."

Nancy (Shirley as the Therapist)

Nancy was adopted from the Philippines by a white Christian family when she was three years old. She came to work with me on her early attachment wounds when she was 38 and going through a divorce. When I told her that I work with touch, she said that she is terrified of touch and did not want to work in that way. I completely respected her hesitation. We started to unpack what it meant for her to say no to touch work, which led to an important process around consent, power, oppression, and boundaries. Together, we became aware of how nobody had asked her whether she wanted to be adopted, leave her nurturing caregiver at the orphanage in the Philippines (who's loving touch she remembered), and move miles away to live with white Christian parents in America (with whom she had few memories of nurturing touch).

Although I do not identify as a white woman but as a woman of color (Jewish Arabic descent), in Nancy's eyes I not only represented a parental figure who naturally has more power than her but also a white woman who has more cultural and systemic power. This created an inequitable power dynamic that needed to be addressed to create a sense of safety in the relationship. It took us a year of deep exploration (and a lot of my own internal work around power and oppression) until one day Nancy told me she was ready to start touch work. When she initiated the invitation, I asked her how she knew she was ready. She said she felt safe with me. When we moved to the table, I continued to ask for her consent every time I considered shifting positions to ensure she had full control.

Ganesh (Shirley as the Therapist)

Ganesh was a 10-year-old boy of Russian and Indian descent who presented with severe anxiety that prevented him from attending school. His mother asked me to work with him using touch work on the table. I wanted to make sure I got full consent from Ganesh before I applied touch. I took my time to explain exactly what I was going to do and why. I then asked him, "How about when you're ready, I will put my hand under your left shoulder?" In addition, I found creative ways to teach him about the idea of consent, "Let's have a little sign play between us; when you are ready, tell me—green light. When you don't want touch, tell me—red light, and when you are not sure—orange light." He loved our sign play and felt empowered to tell me red, orange, or green. I only engaged touch when it was a full green light.

Professional Touch

The USABP ethical guidelines help us to answer the following question: *How can we shift from a world in which touch in psychotherapy is stigmatized and seen as unprofessional to one where it is perceived as an ethical and effective component of psychotherapy?* To support that shift, the therapist's state of body–mind–emotion and the quality of touch need to be at the center of the discussion of what constitutes professional touch.

We identify four main themes that underlie legitimate professional touch in psychotherapy.

1. The selfhood and internal state of the therapist: therapists need to develop attuned awareness and know themselves well, and know where they are touching from

and what their intention is. Are they touching from their own needs or desires, or are they attuning to the client's needs? Are they touching from their heart or just the palms of their hands? Can their intention rest in being present with the client, or are they striving to make something happen?

2. Boundaries and consent: therapists need to have good, clear boundaries; ask for consent and re-consent every time they touch; and renegotiate boundaries in each moment, always centering the client's needs. They need to communicate clearly about their intention when moving into touch work, when to initiate touch, and when to stop touching. They need to know how to track and respect any clues of the client's body not wanting to be touched.

3. The quality of touch: in our model, therapeutic touch is mindful, present, embodied, and without agenda; it is listening, connected, loving, gentle, slow, light, and steady.[2]

4. Training and education in professional touch: touch is an art to develop—it takes time, space, and practice to master. Therapists offering touch in psychotherapy should have spent significant time both studying and receiving professional touch. Whether or not therapists are going to use therapeutic touch in their practice, touch is part of daily life and often arises in regular talk therapy. All therapists need to be skilled in negotiating situations, in which a client asks to be hugged or held, particularly those working with psychedelic medicines, which frequently evoke a desire for physical contact.

Touch, Regulation, and Healthy Development

In the first few years of life, humans are completely dependent on their caregivers for safety, security, and nourishment. These early relationships are foundational to the child's psychological development and representations of self, other, and self in relation to other. The child's early models of relationship reflect and shape their basic capacities for safety and regulation, distress tolerance, curiosity, sense of agency, and communication (Cook et al., 2005). To understand the neurophysiological foundations of safety, regulation, and connection, we will provide an overview of the autonomic nervous system and polyvagal theory.

As described in Chapter 6, the autonomic nervous system has two branches. The sympathetic branch prepares the body for action, such as exercise, play, and the survival responses of fight or flight. The parasympathetic branch prepares the body for rest, digestion, pause, and the survival response of immobilization. The two systems work together in a reciprocal way to keep the relaxation and activation functions in balance (Kain & Terrell, 2018; Porges, 2011, 2017). According to *polyvagal theory* (Porges, 2011, 2017), the parasympathetic branch mediates the sympathetic branch through the vagus nerve. The vagus nerve is a major cranial nerve in the body that connects the brain stem to essential organs, such as the lung, heart, and digestive system. The function of the vagus nerve is to regulate the heart and therefore the autonomic nervous system. Having a *high tone* vagus nerve means that one has a strong ability to regulate and feel safe.

There are two different ways the vagus nerve regulates the sympathetic nervous system: the dorsal vagus and the ventral vagus. The dorsal vagus branch connects to the organs below the diaphragm through the back of the body and slows down the digestive system to conserve bodily resources. The ventral vagus nerve connects to the organs above the diaphragm, such as esophagus and bronchi of the lungs; mediates the facial muscles and hearing; and supports the activity of social engagement and connectedness.

While the dorsal vagal branch remains unmyelinated throughout life, the ventral vagal is not fully myelinated at birth and becomes myelinated over time. Healthy myelination of a nerve (when the nerve is insulated by a fatty covering) allows it to function quickly and accurately, thereby effectively regulating the sympathetic nervous system. Myelination is influenced by early interactions between a caregiver and an infant, such as touch, eye contact, singing, cooing, and emotional attunement to the infant's non-verbal expressions. Bar-Levav (1998) emphasized that the infant's experience of safety rests in the hands of their caregivers; in his words, "Our sense of safety comes from the softness, firmness, consistency, and steadiness of the mothering body" (p. 53). Through these interactions, caregivers play a crucial role in the development of the ventral vagal nerve and the infant's capacity for autonomic nervous system regulation (Kain & Terrell, 2018; Porges, 2011, 2017).

Regulation is how we manage our emotional and somatic state—that is, how we calm ourselves amid internal or external stress (Kain & Terrell, 2018; Porges, 2011; Schore & Schore, 2007). Co-regulation is "the mutual regulation of physiological states between individuals" (Porges, 2017, p. 9); it is the means by which the caregiver becomes a source of soothing when the infant is stressed (Kain & Terrell, 2018; Schore & Schore, 2007). To regulate the infant's activated nervous system and emotional state, the caregiver needs to make intimate contact with the infant coming from a regulated state within themselves. From this regulated place, they offer soothing behaviors, such as stroking, holding, gazing, singing, skin-to-skin contact, and emotional attunement to the infant's non-verbal expressions (Field, 1998; Kain & Terrell, 2018). Co-regulation involves an interactive exchange that is mutually beneficial for both infant and caregiver (Changaris, 2019; Kain & Terrell, 2018).

According to Schore and Schore (2007), the emotional bond between a caregiver and an infant is the primary medium for co-regulation. In his research, Alan Schore posited that the co-regulation process is an interaction between the right brains of the infant and the caregiver. The right hemisphere of the brain is where non-verbal and social communication, emotional processing and expression (especially facial expression), and implicit learning take place, "as opposed to the more explicit and more conscious processing tied to the left hemisphere" (Happened et al., 2004, p. 7; Schore, 2003; Schore & Schore, 2007). Touch, as a right-brain non-verbal communication, is an effective way to facilitate co-regulation and to convey the message "you are safe" (Tronick, 1995).

Complex and Developmental Trauma

When children do not experience adequate care, connection, touch, or co-regulation during their early years of life, they will not develop the neurophysiological foundation needed for psychological, physiological, and social well-being. This can lead to developmental trauma disorder. According to Spinazzola et al. (2018), the proposed diagnosis of "developmental trauma disorder" provides an integral framework for understanding "children's emotional, biological, cognitive, behavioral, interpersonal, and self/identity dysregulation in the wake of traumatic victimization and disturbed attachment" (p. 631). The term *complex trauma* was adopted in the trauma field to describe the experience of multiple chronic and prolonged developmentally adverse traumatic events, most often of an interpersonal nature (Cook et al., 2005; Van der Kolk, 2005). These experiences often occur within the child's caregiving system and include physical and emotional neglect and child maltreatment beginning in early childhood. Developmental and complex trauma in childhood result in diminishing capacities for self-regulation and interpersonal relatedness (Cook et al., 2005).

To describe how complex trauma impacts development, it is helpful to first illustrate how the brain develops in non-traumatized children. Children who are not traumatized learn to gradually "shift from the right hemisphere dominance (feeling and sensing) to primary reliance on the left hemisphere (language, abstract reasoning and long-range planning), and to an integration of neural communication across the two brain hemispheres (corpus callosum)" (Cook et al., 2005, p. 393). This brain integration helps the child regulate rather than react to stimuli.

Children with complex childhood trauma often exhibit inadequate integration of the two brain hemispheres and are therefore at risk of failing to develop the capacities necessary to modulate emotions in response to stress. Healthy affect regulation requires integration of left and right hemisphere processes, which supports the capacity to identify internal emotional experiences, differentiate among states of arousal, and interpret and safely express these states. Children and adults with complex childhood trauma show impairment in these skills and are therefore at risk of a compromised capacity to self-regulate and self-soothe. Impairments in one's capacity to self-regulate tend to have a significant impact on their ability to form and maintain stable interpersonal relationships.

The Healing Relationship

Many of our clients experience chronically dysregulated nervous systems without memory or understanding of what happened to them. This suggests the presence of developmental trauma, which may have occurred while they were in a preverbal state. Traditional psychotherapy relies primarily on verbal interventions in the form of reflection, education, explanation, and interpretation. However, when a client's developmental trauma arises, these states often require a form of communication that can be preverbally understood. Those in preverbal states do not have the capacity for higher-level processing. In these instances, communications with the client need to emphasize right hemisphere brain interactions (feeling and sensing); we can do this in a way that mimics the co-regulation offered by the caregiver–infant relationship through touch, cooing, or singing. Like the caregiver–infant relationship, the therapeutic relationship can become a reliable source of co-regulation, particularly when therapeutic interventions are rooted in consistent relational and somatic attunement (Schore, 2003).

Unlike some modalities that view the client's experience as separate, we view the therapist and the client as part of a relational field. The relational field is the space between two people where the conscious and unconscious meet, experienced through intuitive impulses, unbidden images, empathetic resonance, and body sensations. Bonnie Bainbridge Cohen coined the term SelfOther to indicate there is no self without other, and there is no other without self (personal communication, June 4, 2018). Creating a healing relationship involves attention to the relational field between two people. By working with the relational field in the present moment, we coalesce with its wisdom and can utilize its pervasive information to refine our approach and offer closer attunement.

When attuning to the relational field, the therapist is invited to BE before they DO anything. "Being" involves connecting with ourselves first, acknowledging and accepting where we are: the state of our nervous system, emotions, and thoughts. From there, we connect to our clients while opening to the underlying space of stillness and loving presence. Bill Bowen, the founder of *Psycho-Physical Therapy*, discussed the importance of cultivating the therapist's presence such that they can be open and receptive to their clients and receive subtle information. He also encouraged therapists to "surrender to what you think you know and be open and receptive to what is there in the present moment. Let go of expectations and the need to be doing the listening correctly. Just listen" (Bowen, 2010, p. 6). Listening happens not only with the ears but also with the body, heart, hands, and almost any other organ in the body (Bowen, 2010). From this place of stillness and listening, we expand our awareness to the relational field. This space, when recognized, is where healing happens. For a further elaboration of the relational field, see Chapter 5.

Relational Touch

Therapeutic touch is rooted in attunement to the relational field, with the awareness that when we touch we are also being touched—the touch circuit is felt between both client and the practitioner. From our perspective, it is the relationship that heals, and touch is an extension of the relationship. Relational touch is a powerful method of making contact that can be felt through the whole body system—it does not solely depend on an idea of connection.

We would like to suggest that relational touch can play an integral role in meeting clients in preverbal states and in helping them to regain safety, access states of co-regulation, and heal developmental trauma. We recommend the integration of hands-on therapeutic touch with both traditional talk therapy and psychedelic therapy and encourage therapists to learn and apply touch skills in their professional therapeutic work.

In our model, clients are clothed and lie on a massage table. There is a lot that needs to happen before we make physical contact. We start by becoming embodied, a process where we sense into our bodies, breath, heart, level of centeredness and groundedness, and boundaries. Only after sensing into our own energetic and physical body can we attend to the client's energetic, somatic, and emotional state.

Next, we bring our attention to the relational field and listen with our whole body. Ilana Rubenfeld, the founder of Rubenfeld Synergy Method, called her touch "the listening hands" (Rubenfeld & Griggers, 2015, p. 879). When we listen with our hands, we are listening to all the "no's" of the client as well as the "yes's." We are listening for and sensing whether the client is open to receiving. If they are closed—for example, their body is contracted or pulling away—we do not force or push any agenda; instead, we rest with the client in embodied presence. Some have had very little experience of being with another person in this way; simply being together in a state of openness and presence facilitates co-regulation. As we discussed previously, we want to ask explicitly for consent before making physical contact. If consent is given, the therapist places their hand on a part of the client's body that they consider safe, such as the shoulder, back, or knee. Throughout, the therapist facilitates this process without holding to any particular agenda, remaining client-centered and avoiding manipulation or persuasion in any way.

Gill (Shirley as the Therapist)

Gill, a 54-year-old white, cisgender man came to see me as he was transitioning to a new career. As a child, he always felt something was wrong with him. He had learning differences, causing him to feel stupid. He was very sensitive and had a notable capacity to feel things outside of himself, which left him overwhelmed with sensory input and confused about how to make sense of this information.

As Gill positioned his body on my table, I took time to feel into myself and my vibrational tone before I touched him. When I was ready to join him, I asked for permission to touch. When he gave me the green light, I gently put one hand under his right kidney and one hand under his right shoulder. I listened with my hands to his vibrational tone, his nervous system, and his emotional body. Watching his body settle, I noticed the muscles around his eyes start to twitch spontaneously. I slowly removed my hands from his back and asked permission to place them on top of his closed eyes. Once there, I stayed with him, listening, connecting to myself and to him, and fully accepting him. We barely exchanged words in that session. We simply enjoyed the experience of being together as he rested in the hands of a safe person. Only in the subsequent session did we talk about how novel it was for him to feel safe in his body with another person.

Quality of Touch

Bringing awareness to the quality of the touch we offer is an essential element of healing relational wounds through touch therapy. Attachment researcher Mary

Ainsworth (1979) explains that the quality of touch caregivers offer their babies is one of the most important components of developing a secure bond. In her words, it is "*how* the mother holds her baby rather than *how much* she holds him or her that affects the way in which attachment develops" (p. 3, italics in the original). Ainsworth's suggestion implies that the quality of holding communicates to the baby a sense of safety and security, or a lack thereof. Concordantly, to communicate safety through therapeutic touch in psychotherapy, attention should be placed on the quality of the touch.

Tending to the quality of our touch involves mindfulness of our internal state and starts when we invite ourselves to fully be in the room with our clients. The hands are an extension of the relational field we are co-creating and should convey a clear, loving, and present attitude toward the client and anything that arises for them. We touch from our hearts. We touch only in places that feel safe for the client and for us, respecting subtle internal hesitations that may arise. We touch from a completely comfortable place, adjusting our position as needed to ensure we are not straining. We touch to communicate directly to the client's body the message, "I am here with you; you are safe."

Firm but gentle, steady, and embodied touch can undo aloneness, helping to cultivate a deep sense of being held in one's pain, fear, grief, and contraction. It has no agenda; it is simply listening, accepting, welcoming, and present. The sensation of our hands can raise awareness in the client's physical and emotional body, allowing the body's organic healing process to unfold. Touch can be a bridge between cognitive and somatic processes, facilitating an integration between the two. Therapeutic touch is always a relational negotiation ("Is there a place in your body that is asking to be touched? How is it? Do you want me to move my hands there? How is the pressure?").

What Are We Touching?

When we work with touch, we are tracking and receiving the client's full somatic, energetic, emotional, cognitive, and relational expression. When we place our hands on someone's knee, we are not only touching the knee but also the whole person—we are touching their childhood, their inner child, their wounded parts, and their resilient parts; we are touching their somatic armor, their emotional body, their ancestral body, and their soul. When we touch, we hold all of these possibilities and open ourselves to the field to show us what needs to be brought to awareness.

Kat (Shirley as the Therapist)

Kat came to me from afar with her therapist to do a longer, one-time session with touch work. She was a 40-year-old white, cisgender woman, a mother of two, and a childhood sexual abuse survivor. She was determined about her healing and reached out to me to do touch work. I spent considerable time getting to know her and made sure she had given fully informed and embodied consent before she shifted onto the table. Once she had settled on the table, I sat next to her left side and took my time until we both felt ready to initiate touch. Kat gave me permission to touch, and I started with one hand only, placing it gently under her shoulder.

I did not know much about Kat's childhood, except that she was severely sexually abused by multiple people when she was very young. I let her body tell me her story as I stayed in the here and now with her, tracking her body closely and watching it release, shake, and unfold. I kept bringing our awareness to the present moment—my hand under her shoulder, me with her, and her therapist watching out for her. I kept asking her questions, such as, "How is this for you? How do you know this touch is okay? How does your body tell you it's safe now? How is this touch different from the past?" It was a very moving session for all of us; her body kept releasing energy, and I kept bringing her awareness to the present moment. In that session, Kat experienced the quality and the ingredients of safe touch: mindful, intentional, without agenda, and with continuous consent. This was an experience she had not felt before. I was touching the whole person—not only Kat's wounded parts but her resilience and strength as well. At the end of the session, she felt empowered and grateful.

Ketamine-Assisted Touch Therapy

We have found that ketamine-assisted therapy in conjunction with touch work can be a profound means of healing developmental trauma, anxiety, and depression. As ketamine specialist Raquel Bennett (2019) states regarding the impact of ketamine-assisted therapy, "Patients convey that their understanding or resolution of a difficult issue moves from being intellectualized into an embodied way of knowing." Clients will experience resolution intellectually as well as somatically, emotionally, and even spiritually.

Ketamine is a psychedelic medicine legally available for therapeutic application. In our practice, we work in conjunction with a medical professional who prescribes the medicine and monitors the course of treatment through regular check-ins with the therapist and the client. The client takes the medicine sublingually in the presence of the therapist at the beginning of the session, which typically lasts between two to four hours. Here, we will discuss the benefits of ketamine-assisted therapy combined with professional touch to treat developmental trauma.

We will focus on psycholytic ketamine sessions, working with low to medium doses of prescription ketamine. A higher "psychedelic" dose generally induces a full psychedelic journey with the potential for ego dissolution and diminished capacity to communicate or interact with the therapist. A psycholytic dose tends to facilitate an expanded state of consciousness while the client retains control over their thoughts, emotions, and relational dialogue. Psycholytic doses of ketamine allow the client to maintain the conscious awareness necessary to administer professional touch, including negotiation of consent and boundaries.

Phil Wolfson (2016) notes that psycholytic doses of ketamine soften defenses, allowing past traumatic memories and emotions to rise to the surface, thereby accelerating the processing of this traumatic material. The client is able to get under their defensive patterns—such as dissociation, distraction, or armoring—and shift into a more resourced state of consciousness. Psycholytic ketamine therapy can facilitate a state of openness, allowing a person to stretch beyond their usual perspective (Wolfson et al., 2019). This process helps the client become a witness to their experience and helps them move beyond identifying solely with the suffering self; it gives relief to a skewed negative mindset and enables the client to shift into a state of presence. A client who is present, with a witnessing mind, begins to develop an open system. When the client's system is open, they are able to take in relational intimacy, assuming the therapeutic relationship has developed into one of safety and trust over time. With an open system, the client has the capacity to assimilate new relational experiences while processing old trauma. A new, reparative experience that went missing in childhood is the medicine we are seeking for our clients.

Sam (Jacki as the Therapist)

Sam is a 40-year-old cisgender, white woman who had been in therapy on and off for years. She often felt unsafe in the world, unprotected, on her own, and responsible for others' protection, which adversely impacted her intimate relationships. Combining ketamine-assisted therapy with touch, Sam and I were able to address her limiting patterns from a deeper level and offer a new experience. At the start of one particularly powerful medicine session, Sam ingested 150 mg of ketamine sublingually. While she lay on a mat, and with her consent, I placed my hand under her right kidney and watched her body and defenses soften as she grew quieter.

Soon after, early memories of Sam's childhood came through effortlessly. She could feel the emotional, psychological, and sensational experiences of her inner child feeling vulnerable and alone, helpless to care for herself so young. In this altered state of consciousness, it was as if her younger self was expressing this wound through all of her senses, enlivening a whole body understanding. From this place, Sam could reach into the longing that lay underneath her defenses—a longing to feel protected and safe within herself and with another person. In Sam's case, the attention to her kidney enlivened her long-held grief, as she realized she had missed out on an essential childhood need for protection.

With the support of the resourcing effects of ketamine, Sam's relational defenses softened, her thoughts slowed down, and she became aware of and more open to me and my loving presence. I welcomed her grief, and she felt safe enough to express her need for me to place my hand on her lower back, which I did. Because Sam's system was open, she had the capacity to feel the support of my hand through the base of her body; she felt what it was like to be protected. I literally had her back. Sam released tears of gratitude as the new experience registered throughout her whole self. Ketamine helped us to forge an open avenue to Sam's unprocessed psychological and relational material, and find connection, expression, and repair.

Leila (Shirley as the Therapist)

Leila is a 49-year-old Caucasian cisgender woman. She had just lost her beloved 8-year-old son to bone cancer. I had worked with Leila for a couple of years before her son died, and I knew her well. A few weeks after the funeral, as her communal support slowly dropped away, Leila found herself in a deep depression with suicidal ideation. She felt no reason to keep living. Meanwhile, Leila was working with a psychiatrist who monitored her antidepressant medication, and he too watched her reach a dead end. Her psychiatrist, who was familiar with my work, suggested we try ketamine in conjunction with touch. With the psychiatrist's guidance, I started ketamine-assisted therapy with Leila, alternating with regular psychotherapy sessions every other week for almost a year.

In the ketamine sessions, Leila was able to make contact with her grief in a way that she had not been able to before. With the support of the medicine, I was able to hold her in my hands as she grieved and connected to herself. The ketamine allowed her to move out of her head, soften her armoring, and surrender to her experience while she was fully held and supported. By the very first session, we both felt grateful and hopeful that we were on the right track. Throughout the ketamine sessions, she was able to drop more and more deeply into her body and into her present-moment experience while staying connected with me. With the support of ketamine and touch, Leila felt safe enough to go to places she had not been able to go before. She connected with her inner child, who was terrified and confused in the world, as well as her mom who had passed away 20 years ago. She slowly developed acceptance of herself and her experiences. The pain of losing a child will never go away; however, Leila started to regain aliveness and re-engage with life. A year later, she was back in school getting her Master's degree.

Ketamine and Developmental Trauma

In our work with psycholytic ketamine, traumatic memories from the early developmental years of life (0–5) often emerge. During this period, a child does not experience life through words and concepts but rather through sensation, feelings, and somatic expression. Often in ketamine sessions, clients share traumatic memories of being in a crib crying; needing to be held; feeling alone, scared, and helpless; and not feeling loved. When clients are immersed in these memories, we do our best to respond to them as the "good-enough parent" in that moment, emotionally attuning to their non-verbal expressions, co-regulating with their body, holding them with safe touch, and gently cooing or singing to them.

If a client goes into their developmental trauma during a ketamine session and they are not met with these forms of preverbally attuned communication, they may have insight into their early experiences; however, their preverbal self is not likely to deeply integrate the experience of feeling safe, connected, and loved. Understanding would therefore remain intellectual. To heal the early years of developmental trauma, we need to access the client's youngest parts through non-verbal communication. Through this delicate process, our intention is to work with the memories that arise in the moment and provide a new, healing experience that the whole body can register, rebuilding their capacity to regulate and revising painful core beliefs, such as being alone without the support one needs to thrive.

Juan (Jacki as the Therapist)

Juan is a 35-year-old Asian-European cisgender male who sought therapy to build his self-esteem and develop a greater sense of agency in his life. His challenges became more apparent during the time of Covid, heightening his feelings of loneliness and despair. He had been focusing on intimacy and relationships in his ongoing therapy and came to me for adjunctive ketamine-assisted therapy.

During our ketamine-assisted touch session, I checked for consent to place my hand on Juan's kidney to establish a relational connection. Soon after making contact, the "infant Juan" appeared on the table—a vulnerable, dysregulated infant who felt alone and scared. His body went into hypo-arousal, whereby his face and hands started to go numb. I felt his need to be held and co-regulated, and with his permission, I held his head with my hands and watched his body settle as he felt supported, contained, and secure. I responded to the frightened child with touch, soothing sounds, and a calm nervous system in my own body. The non-verbal communication between us demonstrated that he was not alone, trapped, and helpless in his vulnerable state. Because Juan had a history of frequent activation in a state of hypo-arousal, it was a new and healing experience for him to be held in his dysregulation long enough to move into a regulated state. With my presence, he learned how to hold old feelings of terror with a new sense of safety and trust.

Conclusion

Touch in psychotherapy, when applied professionally, can be effective for healing developmental trauma. In this paper, we emphasize that therapists need to have training in professional touch, consider their own internal state before they touch, know why they are touching, and mindfully negotiate consent. We have found that when professional touch is combined with ketamine in the treatment of developmental trauma, the healing process becomes more efficient and effective. Because ketamine can evoke early childhood memories and experiences of trauma, therapists need to be trained in how to safely hold clients in these states and offer a corrective experience in the here and now. Such corrective experiences are facilitated by safe, attuned, and embodied relational touch from the therapist, which can change the attachment circuitry in the client's brain, body, and nervous system. This relational bonding between a therapist and a client allows the client to expand beyond the confined limitations of their childhood trauma, experience more of their life force, and open to relational intimacy.

Notes

1　This paper is written as a collaborative work of the authors and therefore will use the "we" pronoun, except in case presentations when we will specify who is the therapist and use the "I" pronoun.
2　Other models of therapeutic touch, such as Grof's bodywork, can involve more intensive forms of touch, such as applying active resistance or pressure to parts of the body holding tension.

References

Ainsworth, M. S. (1979). Infant-mother attachment. *American Psychologist, 34*(10), 932–937. https://dx.doi.org/10.1037/0003-066X.34.10.932

Bennett, R. (2019). Paradigms of ketamine treatment. *MAPS Bulletin, 29*(1). https://maps.org/news/bulletin/articles/436-maps-bulletin-spring-2019-vol-29,-no-1/7718-paradigms-of-ketamine-treatment-spring-2019

Bowen, B. (2010). *Somatic resourcing: Psychotherapy through the body.* Bill Bowen.

Changaris, M. (2019). Touch and embodiment. In H. Payne, S. Koch, & J. Tantia (Eds.), *The Routledge international handbook of embodied perspectives in psychotherapy: Approaches from dance movement and body psychotherapies* (pp. 379–388). Routledge.

Cook, A., Spinazzola, J., Ford, J., Lanktree, C., Blaustein, M., Cloitre, M., DeRosa, R., Hubbard, R., Kagan, R., Liautaud, J., Mallah, K., Olafson, E., & van der Kolk, B. (2005). Complex trauma in children and adolescents. *Psychiatric Annals, 35*(5), 390–398. https://doi.org/10.3928/00485713-20050501-05

Feldman, R., Singer, M., & Zagoory, O. (2010). Touch attenuates infants' physiological reactivity to stress. *Developmental Science, 13*(2), 271–278. https://doi.org/10.1111/j.1467-7687.2009.00890.x

Field, T. (1998). Touch therapy effects on development. *International Journal of Behavioural Development, 22*(4), 779. https://doi.org/10.1080/016502598384162

Field, T. (2014). *Touch.* Massachusetts Institute of Technology.

Happened, K., Zelazo, P. D., & Stuss, D. T. (2004). Development of orbitofrontal function: Current themes and future directions. *Brain and Cognition, 55*, 1–10.

Jean, A. D., Stack, D. M., & Arnold, S. (2004). Investigating maternal touch and infants's self-regulatory behaviours during a modified face-to-face still-face with touch procedure. *Infant and Child Development, 23*(6), 557–574.

Kain, K., & Terrell, S. (2018). *Nurturing resilience helping clients move forward from developmental trauma, an integrative somatic approach.* North Atlantic Books.

Linden, D. J. (2015). *Touch: The science of hand, heart, and mind.* Penguin Books.

Marcher, L., Jarlnaes, E., & Munster, K. (2015). The somatic of touch. In G. Marlock & H. Weiss (Eds.), *Handbook of somatic psychology* (pp. 494–508). North Atlantic Books.

Milakovich, J. (1998). Differences between therapist who touch and those who do not. In E. Smith, P. Clance, & S. Imes (Eds.), *Touch in psychotherapy: Theory, research, and practice* (pp. 74–91). The Guilford Press.

Montague, A. (1986). *Touching: The human significance of the skin.* Harper. (Original work published in 1971)

Polan, H. J., & Ward, M. J. (1994). Role of the mother's touch in failure to thrive: A preliminary investigation. *Journal of the American Academy of Child & Adolescent Psychiatry, 33*(8), 1098–1105.

Porges, S. W. (2011). *The polyvagal theory: Neurophysiological foundations of emotions, attachemnt, communication and self regulation*. W. W. Norton.

Porges, S. W. (2017). *The pocket guide to the polyvagal theory: The transformative power of feeling safe*. W. W. Norton.

Rubenfeld, I., & Griggers, C. (2015). Somatic emotional release work among hands-on practitioners. In G. Marlock & H. Weiss (Eds.), *Handbook of somatic psychology* (pp. 494–508). North Atlantic Books.

Schore, A. (2003). *Affect regulation & the repair of the self*. W. W. Norton & Company.

Schore, J. R., & Schore, A. N. (2007). Modern attachment theory: The central role of affect regulation in development and treatment. *Clinical Social Work Journal, 36*(1), 9–20. https://10.1007/s10615-007-0111-7

Spinazzola, J., Van der Kolk, B., & Ford, J. D. (2018). When nowhere is safe: Interpersonal trauma and attachment adversity as antecedents of posttraumatic stress disorder and developmental trauma disorder. *Journal of Traumatic Stress, 31*(5), 631–642. https://doi.org/10.1002/jts.22320

Stenzel, C. L., & Rupert, P. A. (2004). Psychologists' use of touch in individual psychotherapy. *Psychotherapy, 41*(3), 332–345. https://dx.doi.org/10.1037/0033-3204.41.3.332

Tronick, E. Z. (1995). Touch in mother-infant interaction. In T. Field (Ed.), *Touch in early development* (pp. 53–65). Routledge.

USABP. (2018). *The science of connection, honoring our somatic intelligence*. https://usabp.org/USABP-Conference-2018

Van der Kolk, B. A. (2005). Developmental trauma disorder. *Psychiatric Annals, 35*(5), 401. https://doi.org/10.3928/00485713-20050501-06

Wolfson, M. D. (2016). *Ketamine assisted psycotherapy (KAP), Sublingual and IM: A potential model for informed consent*. The Ketamine Papers: Science, Therapy and Transformation, MAPS.

Wolfson, P., Dore, J., Turnipseed, B., Dwyer, S., Turnipseed, A., Andries, J., Ascani, G., Monnette, C., Huidekoper, A., & Strauss, N. (2019). Ketamine assisted psychotherapy (KAP): Patient demographics, clinical data and outcomes in three large practices administering ketamine with psychotherapy. *Journal of Psychoactive Drugs, 51*(2), 189–198. www.tandfonline.com/doi/full/10.1080/02791072.2019.1587556

Chapter 8

Coming Home

Psychedelics, Symbolic Images, and
the Innate Intelligence of the Psyche

Jason A. Butler and Evan Sola

The Dreaming Psyche (JB[1])

My father was a Vietnam veteran who suffered from untreated post-traumatic
stress disorder (PTSD). Like many vets, he coped with his pain through the insa-
tiable use of alcohol. He died of cirrhosis one week before I turned 16 years old.
As an angry adolescent, I lacked the emotional resources to grieve my father's
death. Unconscious defenses took hold, building an impenetrable wall around the
chaotic confusion of my emotional world. Although these walls allowed me to
go on living, they also alienated me from myself and from intimate connection
with others.

Four years after my father's death, I took a college course at Humboldt State
University, in which I was asked to keep a dream journal. I began writing down my
dreams each morning so that I could share them in the dream group we had formed.
One sunny day, sitting out on the grassy lawn outside the classroom, I shared the
first dream I had written in my journal. As I read the words aloud to my dream
group, I began to see my inner world shaped into distinct, meaningful, and emotionally revelatory images. In just a few paragraphs of text, the dream disclosed so
much—my longing to be fathered, as imaged by my professor teaching me to fish;
the sudden eruption of my repressed rage, as imaged by a brutal fight with an old
high school friend; and the penetrating sting of my emotional pain, as imaged by
a swarm of bees forcefully stinging my hand, ensuring that the stinger went deep
into my finger. The emotional truth disclosed by the dream woke me up out of a
long period of dissociation and brought me into a relationship with the deep healing
intelligence of the imaginal world.

Like dreams, psychedelics amplify the psyche's innate healing intelligence, ushering in abundant visions, images, memories, and sensory experiences that weave
together our inner and outer worlds into meaningful expressions—reflective pools
for consciousness to witness itself. The dreamlike experiences generated by psychedelics illuminate a range of imaginal expressions, from the majestic and sublime
to the terror-filled images and sensory experience of the traumatized psyche. This
chapter aims to light a path that can help us to move through painful constrictions
and splintered fragmentations, evoked by generations of compounded trauma. We

DOI: 10.4324/9781003167976-8

hope this elucidation will demonstrate the great potential that psychedelic medicines paired with a solid therapeutic relationship hold in facilitating reconnection with the innate intelligence of the dreaming psyche.

Creative Possibilities: A Ketamine-Assisted Therapy

We must follow nature as a guide.

Then what we do is less a question of treatment, but one of developing the creative possibilities latent in the patient.

—Carl Jung (1931/1966a, p. 41)

Michael was a 40-year-old queer, white, cisgender man who worked as a video and sound artist and teacher. He contacted me after the tragic death of a close friend. In our first conversation, he described how this loss added an unbearable layer of grief to the weight of losses he had experienced in recent years. Our work together soon brought forward his long-standing struggle with periods of depression characterized by low motivation, a sharp and punitive inner voice, and a deep-seated fear of sharing his creative work with the world. After meeting weekly in psychotherapy for about two years and developing a strong therapeutic alliance, we decided to introduce ketamine into our work to help soften the strong grip of depression that had constricted his vibrant and creative spirit and inhibited his ability to step fully into his work as an artist.

In preparation for our first medicine session, Michael and I worked with the persecutory internal voice that exerted a dominating force on his inner world. Michael described his pattern of protecting himself from this inner oppression by escaping from the reality of his life (through smoking cannabis and endless scrolling through social media). Naming this pattern of withdrawal from the world evoked Michael's deep-seated fear that he would not fulfill the creative potential he knows he has. As a sense of dread saturated the session, I slowed our pace and asked if these feelings had an associated image. Michael paused for a moment and let his imagination speak. *The image, he said, was a sealed-up tree, all the leaves folding inward toward itself, trapping the birds within the tree, muting their song, killing the life inside.*

Two weeks later, as Michael and I settled into the commencement of our first ketamine session together, we reflected back on the image of the sealed-up tree and his desire to share his creative expression freely. With the tree in mind, he expressed the intention for the medicine session, "I don't need to turn away from people. It's time to face the world again. I want to create a life that is more engaged. I want to be part of the world of people, not run away."

After taking 250 mg of ketamine sublingually, Michael maintained an inward focus for the first two hours of the session. Near the end of his ketamine experience, he began to speak. With the slow pace of someone crafting words out of the ineffable, he described an experience of becoming "a field of grass in the bright sun, blown by the wind, releasing seed into the wind." He added,

> I feel my ripeness, as though I was an egg that cracked. I'm ready to scatter and disseminate, propagate, let things go. I feel like the germ—small, and bent, the introverted part of the wheat seed, a coiled potency of structures folded inwards, waiting for a chance to open. The sun's heat makes me open. My palms are golden with sun. It opens me, unfolds me. I just want to pass along something good, like a warm cup of tea to you. That's a seed.

Michael and I were both deeply moved by the potency of his experience. His generous gesture of passing the warm cup of tea to me was felt and appreciated. We sat together in the openness he had unveiled and appreciated the depth of this psyche's response to his desire: to address his primary struggles and live a more fully engaged life.

The ketamine session opened into an imaginal world, a waking dream, that recontextualized the sealed-up tree and his internal police. The new images of grass, sun, and "releasing seed into the wind" stood in stark counterpoint to—yet in obvious dialogue with—the sealed-up tree. Through the ketamine journey, Michael's psyche evoked an imaginal landscape that cast a new light on the oppressive limits of his constricted self. In our integration sessions, we explored both sets of images—the way the images felt in his body, as well as the emotional and relational expressions of each image. He brought two sides of himself into close contact, facilitating a strong movement toward a symbolic marriage between his wounded shadow side and the psychospiritual potentials of his creative self. From an alchemical perspective, Michael was moving toward a *coincidentia oppositorum* or unity of opposites. His active participation in the psychedelic vision and the integration process facilitated a union with his unconscious process, joining the conscious to the unconscious. "The result," Jung (1928/1953) noted, "is ascension in the flame, transmutation in the alchemical heat, the genesis of the 'subtle spirit.' That is the transcendent function born of the union of the opposites" (p. 223).

In his journey, Michael experienced an alternative sense of self—a more expansive identity that was introduced into awareness by the amplification of his dreaming mind evoked by the ketamine. The ketamine dream extrapolated from and extended the earlier imagistic metaphor of "his tree self," standing as a powerful rebuttal to the imagery of being suffocatingly contracted. Michael's symbolic-self shifted from a singular static tree to a nearly edgeless expanse of wind-stirred grass that was now effortlessly taking in vital life force from the sun and in turn purposefully giving his own life force to the wind and spaces beyond. He experienced himself as an inherently integral component of the larger natural world.

The stark counterpoints of the two sets of symbolic images are provocative and useful: from airless suffocation to the wind itself (the free-flowing breath of the larger natural world) and from a contraction that smothers life to an exalted expansion that freely gives life by sending its fertile seed essence naturally, effortlessly into a welcoming receptive world.

Imaginal Expressions of the Psyche's Inner Healing Intelligence[2]

Like dreams, psychedelic medicines energize and amplify imaginal content and generate significant amounts of emotional material (Carhart-Harris, 2007, p. 198). This catalyzed content gives symbolic form to otherwise formless sensations, emotions, memories, ideas, intuitions, and latent potentials. When met with curiosity and thoughtful engagement, these imaginal forms can provide a foundation for powerful psychospiritual transformation. Like the dormant energy released by a coiled spring, the images of dreams and psychedelic experience launch forth, bringing rapid expansions of perspective; like a meaningful poem, the dreaming psyche "awakens our senses, frees us from the tyranny of literal meaning and assures us of the credible reality of emotional truth" (Smith, 2018, para. 2), and like a great work of art, the emotional truth generated by the psyche is most poignant when it casts a light on the dark constrictions of defensive recoil born from psychic pain.

From the perspective of depth psychotherapy, the psyche's capacity to construct complex self-protective reactions and routines is borne from our innate psychological intelligence, activated by traumatic experience. However, under the influence of untreated trauma, our psyche's shrewd defenses can prove themselves to be debilitating when it comes to long-term adaptability. Traumatic wounding constricts the imagination with the strangling grip of ruminations, repetitive reenactments, and flashbacks. Like an autoimmune disorder, the wounded psyche turns on itself by "over-performing" its basic healthy function of self-protective attentiveness. Consequently, the ability to creatively dream—to imagine and embody the diverse complexities and expressions of psychic reality—is eclipsed by single-minded narratives with a single-minded purpose: defensive self-protection.

Opportunities for psychological healing present themselves through the psyche's capacity to dream. Our use of the word "dream" is not limited to the dreams one has when asleep. Throughout this chapter, we extend the word "dreaming" to encompass the psyche's innate ability to generate symbolic and metaphorically rich images and emotionally meaningful sensate experience. These images and sensations present a rich plurality of emotions, identities, subjectivities, and archetypal themes for the self to consider. The dreaming psyche is the wellspring of each person's inner healing intelligence. Just like the intelligence of the body's immune system or of our physical organs, such as the liver—the psyche can be understood as animated by an innate "knowing" far outside of our conscious awareness or control. The liver "knows" what vital elements need to be stored, traded, or filtered out to optimize its own performance and maintain the health of the body—all without our conscious awareness or participation. The imaginal content of the dreaming psyche can be considered parallel to this intelligence, supporting a person's self-regulation of their psychological, physical, social, and spiritual domains and facilitating emotional healing and movement forward into more expansive and encompassing self-realization.

In his essay *Psychological Factors Determining Human Behavior*, Jung (1936/1970a) put forth a notion of five basic instinctual drives: hunger, sexuality, the drive to activity, reflection, and what he called "the creative instinct" (p. 118), variously described throughout his writing as "the urge to wholeness, toward individuation, or personality development, the spiritual drive, the symbol-making transcendent function, the natural religious function, and the drive of the self to be realized" (Hillman, 1972, p. 34). In his commentary on this essay, Hillman emphasized that "the urge to self-realization works with the compulsiveness of an instinct. We are driven to be ourselves" (p. 34).

Imaginal expressions transmitted from the dreaming psyche to the conscious mind function as a primary facilitator of this drive, providing guiding lights, as well as initiatory impulses to progress on a path of conscious evolution and healing. Depth psychotherapy considers the imaginal activity of the psyche as a wellspring of diverse and divergent reflections of our soul life. A useful analogy for how these images reflect our inner conscious and unconscious emotional landscapes is a hand mirror that may be used to observe and to be in relational "conversation" with ourselves about our outer physical appearance. In parallel to the hand mirror analogy, our imaginal reflections strongly influence our "idea" of ourselves—continually reshaping our identity—with long-standing narratives as well as with fleetingly mercurial meaning making.

When inhibited or constricted by entrenched habits or trauma defenses, the imaginal expressions of the dreaming psyche reinforce the default narratives that we live by. Yet, with curious open-minded inquiry, perhaps paradoxically, the very same symbolic reflections can serve as inspiration for a creative process that can expand our perceptions and our meaning making beyond our limited default perspectives. In other words, imaginal phenomena can both reinforce the distorted views of psychological complexes, like when one falls prey to unconscious rumination, thought loops, and projections, and the very same images, when approached consciously, can become pathways to liberating insight. Imaginal experience is both the prison door and the key, the guard at the door and the prisoner begging to be set free. Because psychedelic medicines have unparalleled abilities to activate and potentiate the dreaming psyche—as well as widen and deepen our ordinary interpretative mindsets—these compounds arguably embody unprecedented potentials to catalyze and amplify the transformational nature of the therapeutic processes.

Therapeutic Mechanisms of Action in Psychedelic-Assisted Therapy (JB and ES)

A reemergence of research on psychedelic therapy over the past 20 years has identified benefits from psychedelic compounds for healing a variety of psychological disorders. The research has shown that psychedelics, in the context of psychotherapy, can reduce and even eliminate the most recalcitrant symptoms in participants with treatment-resistant PTSD (Mithoefer et al., 2011; Mithoefer et al., 2013; Ot'alora et al., 2018), as well as depression and anxiety associated with life-threatening illness (Wolfson et al., 2020). Over the last few decades, a general statement on a mechanism of action for psychedelic therapy has been articulated and is gaining in complexity as more research is conducted. This theory of healing action centers around the notion that psychedelic medicines amplify awareness of meaningful emotional content through the temporary lowering of psychological defenses. This effect was noted early in the psychedelic literature. Aldous Huxley (1959) offered a description of the way psychedelic compounds temporarily lift a "reducing valve" that ordinarily restricts one's access to consciousness, enhancing aesthetic value and momentarily allowing us to strengthen our ability to perceive beauty.

Building on Huxley's observation, Carhart-Harris (2010) has investigated the quieting effect psychedelic medicines have on the DMN, a network of interacting brain regions that are thought to be the neurological basis for the Freudian concept of secondary process, or ego. The DMN is most active during periods of self-reflection, rumination, worry, and mental time travel (thinking about the past or the future). The function of the DMN is similar to Huxley's model of mind as "valving off" or reducing access to expanded states of consciousness to adapt to the demands of daily life and the principle of consensual reality. It has been noted that in various states of consciousness, including meditation, rapid eye movement sleep (dreaming), acute psychotic states, temporal lobe epilepsy, and under the effects of psychedelics (Carhart-Harris & Friston, 2010), this protective "default" function is temporarily diminished. Neurobiologically, psychedelics initiate an "entropic" process in relation to typical brain functioning, a disruption of the otherwise highly organized activity of the brain (Carhart-Harris et al., 2014, p. 1). During psychedelic experiences, the order and organization of typical waking consciousness—or secondary process—orchestrated by the DMN, are supplanted by less habituated brain activity and "a greater repertoire of connectivity motifs" (p. 1). Following Freud's model of mind, Carhartt-Harris postulates that psychedelics diminish the brain's secondary process functionality (ego) and amplify primary process (id), a mode of cognition characterized by a free exchange of neuronal energy and an "animistic style of thinking" (p. 1). Whereas the amplification of primary process evoked by psychedelics would serve most of us poorly at a city crosswalk, an over-reliance on the DMN (i.e., an inflexible ego) can lead to problems with rigid control, especially with regard to the allowance of emotional processing in grief, trauma, and intimate relationships.

Carhart-Harris et al. (2014) conceive of a fundamentally entropic brain process, in which a higher order of functioning is established through a routine loss of order, such as that found in nightly dreaming or psychedelic experience. They have corroborated the theory through brain imaging of participants administered psychedelics. Simply stated, healing action may take place via chaos as a means of restoring or creating more complex order by breaking up or overriding calcified neural networks and limited connections. This allows for enhanced "crosstalk" between otherwise disconnected or less communicative brain centers and neural networks (Petri et al., 2014). The phenomenological experience can be rife with "disorder," confusional suffering, and transitional states, including synesthesia, while also containing tremendous growth potential. This research points to psychedelics as powerful agents of psychic disintegration that expand beyond the constrictions of the adult waking mind, increasing access to a diversity of self-states and more fluid imaginal experiencing. Neurological and phenomenal entropy evoked by psychedelic medicine is thought to improve and even expedite the therapeutic process, often leading therapist and client into the depths of shared and lost meaning, with all the concerns and benefits of deepening intimacy.

The implications of these neurological findings are in alignment with a number of depth psychological theories, where one finds multiple models that articulate the relationship between healing order and chaos. These models may be useful for the psychedelic therapist. While we eventually turn to the work of Carl Jung, Winnicott's simple beauty in holding enigma may be a helpful starting place. In his classic work focusing on the psyche–soma, Winnicott (1954) speaks of the *chaos* involved in having a new thought (a healing thought), which he likens to *changing one's mind* (state), involving the ability to think previously unthought ideas, as well as the simultaneous ability to open awareness to experiences situated in the unknown territory of the *soma*. Here lies the deeper wisdom of the body, beyond the strict confines of the mentally situated egoic self, perhaps again accessed through an "open valve," into larger, dimensionless states of consciousness. Winnicott notes that this mode of experiencing, more aligned with the body, also comes with a threshold of chaos, often presenting as psychosomatic pain and confusion. According to Winnicott, this bodily distress, especially headaches, among other discomforts, suggests that the mind is in conflict with the body, struggling to allow the pace, intensity, and natural processes of the oceanic soma. In terms of direct clinical phenomenology in moments of heightened experiencing, healing waves are often confused with cruel drowning. Winnicott describes the agony and terror that are sometimes involved in healing (Winnicott, 1974), giving clinical and historical examples of humanity's confused sense of needing to literally "crack open the head" to heal, reminiscent of Stone Age medicine.

Parallel examples are evident in the way medication and modern technology are used to numb or silence the painfully confused mind in the face of overwhelming chaos. It is as if our mistrust in the unruly aspects of the healing process has us in search of a doctor, who since antiquity has found ways to remove the chaos. We are gripped by the idea that something concrete should be taken from the brain, or more generally that the chaotic and painful aspects of the process should be stopped. Psychiatric medicine has traditionally colluded with this process-thwarting stance, as seen in antidepressant action focused on 5-HT1A serotonin receptors (i.e., Paxil or Zoloft), which often blunt or shut down unwanted symptoms to help one cope with distressing affect. This approach is distinct from the psychedelic process, where neurological action is focused on 5-HT2A receptors known to flood individuals with symptoms, opening the possibility of working with the experience of oceanic entropy in the service of healing (Carhart-Harris, 2017). Winnicott

(1954) describes the experience of childbirth as a parallel example of a painful process, which should by no means be thwarted but rather engaged through trust in bodily wisdom.

The notion of an inner healing intelligence is now common in the field of psychedelic therapy (Grof, 2000; Mithoefer et al., 2018), often introduced to encourage clients to hold unwanted or "negative" aspects of experience with curiosity and non-foreclosure. This approach embraces the assumption that all of the contents that surface in the session are "coming up for healing," including and often especially the harrowing elements of one's emotional process. As with the natural movement of relieving waste from the body or the birthing of a new human body into the world, an attitude of permission and trust facilitates movement through turbulent and uncharted waters during aversive psychedelic experiences. This is perhaps one method through which the client comes to think a new thought, one which comes less from the protective mental constriction of previously *known* thoughts, and more so from the unfolding *unknown*, primordial intelligence of the psyche–soma.

The therapist's overly eager attempts to help, seeking seamless or overly certain and simplified ways of bringing the client into the "good" life full of healing or positivity, may inadvertently condemn deeper and more recalcitrant psychic content to the underworld. The technical notion of negative capability (Bion, 1970), or the capacity to withstand states of not knowing such that the therapist does not push their own tightly certain meaning or agenda, is perhaps all the more necessary in psychedelic therapy. Moments of regression to earlier life-dependency feelings, such as the infant's total dependence on the parent for care and orientation to the environment, may emerge through immediate preverbal needs for provisions (i.e., food, physical closeness, rest, safety, comfort, etc.) (Winnicott, 1974). Meanwhile, cycling into more precocious, defended, or otherwise healthy adult reflectivity may intermittently or simultaneously take the stage in a matter of minutes, leading to levels of confusion in the therapist, as they adapt to the multi-perspectival lens provided by the psychedelic encounter. For this reason, the MAPS protocol, arguably the most comprehensive articulation of psychedelic therapy technique, has upheld the clinical use of "non-direction" or "inner-direction," as well as "beginner's mind" to facilitate healing action (Mithoefer et al., 2018). Rather than a simply passive stance, curiosity and interest lead the way, alongside trust that a gesture will come from beyond any prescribed location, and that this movement is often present in the content of the client's immediately unfolding experience. The need for both therapist and participant to repeatedly surrender pre-established notions of what will help is especially true when working with clients suffering from refractory symptoms, disorganized attachment histories, and developmental trauma, where feeling lost and disoriented is a central component of the relational experience.

In his paper *Images of Initiation*, Joe Henderson (1993) highlights the ancient and symbolically rich image of the spiral, designating the shaky ground an initiate must stand on before a new order can be established. As Henderson expresses regarding artistic renderings of the spiral, labyrinth, or *wave*-like images, which have been perennially represented since Stone Age cultures:

> They seek to erase any consciously acquired stereotypes of order and show the initiate how to lose his or her way symbolically to arrive at an inner center where something new, strange, and primordial may engage his or her interest in order to bring back, along its own winding way, some basic truth about psychic life. However, this truth may not be easily acquired.
>
> (p. 47)

This sense of lostness, or loss of emotional control and mental clarity, often teeming with waves of raw experience, can be understood as distinct from the homeostatic dissociation of usual PTSD symptoms and can perhaps represent a generative form of suffering en route to healing action. This implies that the pain of protection is of a different nature than the pain of healing, although they are often confused and exist side by side—one perhaps a closed loop and the other a spiral that takes on the dimension of depth and directionality. As noted by Masud Khan (1974), "What is most difficult to resolve and cure is the patient's practice of self-cure" (p. 97). Instead of a self-cure leading to a closed loop of armoring against novel experience, authentic suffering may lead the way toward initiatory movement into a healthier, more alive relationship to self and others. However, this "truth not easily acquired" first requires the crossing of a transitional or threshold period, often one of suffering, before reaching the "new" yet "primordial" lesser-known territory rich with "psychic truth," in Henderson's terms.

From Jung's alchemical perspective, the initiation into a piece of soul work is described as the alchemical phase of *nigredo*, or blackness. This soul work is a *beginning* process leading to a deepening relationship with the self through a descent into the blackness of the unconscious, a confrontation with the emotional experience of psychological decay and death (Marlan, 2005). As the *Rosarium Philosophorum* speaks of this alchemical embarkment, "When you see your matter going black, rejoice, for this is the beginning of the work" (McLean, 1980, p. 9). By moving into and through the blackness and the accompanying loss of the known order, a tension of opposites becomes available to be felt and expressed as overwhelmingly painful conflict, confusion, and contradiction before it can be tolerated and experienced as paradox. Blackness is not eliminated; however, it is no longer the singular reality/identity, as was demonstrated in the preceding case example in which the client, Michael, was able to move through the nigredo of repressed grief and transform his depression by holding the paradoxical tension between the sealed-off tree and the expansive gesture of "releasing seed into the wind." This suggests that the suffering of overwhelming psychological content may be a necessary rite of passage, in Henderson's view, implying that conflict and chaos are valuable grounds for losing one's way, catalyzing access to deeper hard-won truths and authentic self-discovery.

Archetypal Meaning in the Psychedelic Experience (JB)

Psychedelic medicines are vehicles of NOSC that can usher in boundless imaginal phenomena, often with sudden exposure to the numinous. The generative power of these medicines calls for the development of a therapeutic approach that makes more room for, and better use of, the flood of imaginal content that can surface in the therapeutic process.

The field of depth psychotherapy provides a strong theoretical and practical foundation upon which we build an imaginal model intended to assist both client and therapist in navigating the profound activation of the dreaming psyche evoked by psychedelic medicines—the abundant flow of archetypal images; inchoate sensations; numinous encounters; and entropic experiences of lostness, mystery, and disintegration. In this section, we will discuss relevant therapeutic approaches that can support the delicate process of orienting to and making meaning from nonordinary states in psychotherapy.

Amplification is a term Jung used to describe a method for working therapeutically with symbolic material by drawing out connections between the client's imaginal material and archetypal, transpersonal, and culturally historical themes and images. Jung (1937/1968) argued that the patterns present in collective symbolic systems, like world mythology, alchemy, astrology, tarot, and spiritual traditions, are powerful mirrors for the deep structures of human experience. Amplification involves drawing out associative links between one's lived experience and these symbolic systems—*amplifying* the significance of lived experience by connecting it with a related myth, story, theory, etc., from a wisdom tradition or symbolic system. Amplification connects the particular and personal with the larger cultural and transpersonal context, as Jung wrote, "not as my sorrow, but as the sorrow of the world; not a personal isolating pain, but a pain without bitterness that unites all humanity. The healing effect of this needs no proof" (Jung, 1931/1969, p. 150).

Transpersonal and archetypal phenomena, such as symbolic visions and encounters with entities, are a commonly occurring part of the phenomenology of psychedelic experiences. When the structures of the ego dissolve, as is common in psychedelic experiences, the mythic dimension of the psyche becomes more visible. In the expansive states engendered by psychedelics, our sense of self, "the house we live in," suddenly becomes much bigger, perhaps not recognizable or familiar, and far more permeable the collective unconscious, ushering in expanded potential to experience meaningful encounters with archetypal energies, cultural complexes, aspects of the personal and collective shadow, enactments of intergenerational trauma, as well as expressions of the *anima mundi* (soul of the world) and *anima loci* (soul of the place). It is as if the expanded state makes space that is filled with inner depths and outer mysteries. The following diagram provides a visual representation of the personal and collective psychic structures as conceptualized from a psychodynamic and archetypal perspective.

In the context of psychedelic therapy, a mythic/archetypal sensibility helps the therapist and client orient to the broader context and grand field of meaning

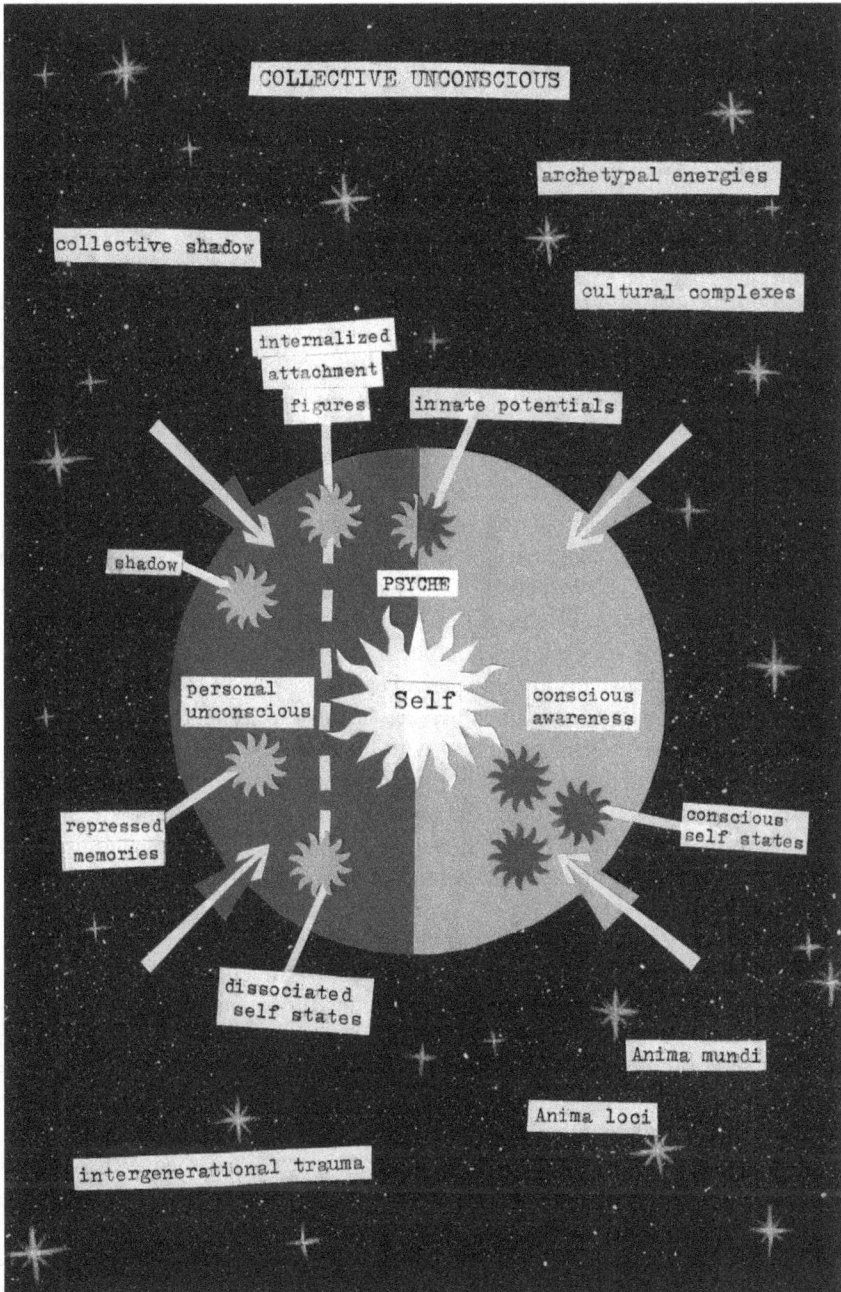

Figure 8.1 Diagram of the personal and collective psyche

Source: (illustrated by Inaê Cintra Mattiazzi)

expressed within psychedelic experiences. For example, one client experienced a strongly painful feeling of emptiness during a medicine session. He described it as a "black lake—a deep body of dark water, not sure where it stopped or if it even had limits." His terror grew as he experienced the limitless quality. He expressed that he was unsure if he could "handle the feeling," but he also felt "desperate to understand it." From an archetypal perspective, the black color, the references to depth, limitlessness, desperation, overwhelming intensity, and the terror evoked by the image were all indicators that this client had moved into the first stage in the process of alchemical transformation: nigredo or blackness. As stated previously, Jung (1956/1970c) underscored the significance of the nigredo, noting "the *magnum opus* begins at this point" (p. 318). Nigredo is marked by chaos, disorganization, deconstruction, and negation, as well as the fecundity of decay. "By deconstructing presence into absence, the nigredo makes possible psychological change" (Hillman, 1997, p. 8).

As I sat with the client in this painful state, my recognition of this archetypal pattern allowed me to orient to his state and empathically imagine into his experience. As I shifted to a more open and receptive state, I was able to gently encourage his curiosity about the experience, inviting him to notice what the empty feeling was like in his body. This helped to shift his attention away from his growing identification with the feeling. He began tracking the feeling of emptiness in his gut. The sensation slowly evolved into numbness, tingling, and an image of dark blue energy radiating through his lower torso and pelvic area. Tears rolled down his face as he shared memories of childhood neglect and shame around his sexuality. Following the color symbolism associated with the stages of alchemical transformation, the client moved through the empty blackness of nigredo into "the blue mood which sponsors reverie" (Hillman, 1981, p. 39). Like a bruise rising to the surface, with the shift from black to blue, "Shadow . . . is not washed away and gone but is built into the psyche's body and becomes transparent enough for anyone to see" (Hillman, 1981, p. 34).

Although archetypal amplifications can be a powerful method for discovering deeper layers of psychospiritual significance, many clinicians who are interested in working symbolically move too quickly into interpretations or abstract formulations of the client's material, resulting in an overly intellectualized conversation or misattunement to what is meaningful to the client. Like any interpretive intervention, amplifications, as in the preceding example, need to be relevant to the emotional context of the moment. Archetypal references, if explicitly shared at all, are best woven into the conversation with a light touch, attunement to the client's interest, cultural humility, and offered as one possible source of meaning within the collaborative play space created by client and therapist.

In practice, before amplifying an image, it is important to meet the imaginal experience on its own terms to stick closely to the image itself while also listening for the way it speaks through metaphor and analogy through word play, pun, double meanings, and reiteration of its presenting context. To this point, Jung (1916/1970b) wrote, "The unconscious contents want first of all to be seen clearly, which can only be done by giving them shape, and to be judged only when everything they have to say is tangibly present" (p. 86). Returning to the image again and again with curiosity and attention to aesthetics, the therapist helps create space for a close read of the imaginal experience, through which the image can disclose its "unfathomable analogical richness" (Hillman, 1977, p. 82). The aesthetic elaboration of the image leads toward further understanding within the context of the client's life. Jung (1916/1970b) noted,

> By shaping it, one goes on dreaming the dream in greater detail in the waking state, and the initially incomprehensible, isolated event is integrated into the sphere of the total personality, even though it remains at first unconscious to the subject.
>
> (p. 87)

In psychedelic therapy, this phenomenological approach of sticking to the image is part of an underlying ethic which aims to preserve the integrity of the psychedelic experience, setting aside and deconstructing preconceptions and listening carefully to what the client's psyche is communicating. When practiced with care, this approach helps safeguard against overly reductive, abstract, or misattuned meaning making.

Working With Images

The range of imaginal experiences generated in psychedelic therapy extends beyond the visual pictures that appear to the mind's eye, as experienced in visions, dreams, and fantasies. Rather, any spontaneously generated content or process becomes an image when it is approached through imagination. An image can be expressed as a bodily sensation, a figure or object in a dream or fantasy, a psychedelic vision, a relational enactment, a spontaneously recalled memory, a significant interpersonal event, a synchronicity, or a symptom. The imaginal perspective generates curious engagement with the psychological significance of these phenomena as seeds for reflection and meaning making.

With an imaginal perspective, one can begin to learn about the image by investigating the qualitative nuances, the specific context, mood, and scene of the image (Hillman, 1977). As these features are elaborated, the descriptions are often revelatory in and of themselves and provide generative seeds for further reflection. Because images speak their significance through the qualitative details of their form, with more precise description comes more insight. In other words, meaning is found through precise portrayal of pattern, the weave and texture of the image, or as Hillman (1979) noted, "the careful aesthetic elaboration of a psychic event is its meaning" (p. 135).

Patricia Berry's insightful writing on dreams is equally relevant to understanding psychedelic experiences. She points out that restating descriptions of the image, with attention to the metaphorical nuance, can help echo or reflect the imaginal experience beyond its literal statement (Berry, 1982). She noted,

> Without restatement we tend to get caught in the dream at its face value and draw easy conclusions from it, never truly entering into the psyche or dream.

When we are completely stumped with a dream, there might be nothing better to do than to replay it, let it sound again, listening until it breaks through into a new key.

(p. 72)

She described two approaches to restatement, "First, by replacing the actual word with synonyms and equivalents. . . . Second, by simply restating the same words but emphasizing the metaphorical quality within the words themselves" (p. 71). The second approach is an engagement with the image through word play, where the multiple meanings of words are illuminated through giving voice to the undertones, double entendre, puns, and idioms that emerge through restatement.

Restatement and word play increase the volume of the image, allowing it to speak more loudly, with expanded possibility for psychic patterns and insights to emerge. As the patterning is elaborated and connections between the image and the client's life take form, the psychedelic experience takes on a greater sense of value, "that all-encompassing sense of importance which we tend to call archetypal" (Hillman, 1977, p. 75). For example, one client experienced an image in which he was painting his face with white makeup. He said, "As *I began applying the white makeup, I was surprised by how quickly it began covering over the features of my face.*" With a few simple restatements of key words in this description, we moved into a cascade of emotional associations: his frequent experiences of shame about who he is, the way he "whites out" his emotional expression to guard himself, and his "white face" as a reflection of his social conditioning as a white man—his unearned power and privilege in a culture that is structured by white supremacy. He noted that when this white face is painted on, it covers over his ancestry as a Jewish person, obscuring his process of "facing" his family history and the cultural trauma his lineage has carried for generations.

Complimenting this personal and cultural reading of the image, an archetypal perspective provides further expansions in the field of associations and an additional source of guidance for his process of transformation. In sticking close to the image, we recognized that the whitening covered over the marks of character on his face—the wrinkled lines of laughter around his eyes and the worry on his brow. This connection led him to insightful reflections about his relationship to both the innocence of childhood (his unconsciousness and naivete) and the more mature innocence that comes from not identifying with experience; times when he has found release "from the nigredo of personal identity into the mirrors of impersonal reflections" (Hillman, 1980, p. 25); the way he can step out of the way, shift into lunar consciousness, reflecting light from beyond himself. As Hillman has noted (1980), lunar consciousness "implies others; it is no sovereign solar king producing its all-important, self-sufficient light out of itself. It reflects light from beyond itself. Devotion to the moon extends to what the moon reflects—a variety of other powers" (p. 48). This archetypal perspective helped lead the client beyond the painful constrictions of shame and the cultural pathology of whiteness toward a generative image of his lunar face—the way he can face the world like the moon faces the sun, reflecting light from beyond himself, devotion to a variety of other powers beyond the self.

In psychedelic therapy, it is important to model curiosity in engaging with the client's internal world, holding empathic receptivity and a symbolic attitude—the capacity to "see in surface phenomena the meaning of deeper realities" (Anzaldúa, 1987, p. 38), including the social realities that both client and therapist are participating in. Preparation sessions are an important time for developing a cooperative relationship with the client's unconscious—encouraging curiosity about the client's present-moment experience and discussing the deeper realities that unfold through close tracking of their experience. These sessions may include basic instructions in mindfulness to support the client in tracking their inner experience from the position of an observing self, describing their moment-to-moment bodily experience to the therapist like a narrator in a novel, with close emotional engagement and thoughtful consideration of the salient details. Once the client is mindfully connected to sensation in their body, the therapist can help the client access their embodied imagination, taking note of any images, colors, moods, memories, or places associated with the sensation, bringing out the imaginal and emotional dimensions of their somatic experience.

Collaborative Meaning Making

In a Johns Hopkins study of mystical-type experiences occasioned by psilocybin, "67% of volunteers rated the psilocybin-occasioned experience as being among the five most personally meaningful and among the five most spiritually significant experiences of their lives" (Griffiths et al., 2006, p. 628). The expansive states evoked by psychedelic medicines place psychedelic therapists in a position of supporting the client in creating the opportune conditions to not only receive these highly significant experiences but to also integrate them into their lives in therapeutically useful ways. This section provides considerations for engaging with, understanding, and integrating psychedelic experiences by creating a collaborative, culturally sensitive, emotionally attuned, imaginative play space for meaning making.

Winnicott (1971) described playing as essential to effective psychotherapy. He noted, "It is in playing and only in playing that the individual child or adult is able to be creative and to use the whole personality, and it is only in being creative that the individual discovers the self" (pp. 72–73). For Winnicott, discovery of the self was predicated on the potential space[3] of creative playing, in which the self and the meaning attributed to the moment are undefined and creatively discovered, not through the interpretive explanations of the therapist but through the client's process of trying out "new solutions and experiences" (Lenormand, 2018, p. 85). In fact, Winnicott (1971) noted that his use of interpretation was "mainly to let the patient know the limits of [his] understanding" (p. 116). In other words, when the therapist shares associations or interpretations as one voice within the creative play of meaning making, the client has an opportunity to build on those limits, like scaffolding, in developing their own creative formulation. Winnicott added, if the client is not able to engage in spontaneous, non-compliant play, then the work of the therapist should be directed toward helping the client find their way "into a state of being able to play" (p. 51). He added that "resistance arises out of interpretation given outside the area of the overlap of the patient's and the analyst's playing together. Interpretation when the patient has no capacity to play is simply not useful, or causes confusion" (p. 68).

Explorative interventions, like collaborative meaning making, need to be built on a foundation of emotional safety to mitigate ruptures in the therapeutic relationship, such as intrusion, projection, coercion, indoctrination, microaggression, and other enactments of harmful power dynamics. Throughout the collaborative meaning-making process, the therapist should remain attuned to the client's response, including whether they are consenting to a deeper exploration of their experience. Lack of consent is demonstrated with both verbal and non-verbal expressions. The client's sense of safety can be tracked in numerous ways but perhaps most directly in the here-and-now verbal and non-verbal emotional expressions of the client. Explorative interventions, like interpretation, should be offered with humility and sensitivity to impact. Given the profoundly sensitive states client's enter into in psychedelic therapy, it is important for therapists to couple explorative interventions with consistent tracking of the client's somatic expressions of nervous system arousal. Interpretive interventions can contribute to overwhelm and cause harm when a client is outside their "window of tolerance"[4] (Siegel, 2012).

Psychoanalyst Antonino Ferro articulated a helpful distinction between two types of interpretive styles: saturated and unsaturated. Unsaturated interpretations are open and tentative, and therefore tend to be more accessible for the client in that they leave space to move and breathe, and for the client to freely associate and make their own contribution to the meaning of the moment (Ferro & Civitarese, 2015). Saturated interpretations are interpretive comments that are already saturated with particular meaning constructed by the therapist. Unsaturated interpretations, on the other hand, tend to be more suggestive and respectful, giving space for the client to develop the meaning-making process as an active partner. It is important for the therapist to maintain caution around stepping into a position of "holding truth" in an authoritative way, and situate oneself as more of a "helmsman" who helps the client "read the nautical charts and make [their] own active contribution" (Ferro, 2009, p. 174).

Interpretations are more impactful and transformative when they speak to the emotional tone of the moment. A good interpretation makes a meaningful link between thinking, feeling, and somatic experience, guiding reflections closer toward emotional truth and deeper engagement with the client's here-and-now process. The effectiveness of an interpretation can be assessed by observing the impact. Does the comment constrict or open access to the client's present-moment experience? Is the client moved to elaborate further on the topic, introduce a new character into the dialogue, deepen into an emotional experience, express a creative and surprising association, and recall a repressed memory? In times of profound emotional anguish, when an interpretation lands for a client, they may simply soften into an expression of relief and repose, as in when a client takes a deep breath—signifying that the tension of an emotional conflict is moving toward resolution.

MDMA-Assisted Therapy and the Intelligence of the Psyche (ES)

This section draws directly from Dr. Evan Sola's (2017) research on the qualitative themes that emerged as combat veterans engaged in MDMA-assisted therapy for PTSD. The themes described as follows provide a differentiated understanding of the psychological effects of MDMA when taken in the context of MDMA-assisted therapy. These themes include:

- Expanded awareness of the protective–persecutory parts of the psyche and a diminishment of their controlling dominance
- A sense of safety and expanded capacity to process complex emotions and traumatic memory
- Spontaneous occurrence of symbolic images and somatic metaphors related to the trauma
- Expanded curiosity, meaning making, and interest in life

Together, these themes were significant factors in the participants' process of recovering from the harrowing effect of combat trauma and restoring their relationship to the innate intelligence of the psyche.

MDMA-assisted psychotherapy enhances the therapeutic container, alliance with therapists, and sense of safety, thereby expanding the ability to tolerate and hence engage and process difficult affects and self-states related to PTSD. Guided by the innate healing intelligence of the participant's psyche in MDMA-assisted psychotherapy, the healing process moves through a series of stages, often in a non-linear and overlapping fashion. The process frequently begins with the protector parts of the psyche surfacing; following this is a conflicted initiatory stage marked by tension, conflict, and overwhelm; once this threshold is passed through, the participant experiences a stage of release and surrender, leading to enhanced curiosity and meaning making and sense of connection with self and others.

Expanded Awareness of Protectors

With the support of MDMA and the close therapeutic holding of Michael and Annie Mithoefer, lead therapists in the MAPS study of MDMA for PTSD, the participants in this study were able to significantly expand their awareness of the protective parts of their psyche and make use of the observing self to witness and reflect on these parts without being taken over by them. Several veterans described the way they have been ensconced in once-safe now-confining defensive strategies, lacking contact with the external environment, especially deep interpersonal relationships. They described themselves as feeling divided or disconnected both internally and externally from aspects of their own vulnerability, creative growth, and healing process. For example, one study participant, an Army combat engineer who served in Iraq, noted, "After we came back, many of us were only back in body. Our souls stayed over there." This participant's experience of alienation, of soul vacancy, stems from his need to rely on dissociation and splitting to ward off aspects of self in service of establishing long-term preservation. He was able to shut down the overwhelming intensity of trauma reactions as a means to survive; however, this shutting down came at a high cost. Mike, a Marine who served in two tours in Iraq, poignantly described the alienation of this inner division:

> I honestly used to always think that I never came home from the desert. I always felt like I was lost over there. That I never really came home. . . . I took that person, and I caged him up, and threw him away.

During MDMA sessions, participants frequently encountered spontaneous images of protector and persecutory figures: warriors, guardians, jail keepers, jail cells, and figures imprisoned within. Vulnerable aspects of the self, often described as the "child," are central targets for the protector–persecutor defenses, as they represent an amplified threat of psychic annihilation due to their permeable and unprotected nature, and must therefore become locked up, hidden, or "sucked up," as Mike articulates:

> And thinking about it now, after firefights, and watching friends die, and every-thing, I would go duck behind the hootch, which is what they call this building, and I would go smoke a cigarette. It's like thinking about it now, that little aspect of me that was a kid was scared, and crying. And I would just be mean to it, and tell him to suck it up.

The refractory nature of this protector–persecutor system cannot be underestimated for its ability to keep the peace, maintain stasis, and in many cases create an isolation that contradicts its original purpose of protection. The distinct appearance and intensification of the protector parts in MDMA sessions are a common theme, especially as the client attempts to move from isolation into connective relationship with self and others. With care and patience, participants are able to move through the waves of protection and the painful deadening of these defenses, accessing meaningful connections with lost parts of self, especially the vulnerable child parts and the accompanying sense of being fully and courageously alive.

Safe Enough to Feel Unsafe

Often, participants' reflections and stories have not been shared before and have up to that point been lived as unspoken discomforts, dissociated from conscious thought, unsafe to bring into conversation. With the support of MDMA, previously unspoken stories may feel safe enough to share and often bring a sense of direct experience, or reexperiencing of the trauma through the more expanded perspective of the observing self. Participants frequently relive visual and somatic memories and affect states taking the form of waking dreams that facilitate an active engagement with visualized emotions, as opposed to mere abstract cognitive reflection.

In the following transcript, Aiden shares a trauma narrative for the first time with his co-therapy team, Michael and Annie Mithoefer:

Aiden: Sometimes people died, and it could've been prevented. But, you know, it wasn't. Right before we came home, the people that were doing our relief in place, they lost like six guys in two weeks, and it was just doing stupid stuff. Like, so we were rolling down to [a city] one night, and it was a mixed convoy; it was us and them. And they had been running drills all day long during the heat, and then of course, we would never leave until about midnight. The driver of the Humvee in front of mine fell asleep at the wheel. And the Humvee veered off down this path because we were on an alternate supply route, so it had, like, a 40-foot shoulder. And it started tumbling. And I could see the machine gunner in the turret. I mean, tumbling with it, it damn near broke them in half. And three of the people in the vehicle died. One of them didn't. But I remember having told their lieutenant that day, "You know sir, you're gonna want to take the afternoon off and let them get some shut-eye, because it's a long drive. That's what we do. Because we would run some drills and then we'll take the afternoon and the evening off." And he more or less told me he didn't need a lance corporal's opinion. And then I got in trouble. I thought, "Well what the fuck would I know, I've only been here for like eight-and-a-half months."

Annie: He didn't follow your advice.

Aiden: No. And it's not like I was the only one, several of us. . . . Yeah. I guess when you get into your head that you can do anything, when you can't it's really hard.

Michael: Especially when people are dying needlessly.

Aiden: Yup. That Humvee just rolled and rolled and rolled. That boy was flopping around like a fish in the turret. Already dead. That's the first time I've ever talked about that.

Michael: Glad you could talk about it.

Aiden: Me too. It feels good to talk about it. It was just a really defining moment in my young life.

During this process of sharing stories, spontaneous visions or inner imagery arise simultaneously with metaphorical meaning, often signaling an embodied sense of reliving events from the past. While Aiden's style often appears cool and cognitive, it could be said that in this sequence he reexperiences this untold story in a way that is not too close nor distant. He successfully holds a complex of anger and disdain for superior officers who negate his perspective while simultaneously expressing tenderness and regret for the lifeless "boy" in the turret. Although the feelings are rife with meaning that would ordinarily be confounding for him, he is able to experience and express relief by telling the story in all its emotional layering. Aiden's immersion in a highly significant experience is considered important for the healing process due to its ability to encapsulate and express difficult emotions through the narrative arc of a story. Through the participants' engaged interest with vivid imagery and the simultaneous disidentification with the affectively charged content, dissociated experiences and deeply felt conflicts can be expressed at a distance comfortable to the participant and recontextualized through the more expansive perspective offered within the MDMA-assisted therapy, as Mike so vividly experiences in his MDMA session:

> Now, when I got blown up myself . . . I don't know. I see it completely different now, thinking about it. That moment that I got blown up, and it was happening, and everything was moving so slow. And my mind was just racing at the speed of light. I can really go back and visualize it. I've never been able to visualize it so hard before. The way you feel. There was this calmness about it all. And I was watching it happen. I knew I was in my body.

The significance of *reexperiencing* phenomena in psychotherapy was noted in the early literature in Freud's discussion of *nachtraglichkeit*, or "deferred action," in which history is reactivated and rewritten based on an experience of containment in the present moment of the session (Freud, 1933/1964; Bollas, 2012; Ferro, 2013). Deferred action in the present context means that the processing of traumatic material is deferred until a future time in which conditions are safe enough to reestablish connection with split-off aspects of self in an attempt to heal the psyche. The results of the MAPS MDMA studies thus far have shown great promise (Mitchell et al., 2021; Ot'alora et al., 2018), suggesting that daylong MDMA-assisted therapy sessions provide the conditions for deferred processing to take place, signaling to the psyche that *a safe environment has been found in which to feel (remember) unsafe feelings*.

In MDMA-assisted therapy, the raw experience of trauma or breakdown can be "caught," so to speak, by the care of the therapeutic relationship in daylong sessions, which invite ego defenses to surrender and regression to dependence. From a safe and supportive environment, the breakdown can be reexperienced as a breakthrough of transformative learning experience regarding core existential dilemmas surrounding the experience of trauma (Bollas, 2012). The breakdown itself represents not only the psyche's attempt to repeat, remember, and work through perplexing scenarios of loss and disillusionment (Freud, 1914/1958) but also to revision these experiences in the context of a sound and caring relationship, in this case facilitated by the bonding action of MDMA. Thus, an enhanced reimagining of traumatic material is established in the therapeutic situation, as difficult content is not removed but experienced fully amid an addendum of support and care, which allows prolonged experiencing of the trauma from a new perspective, as opposed to the obliteration of the self via judgment, numbness, and splitting.

Expanded Capacity to Tolerate Difficult Emotional Experience

Several participants in this MDMA study demonstrated reduced reactivity to discomfort and an expanded capacity to engage with aversive thoughts, memories, and emotions—a kind of "calm within the storm," as previously dissociated emotional conflicts emerged into conscious awareness. The waves of tension evoked by the conflict frequently gave way to release and relaxation, accompanied by clarity of mind and a general sense of well-being. Participants were then able to give voice to their traumatic experience in narrative form, often using images and metaphoric language to describe experiences that were previously unspeakable.

Early in one participant's session with the Mithoefers, a young man named Chris began experiencing intense and overwhelming feelings of anxiety and paranoia as the MDMA began to take effect:

Chris: I feel really messed up, like I'm hallucinating right now.
Michael: You mean like you're actually seeing things that aren't there?
Chris: I just feel out of it. I feel, like, a fear.
Michael: You feel like a fear. . . Yeah.
Chris: It's like . . . I feel like something's, like, taking over me right now. That's what I keep fighting in my head. I keep telling myself you don't like this because you're not in control. It feels like I am having an inner battle with myself.
Annie: Maybe that's part of what it's showing you, that it's still there all the time.
Chris: I'm just feeling like I want this to end right now.
Michael: Yeah.
Chris: I don't like how I feel.
Michael: Can you say what it's about?
Chris: I feel like I'm losing my damn mind.
Michael: Yeah. Are there images and thoughts coming up?
Chris: I'm just going back and forth. I just feel really, really anxious right now.
Michael: Back and forth between relaxed and anxious?
Chris: Yeah.

As the MDMA takes effect, the layers of numbed protection and rigid control over emotional experience often drop away, giving rise to an eruption of intense emotional content. With the assistance of the MDMA and the gentle guidance of the therapists, a painful conflict can begin to be felt and tolerated, giving way to a sense of containment and higher-order relief. As the waves of emotional intensity build, Michael and Annie help Chris stay engaged with the experience by guiding him toward a position of curiosity and aesthetic perception. Annie wonders if the experience is showing him something, relating to the wave of emotion as revelatory. Michael invites Chris to direct his attention to the imaginal dimension of his experience, asking if he notices any images accompanying the fear of losing his mind. These interventions help Chris to hold the tension of his "inner battle," the back and forth between his impulse to shut the experience down and his intention to work through the trauma, which feels like losing control.

Although Chris experienced the cycles of profound anxiety and relaxation as intolerable early in the session, they continued to occur at a growing frequency and proximity to each other, until they were eventually felt as a tolerable tension, with wavelike movements between two opposing states:

Chris: I just feel really relaxed. I'm going back and forth between anxiety and relaxed. I feel really relaxed. I felt really, really anxious. Now, I feel the exact opposite.

Michael: Really? So it comes back and forth really quickly?

Chris: I felt like I was really scared, and now I feel so relaxed. This is the . . . I haven't felt like this in forever. It was the exact opposite just a minute ago, like I was regretting that I took [the MDMA]. I don't have control of my mind. Well, like I just feel relaxed. I'm so used to . . . I haven't felt like this in a long time.

Later in his session, Chris describes the overall trajectory of his experience pendulating between anxiety and relaxation, saying, "It definitely went like waves. So it went like anxiety, relax, and the amount of anxiety would equal how relaxed I got. And then after I passed that point it was just more relaxation than anything."

Waves of intense emotional experience and imagery are a major component of MDMA therapy session, so much so that they are noted in the MAPS treatment manual (Mithoefer et al., 2018), where it is recommended that therapists introduce the concept of "waves of emotion" to participants, using the metaphor to anticipate, trust, and create context for big emotions, which may bring tension and discomfort but may shift into relaxation and blissful feelings or deep work with trauma-related affect.

In successfully moving through the emotional waves of anxiety and relaxation without shutting down, Chris was able to build his tolerance for navigating emotional complexity. This increased capacity to hold previously intolerable tensions corresponds with an ability for thinking thoughts previously unthinkable—links and narratives may spontaneously take shape as the dreaming psyche is activated. However, the processes of MDMA-assisted therapy are best understood as nonlinear, simultaneous, and cyclical (spiral-like), as defenses and waves of discomfort will often rear back up before giving way again to a deeper sense of organization, relief, and meaning making (Sola, 2017). In this manner, a healing transition occurs in which the injury or breakdown is returned to (Winnicott, 1974), not as a means of delivering further cuts, as the confusion of traumatic perceptions may suggest, but as a breaking-back-into and through the defensive structure, beyond willful solutions merely co-opted by the defensive structures.

This transition calls for a necessary balance between relational safety and risk (Bromberg, 2003), with a requisite of surrender to the raw emotional truth that is dynamically unfolding (Ghent, 1990). Surrender in this sense could not be further from giving up, but rather it implies a giving in, or giving over the gift of the richly heartened tender feelings and reparative pleas. Surrender involves laying down willful constrictions and posturing against the inevitability of suffering, a step in the direction of building faith in the unknown emergent process of one's healing. With surrender, one might come to trust the conflict, which mitigates the feedback loop of generating conflict about the conflict. Rather than fighting or fleeing the conflict, a place of allowance, compassion, and curiosity must be found as a viewpoint, if initially only existing in the therapist.

Daylong sessions offer significant opportunities for the therapeutic dyad (or triad) to learn from and work through the emotional unfolding in real time. In these transformational sessions, the "known order" of protection is lost (Henderson, 1993), and a new order of learning and meaning making is initiated from deep within the psyche–soma temporarily freed of mental posturing (Winnicott, 1954). It is notable that daylong sessions often last eight or more hours and provide a significant shift in therapy paradigm from the 50-minute session. In one MDMA study, 25% of the placebo group no longer met the criteria for PTSD after the study, although no psychedelic was administered (Mithoefer, 2011). This finding implies that a substantial amount of consecutive time in a healing environment can itself have a significant impact on clients. From a Jungian perspective, the *indefinite* quality of time afforded by a daylong session extends a clear invitation to the deeper contents of the psyche. The feeling-shape of a 50-minute session may be more so one of a closed loop, too tight to open fully, before having to shut it all down again just as the client starts to ease open. The timeless quality of a daylong session may allow participants to forget the feeling of closure, drifting more toward a Sunday afternoon feeling, or as one client said, "nothing to do, nowhere to go."

Spontaneous Occurrence of Symbolic Images and Somatic Metaphors

As noted throughout this chapter, Jungian depth psychotherapy frequently makes use of imagery for eliciting and facilitating the therapeutic processing of strong emotion (Jung, 1934/1966b), a clinical technique that has been supported by cognitive neuroscience, suggesting the organizing function of dream and mental imagery (Fosshage, 1997). Spontaneous use of imagery can be considered highly important for displaying rich and layered meaning. In MDMA-assisted therapy, participants are encouraged to allow the imaginal experience to develop while staying close to direct embodied experience. In Marshall's narrative, sudden imagery tells a rich story:

Annie: What are you noticing?
Marshall: So I was breathing into that, and trying to process it. And then I was having images of mutilation, and destruction of flesh.
Annie: Mm-hmm.

Marshall: Then for the last five minutes, all I can think about is . . . sounds nerdy, the 3D structure of an atom.
Annie: Of a what? Atom?
Marshall: Yeah, an atom, plus the coenzyme. I just keep imagining it folded on itself now, so I could probably use a push in the right direction to . . .
Michael: The images of things that you saw in the war?
Marshall: No, they were real abstract. It was like not really people as much as it would be just a template of flesh being destroyed, punctured, blown away.

In this passage, after the surface flesh of the human body is "blown away," a deep and essential structure reveals itself. The image carries connotations of destruction but also deconstruction and a means of building something new out of the basic building block of life, the atom. Marshall's abstract representation of a destructive force holds intense emotion, reflecting fear and loss but also the hope of what may happen if he can trust a process of renewal, or reformation.

Soon after this moment, Marshall encountered his ambivalence about rebuilding his connections to people. He notes, "I think it's like a fear I have, to touch people," and "it's like I have this feeling that I'm going to hurt you." This was followed by an experience of paralysis in his arms, a distinct psychosomatic reaction "loaded" with the symbolic implications of "laying down his arms," as in the cessation of fighting, in this case signifying his desire to protect the therapists from his own destructive impulses.

Rich images, such as those experienced by Marshall, hold an immense amount of preverbal emotion and symbolic material, and over the course of daylong sessions this material can be brought into a verbal expression where healing narratives are developed. It should be reemphasized that priority cannot be firmly placed on a linear movement toward verbal narrative or more integrated states, as continual shifts back into waves of chaos and tension—and encounters with defenses and protector figures—remain integral to the healing experience in which words are temporarily unhelpful and sensory experience must first be reencountered (Balint, 1979).

Expanded Curiosity, Meaning Making, and Interest in Life

Part of the process of recovery from trauma is about fully feeling lost and the loss of foreclosed certainties this signifies. Feeling "lost" puts one in touch with the parts self that have been lost since the time of the trauma. Restoring interest in life, especially in one's emotional experience, was a prominent theme in the MDMA-assisted therapy for PTSD research (Sola, 2017). The general trend followed here is a movement that involves confrontation with intense sensory and affective experience toward a release into a more spacious mental quality. From this mental space, participants frequently experienced either a peaceful repose from mental activity or access to a set of powerful associations, linkages, or memories with new meanings. Participants gained greater access to helpful forms of abstract thinking, imagination, reflection, mentalization (Fonagy, 1997), reverie, and meaning. In restoring this capacity, participants were able to engage their inner experience with curiosity resulting in powerful emotional insights and perspective taking with regard to helpful and unhelpful relational patterns.

In the following transcript, Aiden describes his process of losing interest, curiosity, and capacity to think intelligently due to PTSD, as well as his reclamation of these attributes in response to MDMA-assisted therapy:

> I've always intuitively understood things. And I have this really, really intense curiosity, I just wanna know everything. And it was, it was just kinda gone. I wasn't curious. . . . I was just sort of fading into . . . I don't even know how to describe it. I mean, it felt like nothingness. It really did. But yeah lately, I mean, I've been reading a lot. Math has gotten easy again.

Later in an MDMA session, Aiden is able to safely relate and make meaning about the role he plays in his family, which was recreated in the military and consisted of controlling the situation as much as possible and trusting only himself.

Increased ability to think and reflect on personal dilemmas may be a product of MDMA's known increase in prefrontal cortex activity (Gamma et al., 2000), as well as the release of prosocial facilitators oxytocin and prolactin (Bedi et al., 2010; Johansen & Krebs, 2009). The increased sense of safety brought on by these human-bonding hormones is a significant boon for creating the conditions in which the intensely charged unformulated emotional energy associated with trauma can be translated into imaginal elements that can be used for reflection and recontextualization of the traumatic experience. In this sense, bringing non-verbal, unconscious emotional processes into the realm of language and thought is itself a healing action in terms of self-integration.

"Like the Telescope for Astronomy"

After many years of facilitating LSD psychotherapy, Stanislov Grof (1980) confidently noted that "psychedelics, used responsibly and with proper caution, would be for psychiatry what the microscope is to the study of biology and medicine or the telescope for astronomy" (p. 299). With the inclusion of psychedelic medicines, psychotherapists gain access to tools that have the potential to exponentially enhance our knowledge and capacity to assist clients in their processes of psychic healing and transformation. Psychedelic medicines taken in the context of an emotionally attuned and culturally sensitive therapeutic relationship offer a profound support to the psyche's innate creative drive to heal and to unfold into more expansive expressions of self-realization. With the gradual recession of the psychedelic prohibition era, psychotherapy is poised to undergo the most significant expansion of scope and efficacy since its inception.

Psychedelic therapy expands the paradigm of standard psychotherapy by ushering in an exponentially amplified volume and intensity of imaginal content. The approach outlined throughout this chapter is intended to provide a framework for respectfully receiving and responding to the eruption of richly symbolic imaginal material and inchoate sensory experience that are generated in psychedelic therapy. This model situates the therapist as a co-navigator, following the direction of the client's inner healing intelligence and collaboratively engaging with the creative procession of imaginal experiences that flow like a river through the psychedelic journey. With sensitive holding and containment, the dreamlike nature of psychedelic experience can help repair the severed connections between body, heart, mind, and the deep imagination, helping those who have been shattered and alienated by the ravages of trauma to restore their connection to the inner healing intelligence of the dreaming psyche—*to find their way home.*

Notes

1   Throughout the text, we indicate the name of the author with their initials. Sections written by Jason A. Butler are marked with the initials (JB), and sections written by Evan Sola are marked with the initials (ES).
2   The "inner healing intelligence" is a central concept used in the Multidisciplinary Association for Psychedelics Studies (MAPS) MDMA-assisted therapy for PTSD treatment protocol. The MAPS model defines this concept as "a person's innate capacity to heal the wounds of trauma" (Mithoefer et al., 2018, p. 7).
3   Potential space is a term Winnicott used to conceptualize "the intermediate area between psychic reality and 'actual' or external reality" (Inman, 2013, para. 1).
4   In describing this concept, Siegel (2012) noted, "Each of us has a "window of tolerance" in which various intensities of emotional arousal can be processed without disrupting the functioning of the system. . . . *One's thinking or behavior can become disrupted if arousal moves beyond the boundaries of the window of tolerance"* (p. 281).

References

Anzaldúa, G. (1987). *Borderlands/la frontera: The new mestiza.* Spinsters/Aunt Lute.
Balint, M. (1979). *The basic fault: Therapeutic aspects of regression.* Tavistock.
Bedi, G., Hyman, D., & de Wit, H. (2010). Is ecstasy an "empathogen"? Effects of ±3,4-methylenedioxymethamphetamine on prosocial feelings and identification of emotional states in others. *Biological Psychiatry, 68*(12), 1134–1140.
Berry, P. (1982). *Echo's subtle body: Contributions to an archetypal psychology.* Spring.
Bion, W. R. (1970). *Attention and interpretation: A scientific approach to insight in psychoanalysis and groups.* Tavistock.
Bollas, C. (2012). *Catch them before they fall: The psychoanalysis of breakdown.* Routledge.
Bromberg, P. (2003). Something wicked this way comes: Trauma, dissociation, and conflict: The space where psychoanalysis, cognitive science, and neuroscience overlap. *Psychoanalytic Psychology, 20*(3), 558–574.
Carhart-Harris, R. (2007). Waves of the unconscious. The neurophysiology of dreamlike phenomena and its implications for the psychodynamic model of the mind. *Neuropsychoanalysis, 9*(2), 183–211. https://doi.org/10.1080/15294145.2007.10773557

Carhart-Harris, R., & Friston, K. (2010). The default-mode, ego-functions and free-energy: A neurobiological account of Freudian ideas. *Brain, 133*(4), 1265–1283. doi: 10.1093/brain/awq010

Carhart-Harris, R., Leech, R., Hellyer, P., Shanahan, M., Feilding, A., Tagliazucchi, E., Chialvo, D., & Nutt, D. (2014). The entropic brain: A theory of conscious states informed by neuroimaging research with psychedelic drugs. *Frontiers in Human Neuroscience, 8*(20), 1–22. https://doi.org/10.3389/fnhum.2014.00020

Carhart-Harris, R. L., & Nutt, D. J. (2017). Serotonin and brain function: A tale of two receptors. *Journal of Psychopharmacology, 9*(31), 1091–1120. https://doi.org/10.1177/0269881117725915

Ferro, A. (2009). *Mind works: Technique and creativity in psychoanalysis.* Routledge.

Ferro, A. (2013). *Seeds of illness, seeds of recovery: The genesis of suffering and the role of psychoanalysis.* Routledge.

Ferro, A., & Civitarese, G. (2015). *The analytic field and its transformations.* Karnac.

Fonagy, P. (1997). Attachment and reflective function: Their role in self-organization. *Development and Psychopathology, 9*(4), 679–700.

Fosshage, J. L. (1997). The organizing function of dream mentation. *Contemporary Psychoanalysis, 33*(3), 429–458.

Freud, S. (1958). Remembering, repeating, and through: Further recommendations on the technique of psychoanalysis II. In J. Strachey (Trans. & Ed.), *The standard edition of the complete psychological works of Sigmund Freud, Volume 12 (1911–1913): The Case of Schreber, Papers on Technique and other works* (pp. 145–156). Hogarth Press & The Institute of Psycho-Analysis. (Original work published 1914).

Freud, S. (1964). New introductory lectures on psychoanalysis. In J. Strachey (Trans. & Ed.), *The standard edition of the complete psychological works of Sigmund Freud, Volume 22 (1932–1936): New introductory lectures on psycho-analysis and other works* (pp. 1–182). Hogarth Press & The Institute of Psycho-Analysis. (Original work published 1933).

Gamma, A., Buck, A., Berthold, T., Liechti, M. E., & Vollenweider, F. X. (2000). 3,4-Methylenedioxymethamphetamine (MDMA) modulates cortical and limbic brain activity as measured by [H(2)(15)O]-PET in healthy humans. *Neuropsychopharmacology, 23*(4), 388–395.

Ghent, E. (1990). Masochism, submission, surrender: Masochism as a perversion of surrender. *Contemporary Psychoanalysis, 26*(1), 108–136.

Griffiths, R. R., Richards, W. A., McCann, U., & Jesse, R. (2006). Psilocybin can occasion mystical-type experiences having substantial and sustained personal meaning and spiritual significance. *Psychopharmacology, 187*(3), 268–292. https://doi.org/10.1007/s00213-006-0457-5

Grof, S. (1980). *LSD psychotherapy.* Hunter House.

Grof, S. (2000). *Psychology of the future.* State University of New York Press.

Henderson, J. (1993). Images of initiation. *Journal of Sandplay Therapy, 3*(1), 45–55.

Hillman, J. (1972). *The myth of analysis.* Northwestern University Press.

Hillman, J. (1977). An inquiry into image. *Spring, 44*, 62–88.

Hillman, J. (1979). Image-sense. *Spring, 46*, 130–143.

Hillman, J. (1980). Silver and the white earth. *Spring, 47*, 21–48.

Hillman, J. (1981). Alchemical blue and the unio mentalis. *Sulfur: A Literary Tri-quarterly of the Whole Art I*, 33–50.

Hillman, J. (1997). The seduction of black. *Spring, 61*, 1–15.

Huxley, A. (1959). *The doors of perception and heaven and hell.* Penguin Books.

Inman, L. D. (2013, October 28). Potential space: Psychoanalysis and creativity in the Winnicottian spirit. *Unlocking Creativity Through Psychoanalysis*. https://ldf. org/1999-potential-space-psychoanalysis-and-creativity-in-the-winnicottian-spirit/

Johansen, P. Ø., & Krebs, T. S. (2009). How could MDMA (ecstasy) help anxiety disorders? A neurobiological rationale. *Journal of Psychopharmacology*, *23*(4), 389–391.

Jung, C. G. (1953). The technique of differentiation between the ego and the figures of the unconscious. In H. Read, M. Fordham, G. Adler, & W. McGuire (Eds.), *The collected works of C. G. Jung* (R. F. C. Hull, Trans.) (2nd ed., Vol. 7, pp. 123–244). Princeton University Press. (Original work published 1928)

Jung, C. G. (1966a). The aims of psychotherapy. In G. Adler & R. F. C. Hull (Trans. & Eds.), *The collected works of C. G. Jung, Volume 16: The practice of psychotherapy* (2nd ed., pp. 36–52). Princeton University Press. (Original work published 1931)

Jung, C. G. (1966b). The practical use of dream analysis. In G. Adler & R. F. C. Hull (Trans. & Eds.), *The collected works of C. G. Jung, Volume 16: The practice of psychotherapy* (2nd ed., pp. 139–162). Princeton University Press. (Original work published 1934)

Jung, C. G. (1968). Individual dream symbolism in relation to alchemy. In H. Read, M. Fordham, G. Adler, & W. McGuire (Eds.), *The collected works of C. G. Jung* (R. F. C. Hull, Trans.) (2nd ed., Vol. 12, pp. 102–223). Princeton University Press. (Original work published 1937)

Jung, C. G. (1969). The structure of the psyche. In H. Read, M. Fordham, G. Adler, & W. McGuire (Eds.), *The collected works of C. G. Jung* (R. F. C. Hull, Trans.) (Vol. 8). Princeton University Press. (Original work published 1931)

Jung, C. G. (1970a). Psychological factors determining human behavior. In H. Read, M. Fordham, G. Adler, & W. McGuire (Eds.), *The collected works of C. G. Jung* (R. F. C. Hull, Trans.) (2nd ed., Vol. 8, pp. 114–128). Princeton University Press. (Original work published 1936)

Jung, C. G. (1970b). The transcendent function. In H. Read, M. Fordham, G. Adler, & W. McGuire (Eds.), *The collected works of C. G. Jung* (R. F. C. Hull, Trans.) (2nd ed., Vol. 8, pp. 67–91). Princeton University Press. (Original work published 1916)

Jung, C. G. (1970c). Mysterium coniunctionis: An inquiry into the separation and synthesis of psychic opposites in alchemy. In H. Read, M. Fordham, G. Adler, & W. McGuire (Eds.), *The collected works of C. G. Jung* (R. F. C. Hull, Trans.) (2nd ed., Vol. 14). Princeton University Press. (Original work published 1956)

Khan, M. (1974). *The privacy of the self* (pp. 93–98). International Universities Press.

Lenormand, M. (2018). Winnicott's theory of playing: A reconsideration. *International Journal of Psychoanalysis*, *99*(1), 82–102. doi: 10.1080/00207578.2017.1399068

Marlan, S. (2005). *The black sun: The alchemy and art of darkness*. Texas A&M University Press.

McLean, A. (Ed.). (1980). *The rosary of the philosophers*. Magnum Opus Hermetic Sourceworks.

Mitchell, J., Bogenschutz, M., & Lilienstein, A. (2021). MDMA-assisted therapy for severe PTSD: A randomized, double-blind, placebo-controlled phase 3 study. *Nature Medicine 27*, 1025–1033.

Mithoefer, M., Mithoefer, A., Jerome, L., Ruse, J., Doblin, R., Gibson, E., Ot'alora, M., & Sola, E. (2018). *A manual for MDMA-assisted psychotherapy in the treatment of post-traumatic stress disorder*. MAPS.

Mithoefer, M., Wagner, M., & Mithoefer, A. (2011). The safety and efficacy of ±3,4-methylenedioxymethamphetamine-assisted psychotherapy in subjects with chronic, treatment-resistant posttraumatic stress disorder: The first randomized controlled pilot study. *Journal of Psychopharmacology*, *25*, 439–452.

Mithoefer, M., Wagner, M., & Mithoefer, A. (2013). Durability of improvement in post-traumatic stress disorder symptoms and absence of harmful effects or drug dependency after 3,4-methylenedioxymethamphetamine-assisted psychotherapy: A prospective long-term follow-up study. *Journal of Psychopharmacology*, *27*, 28–39.

Ot'alora, G., Grigsby, J., Poulter, B., Van Derveer, J., Giron, S., Jerome, L., Feduccia, A., Hamilton, S., Yazar-Klosinski, B., Emerson, A., Mithoefer, M., & Doblin, R. (2018). 3,4-Methylenedioxymethamphetamine-assisted psychotherapy for treatment of chronic posttraumatic stress disorder: A randomized phase 2 controlled trial. *Journal of Psychopharmacology*, *32*(12), 1295–1307.

Petri, G., Expert, P., Turkheimer, F., Carhart-Harris, R., Nutt, D., Hellyer, P., & Vaccarino, F. (2014). Homological scaffolds of brain functional networks. *Journal of the Royal Society Interface*, *11*, 1–10.

Siegel, D. J. (2012). *The developing mind: How relationships and the brain interact to shape who we are*. The Guilford Press.

Smith, T. K. (2018, May 29). Staying human: Poetry in the age of technology. *Washington Post*. www.washingtonpost.com/entertainment/books/tracy-k-smith-staying-human-poetry-in-the-age-of-technology/2018/05/29/890b6df2-629b-11e8-a768-ed043e33f1dc_story.html

Sola, E. (2017). *MDMA assisted psychotherapy for PTSD: A thematic analysis of transformation in combat veterans*. California Institute of Integral Studies.

Winnicott, D. W. (1954). Mind and its relation to the psyche-soma. *British Journal of Medical Psychology*, *27*, 201–209.

Winnicott, D. W. (1971). *Playing and reality*. Basic Books.

Winnicott, D. W. (1974). Fear of breakdown. *International Review of Psychoanalysis*, *1*, 103–107.

Wolfson, P., Andries, J., Feduccia, A., Jerome, L., Wang, J., Williams, E., Carlin, S., Sola, E., Hamilton, S., Yazar-Klosinski, B., Emerson, E., Mithoefer, M., & Doblin, R. (2020). MDMA-assisted psychotherapy for treatment of anxiety and other psychological distress related to life-threatening illnesses: A randomized pilot study. *Nature*, *10*, 20442.

Chapter 9

The Mystery of the Unconscious

Non-Ordinary States in Psychedelic-Assisted Therapy

Karen Peoples

Introduction

It is late December 2020. I wake from a dream in which I am grieving with other women. The sorrow I feel is palpable. Opening my computer, I read, "A season typically defined by joy is increasingly defined by grief." And further, "The pandemic continued its deadly ascent in America this week, shattering once-unthinkable numbers. . . . The national death toll soared past 300,000 this week."[1] A mere week later, another 30,000 died. As 2021 neared its end, that number climbed to over 750,000, more than the combat deaths in all major U.S. wars of the 20th–21st centuries combined.

From the vantage of this year of extraordinary collective suffering, environmental wreckage, economic instability, and political extremism, I am reminded of how chastened we are by tragedy, how fragile. In the face of immense suffering, I draw strength from the feeling memory of infinite love discovered in the ineffable silence of expanded moments of consciousness. Such expansive states, especially those that dissipate the sense of my separate awareness, have been like an invisible net holding not just my small consciousness but all of creation. They instill a deeply rooted experience of faith: faith that something beyond ourselves—something of Spirit—is available to restore loving connection, transformation, and redemption when our egos are gripped by fear or doubt.

Faith of this deep sort is not ideological but experiential. We know it in our bones. It is the basis of our ability to recover from, make meaning of, and engage our human sojourn with suffering. Faith provides a "containing function" that enables one to not only bear the stress and trauma of suffering but to transform one's relationship to it. It often gives rise as well to faith in the collective healing potential of humankind.

It would be wonderful if psychedelic-inspired mystical experiences could replace the oftentimes arduous process of therapeutic growth. But for those of us working in the reemerging field of psychedelic-assisted therapies, it is important to remember that the acceleration of healing that psychedelics can provide should not obscure the fact that psychospiritual growth is a lifelong process. Healing and self-realization involve ever new iterations, including the often-frustrating revisiting of

DOI: 10.4324/9781003167976-9

old issues. The transformation process involves both waking up and waking down (Bonder, 2004), recognizing that psychospiritual growth comes about as much through maturation of the personal self as it does through experiencing infinity.

In this chapter, I offer a glimpse into how non-ordinary and mystical experiences occasioned either by depth psychoanalytic therapy, by psychedelic-assisted therapy, or by their braiding together can strengthen the containing function of faith for both client and therapist amid the storms and eddies of life and of the therapeutic process. I first provide a general definition of mystical states and the umbrella of NOSC to which they belong. I then draw together contemporary psychoanalytic (CP) and CJ perspectives to formulate a model of the unconscious that encompasses and integrates non-ordinary states. Finally, I explore the clinical implications of this model and highlight the unique value of a psychoanalytic approach for optimally working with psychedelically inspired material.

Depth Analytic Therapy and Psychedelics

When well stewarded, psychoanalysis or depth analytic therapy, like the process of meditation, opens windows into the sequestered rooms of clients' childhood fears; of conscious and unconscious self-protective strategies; and of unmodulated, split-off, or dissociated psychic experience. Patterns developed in early relationships necessarily surface in patterns of interaction with the therapist, making them available for a new experience in the transference–countertransference. Highlighting the importance of access to the unconscious depths that psychoanalysis offers, Adams (1995) states:

> It seems clear that we perpetuate our own suffering through our habitual and defensive alienation from the depths of self and world. Thus we exist as a partial self reacting to a partial world, a self anxious or deadened, cut off from a profound source of awareness, healing, and aliveness.
>
> (p. 467)

Lying on an analyst's couch, first one day then the next soon after, and for several days a week, is like no other encounter. A pregnant waiting occurs, an uncertainty, a dropping into the slipstream of something that captures and carries one to unexpected places within oneself. All the while, your analyst is intimately attuned to you, listening and speaking in ways that the words you exchange can never adequately encompass. Even so, words uttered in this charged crucible can move and spread within to touch many layers of your psyche, emotions, even your body. Dreams begin to announce themselves with greater insistence. Deeply rooted pain begins to surface, while the need for trust in self and other becomes clear. The analyst's attention becomes an internal presence that accompanies, supports, and also heightens the acuteness of one's thoughts, feelings, and sensations. Frozen psychoemotional capacities begin to thaw, restoring neuroplastic capacity to the brain as intuition and symbolic imagination come more alive.

Not least, spiritual sensibilities may flower in the heart, as the needs of the soul to creatively discover deeper meaning, purpose, and aesthetic expression find a receptive space for exploration within the therapy relationship. The journey over months and years of time is multilayered, fraught, arduous, and—one hopes—profoundly enriching. After analysis has ended, the good-enough analyst's presence continues to abide within like the devoted "second" who accompanies you into the struggle with your own suffering, making sure your body—and mind—return home from the fray intact. This is the meaning of the Greek word "therapon" from which the word "therapist" derives: the "second" who is both witness and ritual minister to the psychic life, death, and rebirth of the client (Davoine & Gaudilliere, 2004).

Similar to a good analytic therapy, a good psychedelic-assisted therapy unfolds in a multilayered process of discovery, intimacy, and revelation as the client's psychic life becomes amplified with the aid of the psychedelic. Psychedelics enhance and accelerate access to primal or unprocessed psychic material (Grof, 2008), intensify emotional experience, and often activate dissociated somatic experience. Even though trust in the therapeutic relationship may not be as firmly established as in analytic therapy, over the course of a psychedelic session lasting six to eight hours the emotional intimacy between client and therapist deepens considerably. Layers of fearful resistance tend to soften, and conscious and unconscious material becomes available for exploration as client and therapist steep in the intensified psychic field. Although psychedelic therapy is typically condensed into one or a few very long, intense sessions, and analytic therapy is spread out over many closely linked ones, the two endeavors share important similarities in their flow, depth, and intensity.

I feel strongly that psychoanalytic conceptions of the dynamic workings of the unconscious add great value to what psychedelic medicines have to offer. Psychoanalytic understanding and skill—especially the capacity for reverie and focus on the relationship between client and therapist—have the potential to facilitate the integration of unconscious material as it unfolds over the arc of a treatment, foster the vital component of therapeutic trust, and provide adequate psychological containment of the individual so crucial to the client's faith in the healing process. In a reciprocal fashion, psychedelics have the potential to reduce the arduously time-intensive nature of analytic therapy through the loosening of ego defenses that inhibit the client's access to their inner life. Psychedelics can also initiate NOSC that may soften clients' more entrenched beliefs about themselves, often making psychic movement possible when it has stalled. The current emphasis in psychedelic therapy to make treatment accessible to a diverse range of clients coincides with a growing recognition by psychoanalysts of the need for analytic treatment to be affordable and relevant to underrepresented groups. Together, analytic and psychedelic approaches offer a uniquely efficacious therapy that promises to significantly advance mental health care (Rundel, 2020).

Mystical and Non-Ordinary States of Consciousness

The descriptions in this chapter of mystical and non-ordinary states are situated in, and draw from, Anglo-European traditions that date back to the Greek Hellenistic

Age from 323 to 330 CE. Alongside this Western view, there exists extensive literature on mystical experience from Eastern and South Asian traditions, dating as early as 1500 BCE. Separately, Indigenous traditions have their own rich descriptions of these states reflecting their unique cultural truths. In short, the literature on mysticism is voluminous, and what constitutes a mystical experience has been broadly debated. My accounting here of mystical and non-ordinary states is unavoidably limited.

Mystical experiences are one form of non-ordinary state among many. NOSC represent a marked departure from the known and familiar into new, more ineffable territory. Entrance into non-ordinary reality can stir a hair-tingling quality of uncanniness and otherness (Peoples, 2021a). Classical psychedelics, like psilocybin, LSD, and ayahuasca commonly engender these states, which may evoke profound feelings of awe and wonder as "something sacred shows itself to us," an experience religious historian Eliade called a "hierophany" (Eliade, 1959, p. 11). Non-ordinary states may also stir terror, especially when evoking the perception of imminent ego dissolution.

Central characteristics of non-ordinary states, first described in Western psychology by William James, include 1) ineffability, 2) noetic or revelatory truth quality, 3) transiency, and 4) passivity or surrender to the transformative power of the experience (James, 1902/1982). Charles Tart, a contemporary researcher in NOSC, specifies that they are not simply a quantitative change in a single cognitive function, such as arousal level, but rather a qualitative alteration in the overall pattern of mental functioning recognized by the experiencer as a significant deviation from ordinary waking consciousness (Tart, 1972).

Non-Ordinary States

NOSC are not uniform, but they manifest in a variety of ways, such as:

- Uncanny synchronicities of a powerfully startling nature
- Telepathic communications, often through dreams
- Hypnagogic trance states that stir visions and waking dreams
- Out-of-body experiences
- Psychic birth/rebirth experiences
- Synesthesia or the experience of one sense perception through another sense
- Subtle sensory or paranormal abilities
- Archetypal infusions of psychic energy through dreams or visions
- Unitive or oneness experiences that appear with or without inner imagery, often accompanied by feelings of intense bliss, awe, or rapture
- Profound alterations in the sense of time and space
- Experiencing the cessation of all phenomena—a "touching of the Void" or experience of "no-thing-ness"

Mystical States

The term "mysticism" comes from the Greek *mystikos*, which means to induct or initiate one into the mystery or "secret" behind the veil of the ordinary. The related form of the verb μυέω (mueó) or "myein" means closing the eyes or mouth to experience mystery, that is, to allow a mystery to be revealed non-cognitively and non-verbally. As noted earlier, mystical experiences are a particular type of non-ordinary state. Many scholars have argued that mystical states of complete oneness are the highest, most refined form of consciousness (White, 2012). However, others have asserted that this hierarchical categorization reduces experiences, like powerful visions of gods or angels, to a lesser status. Belser (2019), for example, critiques the unitive ideal to argue that mystical states vary widely. Given the extensive debate and disagreement among scholars on this topic, I utilize a phenomenological description from Western research that has attempted to capture common, salient, subjective features of mystical states, and which draws as well from William James's categories (Griffiths et al., 2006):

1. Internal unity: loss of one's usual sense of identity that contributes to a sense of freedom from the limitations of one's personal self and a bond with what is felt to be greater than the personal self; experience of pure Being and pure awareness; experience of oneness with an inner world; sense of unity or merger into a larger whole or with ultimate reality
2. External unity: experience of oneness or unity with objects and/or persons perceived in one's surroundings; insight that "all is One;" loss of feelings of difference between oneself and objects or persons in one's surroundings; intuitive insight into the inner nature of objects and/or persons in one's surroundings, including their living presence
3. Transcendence of time and space: loss of one's usual sense of time; feeling that one is experiencing eternity or infinity; experience of timelessness; loss of one's usual sense of space, or awareness of where one is or was; a sense of being "outside of" time, beyond past and future or feeling that one has been "outside of" history in a realm where time does not exist; experience of having no physical boundaries between self and environment
4. Ineffability and paradoxicality: sense that the experience cannot be described adequately in words; feeling that it would be difficult to communicate one's experience to others who have not had similar experiences; paradoxical awareness that two apparently opposite principles or situations are both true; sense that to describe parts of one's experience, one would have to use statements that appear to be illogical, involving contradictions and paradoxes
5. Sense of sacredness: experience of amazement, awe or awesomeness; feeling that one has experienced something profoundly sacred and holy; sense of profound humility before the majesty of what was felt to be sacred or holy; sense of being at a spiritual height; sense of the limitations and smallness of one's everyday personality in contrast to the magnitude of what one has experienced; sense of reverence
6. Noetic quality: feeling that the consciousness experienced was more real than one's normal awareness of everyday reality; gaining of insightful knowledge experienced at an intuitive level; feeling of certainty of an encounter with ultimate reality (in the sense of being able to "know" and "see" what is really real)

7. Deeply felt positive mood: experience of overflowing energy; feelings of tenderness and gentleness; feelings of peace and tranquility; feelings of ecstasy, exaltation, and/or joy; feelings of universal or infinite love

A mystical experience as I am defining it here is thus a powerful opening or state of revelation that significantly expands or even dissolves individual consciousness, bringing about contact with something much greater that feels sacred. Mystical experience marks a "going beyond" or transcendence of personal ego awareness and ego preoccupations, typically referred to as a "transpersonal" experience. Richards (2016) relays the experience of a middle-aged woman with kidney cancer on psilocybin in his clinical study:

> Early on the visuals came and dissolved so quickly I could not verbalize them in time. . . . These images changed lighting, color, and texture. I had no doubt I was in the presence of the Infinite because I felt an overriding peacefulness that carried me through everything, even the very few seconds of "Yikes!" that showed up. I had a sense of losing my observer. I no longer witnessed the images. I was becoming them. . . . My body lit up, all parts in succession. It was the brightest thing I have ever seen. I glowed brilliantly from within. My whole being fluttered. . . . I got that every part of us is sacred. There is no speck of the cosmos which is apart from this breath.
>
> (p. 61)

Personal vs. Transpersonal Experiences

Freud (1930) attributed such mystical or "oceanic experiences" to "the preserved 'primitive ego-feeling' from infancy" that is reexperienced in regression, or which exists alongside the reality-oriented, mature ego (p. 68). Psychoanalytic writings since Freud have tended to perpetuate this view, which reduces mystical phenomena to infantile states of mind. Fortunately, psychoanalytic thinking has evolved, and its theories of mysticism are now grouped into three "schools": 1) classic, which sees mystical experience as regressive (infantile), defensive, and pathological; 2) adaptive, in which pathological organizations are seen to occur, and the transcendent nature of mystical experiences is questioned, but their healing or therapeutic value is recognized, and 3) transformational, where both maladaptive and adaptive features are seen in mystical experience, while scholars maintain an open engagement with the transcendent, noetic claims of mystics (Parsons, 1999). More recently, analytic writers have included meditative and spiritual or "superconscious" states (i.e., the ego-transcendent or transpersonal states noted earlier) within a psychoanalytic model of consciousness (e.g., Bobrow, 2010; Safran, 2003; Suchet, 2016).

While Freud and many analysts in Freud's lineage have viewed mystical experiences as regressive or defensive in nature, Jung (1959/1968) and analysts in his lineage have tended to view them as contact with the soul or Self,[2] a notion Jung used to describe the totality of the psyche, both center and circumference, and the medium through which spiritual experience emerges.

Writers, like Ken Wilber (1995), have argued that it is a mistake to reductively attribute mystical states to personal or infantile ("pre-rational") development, while it is likewise a mistake to inflate infantile or "pre-rational" states to "trans-rational" or transpersonal levels of development. Wilber (1995) termed this conflation of personal and transpersonal levels in both analytic lineages as the "pre-rational/trans-rational" fallacy, calling for a differentiation of material that belongs to less mature stages of ego development from experiences that arise from more advanced, transpersonal realizations.

I suggest that, clinically, it is not so easy to distinguish personal and transpersonal material, because their intertwining in mystical experience is common. Corbett (1996) points out that "it is typical for the numinosum to present itself in a manner that is directly relevant to the developmental history of the experiencer" (p. 7). It is also important for therapists to hold in mind that the client's psychic wounds, and defenses against them, will invariably play a role in how the client integrates their mystical experiences. It is not unusual for non-ordinary states to create upheaval in a client's psyche and also in the therapeutic relationship, particularly when contact with archetypal images and energies occurs. Hill (2019) remarks,

> Again and again, we see Jung coming back to the fundamental insight that unusual, altered, pathological, and even religious states of consciousness—whether reflected in dream images, spiritual visions, psychedelic hallucinations, or psychotic delusions—can be understood as unconscious content arising into and sometimes overwhelming consciousness.
>
> (p. 40)

Grief as a Portal Into Mystical Experience

Seemingly paradoxically, intense non-ordinary states can be both traumatic and transcendent at the same time, as when traumatic experience—including dissociated states—opens a portal into non-ordinary states (Peoples, 2000; Stauffer, 2021; Williams, 2019). For example, the intertwining of personal and transpersonal material is often seen in the association of mystical states of union with profound loss. For example, Aberbach (1987) notes, "The climactic stage in the mystical process, union with the divine presence, also has a parallel in the grieving process, in the form of identification with, or in some cases, an actual sense of union with the lost person" (p. 514). Citing the unitive experiences of such diverse individuals as Sister Teresa, Wordsworth, Jean-Paul Sartre, Martin Buber, all of whom suffered early loss of a parent, Aberbach adds:

> Hardly a single characteristic of the grief process—such as withdrawal, yearning and searching, depression and despair, "finding," union, gaining a "new identity," return to normal social life—does not have a parallel in the mystical

process. While *mysticism cannot be equated with grief*, it might provide a framework within which unresolved grief, especially that deriving from child-hood loss, can be worked through and overcome. In some cases, presumably, grief might lead to mysticism.

(p. 524, emphasis added)

I highlight Aberbach's words that mysticism cannot be equated with grief because, even though experiences of loss, conflict, and trauma may give rise to mystical experiences, their "fruits" matter as much as or more than their "roots" (James, 1902/1982; Yaden et al., 2017). For example, in my mid-20s, I was involved in intensive study and meditation practice within the theosophical tradi-tion. I shared in this study with two close, older colleagues and friends, meeting five hours a week for meditation and spontaneous visualization practice. At the time, I was doing my doctoral research attempting to distinguish narcissism or inauthentic self-actualization from authentic self-actualization within the human potential movement. After three years of this intensive meditation practice with my colleagues, the strain of my own narcissistic idealizing tendencies was begin-ning to show. I felt I could not keep up with my friends, and that I was inadequate and not sufficiently spiritually developed. Our work together ruptured, and I was plunged into a calamitous spiritual crisis, an utterly bereft dark night of the soul. I felt I could no longer believe in anyone or anything, including and especially my own perceptions and beliefs due to my narcissistic tendencies and projections.

In a moment of inconsolable grief, I was able to let go and accept the hugeness of my loss. I suddenly "saw" and felt an inner vision of vast, infinite space stretch-ing out before me. Central to the experience was a soft, silent emanation—like an invisible texture—a noiseless "sound" that was also a presence. More than a vibra-tion, a feeling of presence emanated within and through this tangible yet intangible fabric of the universe. That presence was love, a "holy mystery"[3] that brought me to my knees in awe. Although impersonal, it seemed to sustain all of existence in such profound compassion that I was moved to further tears, now of gratitude. I knew in the depth of my being that this was real, and that this I could trust. The "fruits" of my grief coming through this expansion of consciousness remain the ground of my faith in the healing power of infinite spaciousness that is compassion or love itself.

Anxiety Relief Through Mystical Experience

Such personal anecdotes are increasingly supported by contemporary research find-ings with psychedelics, which indicate that mystical states of oneness often have a powerful anxiety-reducing effect (Richards, 2016; Carhart-Harris, 2014; MacLean et al., 2013). The individual's personal concerns temporarily dissolve, and a new experience of openness, free from the grip of ego identifications, tends to arise. Perhaps, in particular, states of mystical oneness that generate a feeling of being held by a larger, benign presence are the most salient factor in reducing anxiety.

For example, researchers studying the effects of psilocybin-assisted therapy for individuals with attachment disorders suggested that "psilocybin-induced neural plasticity along with an experience of mystical unity may lead to overall reduced attachment anxiety by establishing a more secure connection to something greater than, or beyond, the self" (Stauffer et al., 2020, p. 528).

Differentiating Psychological Disturbances From Mystical States

While mystical states have often been misattributed to regressive, infantile experience, psychological disturbances can also be mistaken for transpersonal states. Schwartz (2013) notes, "The healthy mindfulness and detachment characterizing spiritual maturity may be difficult to distinguish from symptoms of depersonalization, depression, or ego-inflation" (p. 200). For example, confusion occurred between me and a co-therapist during a ketamine session with a client. The client was in a deep hypnotic trance and mumbled that they were floating higher and higher into the air. My co-therapist, an experienced clinician well versed in spiritual traditions, believed the client was absorbed in an ego-transcendent state. I perceived that the client, with whom I had been working individually for some time, had actually detached from their bodily consciousness in a dissociated state. In subsequent sessions exploring the ketamine journey, my client reported that they had disconnected from their body in their usual way, although more intensely so, and that they felt alienated and adrift.

In dissociation, there is an automatic disconnection from bodily or emotional experience by the ego, signaling an urgent, unconscious rejection of feeling. In contrast, there is a quality of sacredness in mystical states that often instills faith that one is safely held in a larger reality, even as one's sense of "I" and somatic awareness may have faded into the background. In such moments, when ordinary filters of identity, role, and history fall away, what often remains is an abiding presence of consciousness itself in its going on being. This revelation stills the grasping, ego activity of mind, allowing the heart to open to an experience of faith that being survives when doing comes to rest.

The Therapeutic Value of Mystical States

The therapeutic value of mystical and non-ordinary experiences for clients depends on the therapist maintaining a non-judgmental openness in exploring these states in relation to the complex picture of the client's self-development. Some clients may become attached to the awe and excitement of mystical states and their spiritual narratives, wishing to avoid difficult personal issues or mundane reality. The therapist needs to remain open to and engaged with the client's subjective experience while simultaneously remaining aware of possible defensive dynamics in clients' reports of mystical states.

Despite their differences, psychoanalysts from both Freudian and Jungian lineages believe that access to the depths of the psyche provides a quality of inner nourishment essential to human psychospiritual health. Adams (1995) writes about the ways the discipline of psychoanalysis offers "the wisdom and transformative power of a living relationship with these depths" (p. 465). He points out that the psychoanalytic method helps "cultivate a privileged mode of awareness, namely, that of revelatory openness wedded with the clarity of unknowing" (p. 465). In the following, I discuss the importance of the "clarity of unknowing" for the therapist in the integration of non-ordinary states within the therapeutic process, especially when psychedelics are included. For the sake of simplicity, I generally use the term "mystical" in this chapter to mean states of unitive consciousness that feel markedly sacred, as in the examples mentioned earlier. At the same time, my use of the term "mystical" stands in dialogue with Belser's (2019) emphasis on the variability of mystical states and with Jung's equation of mystical states with "experience of the archetypes" (Dourley, 2007, p. 53). Contrary to the reduction of mysticism to states of oneness, archetypal experience may be perceived as a flowering of the diverse multiplicity of the cosmos, as I will explore as follows.

Speculations on a Unified Field Theory of the Unconscious

To have a multidimensional conceptual framework for integrating non-ordinary states in analytic therapy, I find invaluable the combined richness of CJ and CP theories of the unconscious/consciousness. For too long, the two traditions neglected (or refused) to speak with, and thus learn from, each other. Keeping the rich thinking of each lineage siloed deprives clinicians of perspectives that are needed as psychedelic-enhanced non-ordinary states become more prevalent in the therapeutic setting.

The following is a simplified framework of the two traditions toward a model that seeks to encompass the most primordial to the most transcendent mystical states of consciousness in a unified field theory of consciousness, including the unconscious, as seen from these Western systems of thought. I am only able to highlight here, in an overly schematic and linear way, psychic processes and phenomena that are anything but schematic and linear. Visual–spatial metaphors are hard to avoid. Is the unconscious "below" consciousness? Does it surround or imbue it, neither above nor below? "Where" is the collective unconscious relative to the personal unconscious?

Religious and philosophical literature, East and West, has typically distinguished "lower" from "higher" states (White, 2012), framing consciousness in terms of hierarchical schema from less developed and unrefined to more mature and refined. For example, Wilber (1995) asserts that archetypal experiences associated with the collective unconscious are more "primal" or "primordial"—and thus less developed—than mystical experiences; he thus does not see archetypal experience as spiritual. However, Jungian authors, like Kalsched (2013) and Dourley (2007), emphasize that the archetypal and mystical are both aspects of numinous (spiritual) experience that can occur when the rational organizing tendencies of the mind subside. These questions are complex and require clinicians to keep an open but discerning mind about such phenomena when they appear clinically.

In the same vein, we must recognize that linguistic terms, like "numinous," "unconscious," "consciousness," "Self," and "archetype," are merely concepts and symbols that serve as guides for the clinician. For example, I use the phrase "the unconscious" when referring to a limitless impersonal field of the unconscious, and speak of it as synonymous with "Consciousness" writ large. However, when speaking of a "conscious" awareness vs. an "unconscious" one, I am referring to different states of mind within an individual.

Concepts provide a useful, even necessary, map in navigating complex client material, but they can also interfere with the therapist's trust in their own intuitive function so crucial for connection with the client's experience. Pontalis (2003) points out that the German word for concept comes from "claws." He remarks, "the concept has claws. . . . It is a predator, a tyrant," constricting freedom of thought (p. 4). Similarly, Samuels (1985) stresses the phenomenological over the conceptual, arguing that "the archetypal is a perspective defined in terms of its impact, depth, consequence, and grip. The archetypal is in the emotional experience of perception and not in a pre-existing list of symbols" (p. 53, italic added).

Contemporary Psychoanalytic Perspectives: The Infinite Unconscious

Many psychoanalysts hew closely to a "classical" Freudian or Kleinian conception of the unconscious, focusing on dynamic, unconscious object relations within the personal sphere of the psyche or ego. Classical analysis addresses internal self- and other constellations as these come into play in the transference. Clients' minds are often crowded and besieged by reactive self-parts within their unconscious, and therapeutic work with these introjects is essential. In addition to bringing these parts into conscious dialogue and internal acceptance, a key element in healing involves the greater psychic space an analytic process affords within which the client can observe their internal dynamics.

But with the postmodern turn in psychoanalysis (Elliott & Spezzano, 2000), theoretical conceptions of the magnitude of the unconscious have begun to emerge. The envelope of the unconscious is no longer seen as the interaction of the separate unconscious minds of the therapist and client but as a third force encompassing, and greater than, the unconscious minds of each participant (Benjamin, 2004; Ogden, 1994). In addition, CP writers have come to hypothesize the existence of a social unconscious (e.g., Gonzales, 2020; Hopper, 2003) and articulate a field theory model of the unconscious (Stern, 2013; Dithrich, 2021). There is a growing recognition of the unconscious structuring influences of cultural forces, like race, gender, and class (Layton et al., 2006; Guralnik & Simeon, 2010), and of social trauma with its uncanny intergenerational transmissions (Davoine & Gaudilliere, 2004). All of these contributions have expanded CP models to include a potent collective aspect to the unconscious life of the individual, who is now recognized as situated in an extensive field of unconscious influences.

Wilfred Bion (1962, 1970) developed a view of the unconscious that stretched psychoanalytic thinking perhaps more than any other analyst. Regrettably, his contributions have not been widely taken up in their implications for understanding mystical and non-ordinary states in therapy. However, Bion's later writings are central to this purpose precisely because they address the kinds of "numinous" or spiritual realizations long dismissed in traditional psychoanalytic thinking. Grotstein asserts, "Bion . . . launched a metapsychological revolution (in which he) perforated the flat world of Freud's and Klein's positivism . . . and introduced inner and outer cosmic uncertainty, infinity, relativism, and numinousness as its successor" (Grotstein, 2007, p. 114). As an analysand of Bion's, Grotstein (2000) defined the numinous as "the sense of awe and wonder and the inward journey (into the self) associated with the mystical and meditative contact with the ineffable" (p. 255).

Israeli analyst Eshel (2019) emphasizes the clinical importance of Bion's speculations on "O"—the unrepressed boundless dimension of the unconscious, arguing that "profound interconnectedness rather than separateness . . . operates at primary, deep, invisible levels" (p. 267). She calls for a radical shift in how therapists work, moving from "knowing" to "being O"—that is, moving from concepts about the client to intuitive immersion in a clarity of unknowing with the client. This entails a shift from a two-person framework to that of "oneness." She sees the therapist's capacity to surrender into unity with a client's unconscious as an essential means of accessing archaic, pre-symbolized states of unthinkable early breakdown.

I agree that the therapist's openness to such profound interconnectedness is vital to working with severe early trauma. Eshel (2019) poignantly describes the transformation that occurs in the client's mental functions through the analyst's at-one-ment with clients' most terrifying, unsymbolized states of dread. Although she charts a powerful path into new therapeutic territory—"from Knowing to Being"—Eshel focuses exclusively on making contact with infantile states. Her work thus perpetuates the long-standing psychoanalytic orientation toward early development while missing the broader picture of our intrinsic psychic capacity for at-one-ment, namely, that experiences of at-one-ment occur at many levels of development, including mystical and expansive ego-transcendent levels, not just infantile ones. Following Bion (1970), I am proposing that the infinite field of Consciousness, or "O," is unitive or undifferentiated in its nature and is the medium through which direct contact between two minds occurs. It cannot be experienced through "knowing," but—indeed—only through being at-one with it.

It is clear that experiences of analytic oneness, whether of a mystical or infantile nature, often so disassemble ordinary referents of time, space, and self that uncanny, extraordinary forms of knowing can occur. Specifically addressing these phenomena, American analysts Mayer (2007) and Suchet (2016) call for open-minded investigation into non-ordinary states. Suchet asserts,

> When we reduce mystical or religious experiences . . ., we close ourselves to centuries-old wisdom. It is not that mystical ways cannot be used for defensive purposes . . . rather, that we have not sufficiently recognized what they can also

offer: the generative, creative potentials of self experience; the unbounded states that invigorate the mind as well as the extraordinary and extrasensory powers of the mind that have remained untapped.

(p. 748)

Suchet thus goes beyond most current CP writers in calling for the recognition of transpersonal states—including mystical ones—as irreducible phenomena in their own right. This is in line with the thinking of Belgian psychoanalyst Vermote (2021), who charts the unconscious along a continuum from undifferentiation to differentiation. Current perspectives on development recognize that psychological health rests on the capacity to move flexibly between these states, rather than being a linear progression from immature undifferentiated mental functions to mature differentiated ones (Rundel, 2020). The expanded analytic view of the unconscious field that I posit here is consistent with the Jungian notion of a numinous collective unconscious as well as spiritual traditions that assert that consciousness is an infinite ocean, in which individual waves appear and disappear (Hixon, 1992).

Jungian Perspectives: Archetypes and the Collective Unconscious

Adopting the spatial metaphor mentioned earlier, we can conceive of the unconscious as a vast ocean of energy surrounding and permeating each individual's unconscious. Although Bion considered the unconscious to be basically formless, he believed it was filled with unsymbolized "stuff" he called beta elements that bombard the infant's mind, necessitating the parent's mediation of the raw too muchness of reality (Bion, 1962). Jung similarly believed a field of unconscious surrounds the developing ego, an unconscious that is "practically immortal . . . something like an unceasing stream or perhaps ocean" (Hill, 2019, p. 32). However, in contrast to Bion, Jung believed this ocean was populated with "images and figures which drift into consciousness in our dreams or in abnormal states of mind" (Hill, 2019, p. 32). For Jung, this vast ocean was a "mythopoetic" dimension of the unconscious deeper than the personal unconscious with its disguised sexual and aggressive desires toward the parents, as Freud thought (Kalsched, 1996). Later calling it the collective unconscious, Jung saw this as an ancient historical stratum, a primal or primordial dimension of consciousness existing prior to, and influencing, the psyche of the developing individual and the dynamics of the collective. Jung argued that the collective unconscious enacts its powerful influence through the patterned and polyvalent expression of archetypes. In his description of the archetypes of the collective unconscious, Jungian analyst James Hillman (1975) notes, "Let us then imagine archetypes as the deepest patterns of psychic functioning, the roots of the soul governing the perspectives we have of ourselves and the world" (p. xix).

Jung believed this deep mythopoetic or archetypal aspect was indeed a stratum of consciousness reflecting humankind's "original . . . religious experience . . . centered in the numinosum" (Kalsched, 2013, p. 202, italics in original) or spiritual domain. He considered clients' contact with archetypal images and energies as essentially spiritual in nature, impelled by the ineffable "Self" to stir the individual's evolution toward wholeness. Despite its spiritual nature, however, contact with archetypal imagery can have an overwhelming or disruptive impact. As Jung cautioned early on, archetypes can "saturate consciousness 'with uncanny forebodings or even with the fear of madness'" (Hill, 2019, p. 36). For Jungians, it is through contact with the numinous power and mystery of the archetypal realm, with its highly charged opposing elements, such as angelic and demonic imagery, that the personal self is thrust forward in its developmental journey through ego consciousness into the sacred or spiritual dimension of the Self. Remarking on the vital therapeutic function of archetypal imagery in clients with severe trauma histories, Kalsched (2013) argues that many psychoanalysts "fail to understand the crucial role of a mythopoetic second world in saving the trauma survivor's soul from annihilation in the interpersonal world" (p. 4, italics in original). The traumatized psyche "makes use of 'historical layers' of the unconscious in order to give form to, or 'outpicture,' otherwise unbearable suffering—suffering that (has) no expression except in mythopoetic form" (Kalsched, 1996, p. 77).

Archetypal experience is thus not a regressive production of the individual psyche that one must grow beyond but an "everlasting fact of humankind's experience on the planet" (Kalsched, 2013, p. 5). Appearing through dreams and reverie in analytic treatment as well as visions in psychedelic therapy, one sees a dynamic interplay of the personal and collective unconscious. Kalsched (1996) illustrates how "our internal object-relations make use of or shade over into the mythical or 'imago' level" (p. 77). This shading into the archetypal often occurs when a client's internal objects take on a highly persecutory or idealized character that can overpower the ego, often seen in the early stages of therapy.

It is also true that a shading over from the archetypal into the personal unconscious occurs, for instance, in clients where cultural rituals have had a prominent role in their developing psyche. A client who immigrated from Korea to the U.S.A. as a school-age child had nightmares of a horrifying shapeless creature that would roar up from under her bed at night to psychically possess her. This creature reflected aspects of her own harsh superego coming to devour her for breaking with her family's religious strictures. But the creature also reflected two archetypal cultural phenomena: contemporary unintegrated war trauma of her mother's and grandmother's that haunted both women, and a melding of their unsymbolized personal terrors with the frightening "ghosts" and "evil spirits" in the client's original culture's ancient mourning ceremonies. Identifying and exploring how the archetypal ghosts and spirits of her culture shaded into and activated her personal unconscious, and how the generational trauma of her mother and grandmother activated both cultural archetypal and personal fears, gradually led to the subsiding of her nightmares.

Thus, it is important for therapists working with mystical and non-ordinary experiences to recognize there can be a simultaneous expression of personal, generational, and archetypal influences in clients' material, as in the example presented

earlier. As Schwartz (2013) notes, "working with a combination of the psychological and archetypal therapeutic paradigms can be a tricky task for the patient and the
therapist. Each perspective can potentially enhance or disrupt progress" (p. 200).
Therapists can assist clients to creatively engage in what Kalsched refers to as
a "humanizing" of the archetypes through an intentional, evolving relationship
with archetypal imagery. When clients are helped to welcome, befriend, and learn
from the figures that appear in dreams and visions, even of the most disturbing or
unwanted sort, a generative transformational process between the personal self, the
transpersonal Self, and the collective unconscious is set in motion. It is necessary to
remember, however, that archetypal images are guiding metaphors that are meant
to evolve, rather than become fixated identities with "claws" in the client's—or
therapist's—mind. When images, concepts, and self-narratives become repetitive
and reified, they obscure the spaciousness in which Consciousness is present as a
luminous field.

Touching the Void

Beyond the archetypal, writers from transpersonal psychology and mystic Christian
traditions describe a distinctly different non-ordinary state of consciousness that
occurs when all perceptual phenomena, including images and sensations, disappear, sometimes referred to as touching "the Void." Relying on familiar concepts of
hierarchical strata, John Dourley (2007), a Jungian author, emphasizes that Jung's
writings pointed to "the Void" as a presumed layer of Consciousness "behind or
beyond" or "prior" to the primordial, archetypal one. Ken Wilber (1995), also using
a hierarchical framework, calls this the causal level of Consciousness, of "formless and silent awareness" empty of all qualities (p. 304). Hill (2019), recounting
his early experiences on LSD, describes "a pervasive and overpowering sense of
another reality, a terrifying immense stillness that seemed inexplicably and undeniably sacred. The profound, absolute, and seemingly transcendent nature of this
stillness implicitly and mysteriously called my whole life into question" (p. xiv).
Dourley (2007) believes that contact with this numinous dimension "beyond" the
archetypes helps in "moderating the compulsive attractiveness of . . . [archetypal]
powers through an experience deeper than and prior to the source of their frequently irresistible and swamping allure" (p. 72).

The conditioned and constructed nature of the mind filters or occludes our
awareness of Consciousness. Grasping onto or being grasped by our thought forms,
internal object representations, and self identities ultimately perpetuates the troublesome patterns of mental and emotional life that cause so much suffering. While
the process through which the self-construct develops is a normal brain function,
neuroscience research suggests that,

> Psychedelics target mechanisms on which self-binding depends. Psychedelic
> experience degrades these binding processes, enabling subjects to experi-
> ence cognition not bound by self-models. We emphasize that the "self" which

dissolves in psychedelic experience is not an actual entity or an object of perception, interoception, or introspection but an entity inferred by the mind to predict the flow of experience in and across cognitive modalities.

(Letheby & Gerrans, 2017, p. 2)

Thus, when self-constructs fall away in moments of dissolution, a "groundless ground" of awareness is often revealed that transcends dualistic perceptions, demonstrating the fictional nature of our sense of separateness from others, from world, and from Consciousness itself. Realizing the fundamental emptiness of our constructs—perhaps especially when perceived phenomena disappear altogether in "touching the Void"—can have great healing power, bringing peace to the agitated mind.

Summary: "Whose Consciousness Is It?"

Non-ordinary states, like telepathic communication, archetypal visions, and mystical experiences of unitive or transcendent consciousness, challenge the long-held Western assumption that consciousness is individual and separate. Expanding our working models of consciousness to include these complex, alternate realities can help therapists meet clients' experiences more fully and effectively. Suchet (2016) draws on the teachings of a Sufi master to buttress her call for such an expanded framework:

We have subtle subconscious faculties we are not using. In addition to the limited analytic intellect is a vast realm of mind that includes psychic and extrasensory abilities, intuition, wisdom, a sense of unity, aesthetic, qualitative and creative capacities and image-forming and symbolic capacities. . . . This total mind we call heart.

(p. 750)

It is no longer tenable for analytic theorists to ignore these metaphysical aspects of consciousness given the prevalence of non-ordinary states in human experience. Equally important, it is time for the vital contributions of Jungian theories of the collective unconscious and archetypes to be incorporated into mainstream psychoanalytic theories of the unconscious.

Finally, it is necessary to consider what it is that makes many of these ego-transcendent experiences healing in their own right. Is it the quieting of self-focus through deactivation of the brain's top-down organizing functions (Carhart-Harris, 2014) that brings relief from the ego's incessant borrowing from the past and projecting onto the future? Is it the revelation of awareness as a vast, powerful, and uncontaminated presence that conveys a sense of being extending beyond the limited ego-self? Or is it the experience of unutterable, transcendent beauty that evokes love and a feeling of grace, opening the wounded heart, humbling the mind, and restoring faith that the broken self can be made whole? It is likely that all of these aspects of non-ordinary and mystical experience contribute to their healing power. I will explore how these experiences in a variety of forms can be worked with through the therapeutic process.

Clinical Integrations/Applications

It must be noted straightaway that the employment of psychedelics in therapy is not a shortcut or substitute for ongoing depth therapy. To enhance the digestion of psychedelic experiences in the psychospiritual growth process, a trustworthy relationship with a therapist is vital. I believe the therapeutic relationship is the most significant variable in regard to the influence of the setting in psychedelic work.

Although psychedelics were not in widespread use during Freud's time, Carl Jung was opposed to them because he believed they allowed so much unconscious archetypal material to enter consciousness that it exceeded what the mind could integrate (Purrington, 2020). Similarly, psychoanalytic treatments in the 1960s that included LSD sessions were strongly critiqued by Jungian analyst Michael Fordham, who argued that conventional (non-psychedelic) long-term therapy was a safer route. Other Jungian clinicians, like Ronald Sandison, disagreed, noting that clients were able to make good use of their LSD sessions in their analyses precisely because the ongoing nature of the treatment provided a safe holding environment (Hill, 2019, pp. 25–26).

I mention these historical debates about the integration of psychedelics into therapeutic treatments to highlight the importance of adequate preparedness on the part of therapists doing this work. Psychedelic medicines are extremely powerful, stirring intense psychological material while the client is very vulnerable. I strongly believe that adequate training in the early development of the psyche, unconscious defense mechanisms, the dynamics of transference and countertransference, and the complexities of spiritual development is needed to protect clients from harm, especially given how rapidly the field of psychedelic-assisted therapy is developing. Skill in stewarding psychedelic sessions is necessary; skill in helping clients integrate the material activated by psychedelics is essential. I highlight as follows three psychological capacities in particular that I believe therapists need to develop through training and supervision, because these capacities are central to the adequate containment by the therapist of the client and their potent psychedelic experiences.

What Is "Containment"?

First is the therapist's ability to accept, even welcome with curiosity, the client's self-protective (defensive) reactions and the many forms these can take. Clients may be avoidant, intellectualized, passive, dismissive, or challenging with the therapist. Familiar strategies to avoid vulnerability often come quickly into play and may be steered from within by frightened, distrusting, or angry parts of the self. It is incumbent on therapists to provide room for these aspects to speak and become known (Peoples, 2021b). Related to this is the therapist's ability to bear becoming cast by the client as a figure in the client's internal world, such as a critical authority or a weak, useless parent. One cannot avoid stepping into these positions with a client. It is crucial that the therapist not only recognize but tolerate the discomfort of both negative and idealizing projections by the client, for example, being seen as an untrustworthy character or, conversely, as someone who will finally heal the brokenness the client has suffered for so long. These projections frequently trigger countertransference reactions of hate and love, deflation and inflation in the therapist. Whether doing shorter-term psychedelic work in collaboration with an outside therapist or psychedelic sessions with one's own longer-term clients, the capacity to recognize, welcome, help draw out, and work sensitively with these complex transference–countertransference dynamics is often pivotal to the maintenance of a trustworthy therapeutic relationship.

Second, and equally important, is the therapist's capacity to engage the particular psychic process of containment described by Wilfred Bion (1970). Effective containment requires that we recognize we are operating in a dynamic psychic field of the unconscious that has the power to surface material from the co-mingled unconscious minds of both the therapist and the client (Peoples, 2021a). This dynamic field includes archetypal images and energies from the collective unconscious that become constellated at various moments in the therapy.

A therapist's awareness of the field leans on a third capacity: a rather radical, if temporary, ability to surrender or give over one's thinking, feeling, and sensing functions to the field in order for the therapist's intuition—deeply connected with the unconscious—to emerge. Recall that the origin of the word "mystical" refers to a shutting of one's eyes and mouth. For Bion, the therapist's non-conceptual reverie requires patience and faith—and "to repose there long enough" (Eshel, 2019, p. 35) that "out of the darkness and formlessness something evolves" (Bion, 1967, p. 273). This is what psychoanalyst Adams means by "the clarity of unknowing" (1995, p. 465).

The Clarity of Unknowing

Information about the client, their history, their last session, interferes, "Knowledge screens the sound the third ear hears, so we hear only what we already know. *The analytic method—like the poetic one—proceeds through unknowing*" (Kurtz, 1989, p. 6, italics in original). While this state can be challenging for the therapist and is not maintained at all times in a session, it is central to allowing the dynamic intelligence within the field to take shape. The therapist is better able to experience at-one-ment, or being-within the client's psyche rather than attempting to know it, which is particularly important for contacting unformulated, preverbal states of mind in the client. Eshel notes, "In practice this means *not* that the analyst recalls some relevant memory but that a relevant constellation will *be evoked during the process of at-one-ment*" (Eshel, 2019, p. 243, italics in original). I would add that relevant constellations of emotional experience are initially subtly intuited or experientially sensed, emerging slowly into symbolic form through the therapist's tolerance of the inchoate or confusional states that can precede them, sometimes over many treatment hours.

Suchet (2016) concurs,

> The more we are capable of entering the unknown and unknowable aspects of Self, the more we begin to know, but we know through the "heart," we know from the inside. We develop intuitive knowing as if we were inside the object itself.
>
> (p. 753)

The therapist must thus develop the ability to withstand the pull externally from the client or internally from their own anxiety or desire, or to prematurely move toward ascribing meaning or offering associations and interpretations to the client. Mystical and transpersonal experiences in particular have a quality of sacredness for the client, and prematurely putting these experiences into words can render them hollow or mundane.

The challenge of balancing reverie in the service of containment with attention to transference dynamics occurred with a client of mine in her 50s. Because we were doing phone therapy, I was already limited in the subtle and overt sensory impressions I could ascertain in the field. My client's meditation practice and intense search for truth led her to experience a powerful non-ordinary state she shared with me in the next session. Eager to convey how starkly altered her mind had been and how stunning a realization she had had, she nonetheless felt awkward describing it. She wondered if she sounded superficial and silly, because her words could not capture the magnitude or quality of the illuminated state she experienced outside of treatment.

She animatedly described an intense "blowing open" of her entire perspective on reality, spontaneously realizing she had been caught in a belief system about how her mind worked that she kept trying to figure out or fight her way out of. She described this realization saying, "I felt like I lost my ego for a brief moment." She was keenly aware of the expansive openness and freshness that followed her experience, which she earnestly wanted to transmit to me. At the same time, she acutely felt the distinction between the experience itself—which had enormously freed her—and the humbling process of describing it now to me.

Throughout her sharing, I was aware of emptying my mind and tuning all of my awareness to her experience, including everything she was conveying without words. I knew it was important to register the profundity of her realization even though it was now muted by her ordinary state of mind. At the same time, I was very aware of the sensitive relational exchange taking place between us and knew it was important to convey that I was with her in feeling the power of the opening she had had. I responded slowly, minimally, with vocal sounds and quiet breath that expressed through my body that I was palpably affected by her experience. Describing the awe and freedom she felt triggered a momentary defensive cynicism. Noting this, she pressed forward to work through the meanings of her realization to clarify what was illusory and what continued to be real and true now, within her regular consciousness.

Throughout her 50 years of life, this client had been constantly anxious and obsessive. Her deep revelation blew open the doors of ordinary perception and freed her from the way her mind worked like a steel trap to control her thoughts, behaviors, and access to emotional truth. We continued to integrate this experience over following sessions, toggling between moments of touching back into the felt experience and exploring the many layers of meaning it had for her. She was left with "a small amount of faith that my mind was going to work it out, not me."

Grotstein (2000) notes that Bion believed the psyche needs truth as much as the body needs food, adding, "thus *the search for truth, emotional truth, becomes the prime driving force* of every human being, yet the fear of its consequences and realizations become (their) resistance" (p. 291, italics added). Grotstein is describing here the way in which the unfiltered truth of raw existence—or "O"—presses through our psychic as well as somatic filters. When we can meet and contain this encounter with "O," we are reshaped by it. To do so requires the "being within" described earlier, including at times bearing the intensity of chaotic or disorienting states of mind and body. This client experienced a "transformation in 'O' when her mind's clawing conceptions shook loose and dropped away, leaving her suddenly, surprisingly, open and free" (p. 291).

Containing Archetypal Energies

Clinically, the appearance in clients' consciousness of archetypal images and symbols, whether arising in dreams, meditation, psychedelic experiences, hypnotic trance states, or deep reverie, can flood the psyche with intense energy. Because this can feel overwhelming both psychically and somatically to the client, the therapist needs the capacity to conduct the energies that are transmitted by the client into the field, and thus often into the therapist's mind and body. Conducting these psychosomatic states entails dropping into the heart and relaxing the mind to allow energy to flow freely through the body. The therapist can stabilize this process through awareness of the breath, noticing without aversion the flow of sensations, thoughts, and emotions. Mindfulness of this sort strengthens the therapist's witnessing capacity. This does not mean the therapist does not have feelings in response to what the client is engaging in the relational transference–countertransference. Rather, the therapist's ability to observe sensations, thoughts, and feelings without gripping or focusing on them allows the energies in the therapist's body–mind to flow unobstructed while creating internal spaciousness for intuition to emerge. The therapist's deep reverie of this sort gives rise to what Bion (1962) called alpha function, a metabolizing of subtle intuitions that move toward symbolization in the therapist's mind. This process facilitates a transformation of unconscious material within the client through associative links—in thought and feeling—that the client and the therapist engage together.

At times, the therapist's at-one-ment with the unconscious field may stir up primordial or archetypal imagery in the therapist as a way station into the client's personal material. This could be a useful "shading over," to use Kalsched's (1996) metaphor, from archetypal symbols into the internal representational world of the client through the mediating function of the therapist's connection with archetypal themes. However, the therapist's reverie may not always stir imagery. A client's experience may only be registered deeply in the body because clients can feel haunted by unsymbolized pressures in their psyches. For example, a client who I will call Alex described a dream of lying in bed and feeling only an enormous presence, like a heavy weight pinning him down. He could neither move to flee nor voice any cry for help. He had difficulty imaginatively engaging in conscious dialogue with this image—or with any of his negative self-images—to explore his internal object world. The invisible thing holding him down helplessly had no shape, no texture, and brought up no associations to his life. As an "anti-libidinal" part of his self-care system (Kalsched, 2013), it had a familiar, tyrannical feeling to it, as if a "cosmic force" was victimizing him. Alex had been assailed from early childhood by chronic overwhelming conflict in his family environment. His capacity for containment of his own emotions was limited, leaving him subject to panic attacks and hyper-rational attempts to cope. Over the course of intensive therapy, including ketamine work, he was gradually able to enter a more imaginal space and slowly give shape to the disembodied force in his dream as an immovable "boulder" blocking his path in life.

In our regular therapy sessions, I often felt this boulder as a dead weight in my own chest, a stifling, inert, and inanimate mass that could not be engaged with consciously because it was merely a lifeless obstacle with no meaning in Alex's mind. In contrast, in the ketamine-assisted therapy sessions, this object became animated as a massive torrent of black dirt pouring down, burying him. I could sense the movement and power of this stifling energy in my own body, making it harder to breathe. Over time, our ketamine work helped this client experience a sharply contrasting upsurge of vital energy, which he visualized as a vibrant, green plant stalk. The lively presence of the plant stalk that *he became* radiated a vibrant fullness, enhancing my own felt sense of aliveness. Alex readily identified with this energy as his own reclaimed strength. My steady encouragement to allow himself to feel the quality and movement of these energies in his body (as I traced them privately in my own) led him to increasingly recognize them as active processes in his psyche about which he now had some choice.

Sensory–Energetic Transformations in Consciousness: The Subtle Body

An element too often missing from analytic theory and training until recent years is the crucial importance of the body and the therapeutic exploration of clients' somatic experiences. Advances in the neurobiology of trauma have greatly contributed to clinical understanding of somatic aspects of psychological conditions, especially dissociative states (van der Kolk, 2015). In addition to the therapist's skillful attention to bodily experience within the unfolding transference/counter-transference, work with clients' non-ordinary states necessitates what I call "subtle sensing." New models of the unconscious must take into account metaphysical experiences that arise through *somatic* or *energetic* pathways. While this issue cannot be taken up in detail here, it is important for clinicians to recognize that clients reporting non-ordinary states and psychedelic experiences often describe unusual sense perceptions, such as the noticeable expansion or movement of energy from one area of the body to another, including movement up the spine, around the heart, head, or other zones in the body; "seeing" colors and patterns; possibly "hearing" subtle sounds associated with this energy; and sensing or seeing energy transferred from one's own touch to another or from another person's touch, etc.

Meditative and contemplative traditions east and west have identified such phenomena for centuries. Described as kundalini in Indian yogic systems, transformations in somatic energy patterns often arise with mystical transpersonal awakenings. Recall the participant on psilocybin in Richards's study mentioned earlier; she recounted that her "body lit up, all parts in succession. It was the brightest thing I have ever seen" (Richards, 2016, p. 61). Clients with this kind of experience need their therapists' subtle attunement not only to the emotional quality of the experience and to the meanings evoked for the client but also to the movement of energies in the body and how the client's awareness of these energies develops over time.

Drawing from Vajrayana Buddhist practice, psychoanalyst Kirsten Fiorella (2020) notes that the therapist's ability to develop non-conceptual awareness by locating attention in the subtle body is extremely valuable for bearing the chaos and intensity of clients' disturbed psychophysical states. Non-conceptual awareness entails a meditative "emptying out of saturated information," in which concretization of sense information—attaching to, aversion to, and thinking about one's sensory experience—must be released to access the more subtle dimensions described here. For example, Fiorella notes that to listen from the subtle body, "one must refrain from grasping after a sound and attempting to make sense of it" (p. 10). Similarly, with visual experience, "it is possible to open towards the world in which we are imbedded without perceiving in a concretized way" (p. 10).

In this process of focusing on sensory experience through non-conceptual awareness, it is likely that the therapist will feel more permeable to—and thus more sensorily entwined in—the client's experience, even at one with it. On the one hand, this can feel disturbing to the therapist. Fiorella (2020) notes, "Corporeal becoming of (the client's) psychic reality . . . is potentially more destabilizing. Emptying out of saturated knowledge in the body invites in a level of inter-corporeal contact that can feel like being engulfed" (p. 17). For example, when a client reported a dream that so utterly, exactly, and uncannily mirrored my own from the previous night, I viscerally felt our psyches became entwined in the session. The hair on my neck and head stood up, chills went up my spine, and I felt as if the top of my skull expanded to the point that it dissolved. My consciousness seemed to fill up the room and crowd into the ceiling. The experience threw me totally off balance: my implicit belief that consciousness was located in separate, private minds was turned on its head (Peoples, 2021a).

Despite these disturbances to our sense of self, Fiorella (2020) emphasizes that the practice of non-conceptual awareness brings about a realization of the emptiness or *spaciousness* in which all phenomena exist. The therapist's capacity to root consciousness in emptiness allows one an expanded capacity to move toward, rather than away from, and to tolerate being with intense, chaotic, or disturbing psychophysical energies in the therapy.

Developing the Therapist's Capacity for Subtle Sensing

In contrast to the above, Bion (1970) believed it was necessary that the therapist shut out of awareness sensory stimuli from the body to "listen" deeply into the darkness of the unconscious field. Sensory inputs, he thought, too easily distract the mind of the therapist. However, I share Fiorella's (2020) view that the therapist working with non-ordinary states, much like in meditation, must stretch their attention through non-cognitive feeling awareness to open to sensory impressions arising through subtle channels while simultaneously refraining from preoccupation with sensations. As noted earlier, the therapist needs to be able to allow the circulation of sensory energies through the body and psyche without attaching premature conceptions or associations to it. This allows the *sensory containment* of subtle energies to occur silently in the background while the therapist's consciousness awaits the germination of symbolic material through their intuitive alpha function.

Sensory containment, I believe, can have a powerful transformative effect in its own right. Without ever having to put into words what is happening at this subtle level, clients can experience significant shifts in their sense of psychophysical coherence when this kind of containment through energetic at-one-ment occurs. The challenge for therapists is to strengthen and steady a flexible observing capacity while psychically extending their sensory, perceptual, and cognitive field until it is porous. As the essayist Annie Dillard writes, "The secret of seeing is to sail on solar wind. Hone and spread your spirit till you yourself are a sail, whetted, translucent, broadside to the merest puff" (Dillard, 1974, p. 33). In this way, the powerful energies evoked in non-ordinary states can become consciously stewarded in and through the body. The therapist's attention to the tightening and softening of their musculature and to attention on the flow of breath is key. Both sitting and moving meditation practices can support the expansion of these capacities.

Navigating the Tension Between Non-Conceptual Awareness and Associative Play

An important clinical question comes to the fore here: how does the therapist balance the tension between the more receptive position of surrendering into non-conceptual awareness and loosely flowing reverie, allowing alpha function to coalesce through intuition, and the more active position of entering the client's imaginal play space with one's own associations? This question needs to be considered in the context of the therapist's sense of the transference/countertrans-ference relationship in the moment.

By way of example, an astute middle-aged man who had years of psychoanalysis began exploring MDMA, psilocybin, and LSD outside of treatment. As someone who had devoted considerable attention to developing his intellect and his capacity to navigate intense psychic states, his investigations with psychedelics were aimed at opening his heart. He described how on one occasion, on a relatively light dose of LSD, he found himself uncharacteristically tapping into worry and grief for his young adult son, who was struggling with depression and anxiety. In the journey, the man gave himself over to his concern, feeling love for his son that he'd always known but which, in this moment, flooded him with a depth of feeling that was surprising. He could feel and "see" with his inner vision that he was holding his son in his arms.

Grief soon transformed into a river of love. With tears of gratitude for this immense feeling pouring through his open heart, the journeyer then had a vision of two "spirit guides" approaching him. He felt a twinge of fear. An experienced therapist who was assisting in the journey suggested he first steady himself by reconnecting with his body and sense of personal presence. He did so then checked to assess whether the guides felt safe to him. After a moment, he became clear of their benign nature and surrendered himself to what they had to teach him. For a long while, tears of astonishment and overwhelming joy poured through him for the gift of compassion and benevolence that the spirit guides were wordlessly bestowing on him.

What began as a personal exploration through intimate grief and love in the rela-tional sphere of his connection to his son evolved into a profoundly transpersonal encounter with spontaneously emerging sources of imaginal guidance and wisdom. Bourgault (2020), a writer in the Christian mystical tradition, describes the imagi-nal realm as "within—already coiled inside us as subtler and yet more intensively alive bandwidths of experience and perception" (p. 15). According to Bourgault, creative play with imaginal material occurs through "direct perception through the eye of the heart, not through mental reflection or fantasy" (p. 15).

This journeyer made clear that he could not have successfully stayed present enough to explore the transpersonal visions occurring in his experience had he not been accompanied by a skillful therapist throughout. When the image of the two beings stirred his anxiety, the journeyer needed help recognizing that he first needed to reestablish his personal boundaries. After doing so, he trusted that he could protect himself, that he could accurately assess his perceptions, and thus he could safely open to the information coming in. In this kind of multidimensional process, the therapist is tasked with listening to client communications, verbal and non-verbal, with an inner ear in formless reverie and the inner eye of the heart in the imaginal. This locates the therapist receptively in the dynamic flow of the con-scious/unconscious energy field.

Therapists thus need to hold their own associations loosely within, offering them as speculations in moments when the client appears receptive or stalled, sustaining a curious, spacious process of exploration. This models for the client a deep receptivity to material spontaneously arising between the known and the unknown. Likewise, the therapist's steady attunement to the emotional quality of the relationship in the moment is key. Tracking a client's receptivity to engagement vs. their absorption in internal experience, and noticing indirect transference allusions in clients' material, are part of the complex listening required of the therapist. In this respect, developments in both CP and JP theories of the unconscious offer a richly nuanced, comprehensive, and effective mode of approaching "the mystery of analytical work" (Sullivan, 2010, Pearson & Marlo, 2021).

Conclusion

The enriched potential that well-stewarded psychedelic therapy can provide the often lengthy process of depth psychotherapy is a heartening development. I believe an integrative psychoanalytic–psychedelic framework can ensure a deeply effective healing process, especially for clients wrestling with the damaging effects of early relational trauma. The opportunity to have a reparative relationship over time with a therapist is invaluable; the proper stewarding of the sacred space of therapy enables the containment of non-ordinary experiences, from primordial and preverbal to transcendent, including those states which psychedelics facilitate.

Psychoanalytic therapy has traditionally involved helping clients access the motivations, assumptions, and affects of their unconscious internal objects to bring about conscious acceptance of aspects of self that have been repressed, denied, or dissociated. Lessening the tendency toward splitting of "good" and "bad" parts, reducing the tendency to project these onto others, and facilitating the healthy mourning of loss have been seen as key to the psychic healing process, both in CP and JP orientations. Recent developments extending the model of consciousness in Freud's line to include "superconscious" and mystical states is in keeping with analysts in Jung's line who hold that access to the numinous archetypal dimension is part of the self's spiritual evolution.

Therapists in both traditions increasingly recognize the potential healing power of mystical and non-ordinary states. I have highlighted here how unitive mystical states in particular occasion a direct realization of the illusory nature of our constructs of self, other, and world, "evoking the experiential insight that these elements are constructions we dream into existence every moment" (J. Butler, personal communication, February 21, 2021). Dissolving the veil of apparent separation, mystical states provide a spontaneous felt sense of interconnectedness that often gives rise to profound feelings of gratitude and love. Unitive experiences instill faith in the potential for self and collective transformation through the unquestionable noetic, or truth quality, they impart. Similarly, transcendent moments of touching the Void can generate the sense of a containing "safer consciousness" (Dourley, 2007, p. 52) so that the mind can loosen its "claws" on its self-images and surrender into the unknown. "In quieting self-consciousness, we experience a space that is free from the contractions of personality and find our home in the greater freedom of our very being" (J. Butler, personal communication, February 21, 2021).

Connections with the numinous dimension are at the heart of psychospiritual transformation. Carl Jung (1973) believed that "the approach to the numinous is the real therapy," and that "only the experience of the numinous is capable of effecting any real healing transformation" (p. 377). Contemporary psychoanalysts in Freud's line who advocate for the therapist's "becoming O" with their clients' unconscious clearly recognize the uncanny transformative power of the unconscious. I believe both contact with the numinous and a trustworthy relationship with a skillful, depth-oriented "second" provide the containment so needed in our fraught personal and collective times.

I am sobered by awareness of the very real dangers and pitfalls that can be magnified by psychedelic use in therapy settings. It is incumbent on all clinicians who undertake psychedelic-assisted therapy to recognize the great care, seriousness, humility, and openness to learning that are necessary to carry this field safely forward for succeeding generations of therapists. I share the attitude of Rick Strassman (2001), DMT researcher, that, "It is so important for us to understand consciousness. It is just as important to place psychedelic drugs . . . into a personal and cultural matrix in which we do the most good, and the least harm" (p. xvii).

As therapists, when we surrender our desires, fears, and attachments to our identity, the "eye of the heart" tends to open, and we more readily enter the slipstream of the uncanny mystery of the vast unconscious. If fortunate, we become supported by the "holy mystery of love." I am hopeful for the movement toward collective, mutual healing and discovery among therapists working in the newly reopened field of psychedelic therapy, no longer hidden in the underground.

Notes

1   New York Times, Weekend Briefing, Sunday, December 20, 2020.
2   Jung differentiated between the personal self, or ego, and the transpersonal Self, which he defined as the "fullest potential and the unity of the personality as a whole. The self as a unifying principle within the human psyche occupies the central position of authority in relation to psychological life and, therefore, the destiny of the individual" (Samuels et al., 1986, p. 135). In describing his use of this notion, Jung noted, "As one can never distinguish empirically between a symbol of the Self and a God-image, the two ideas, however much we try to differentiate them, always appear blended together. . . . Psychologically speaking, the domain of 'gods' begins where consciousness leaves off, for at that point man is already at the mercy of the natural order" (Jung, 1954/1970, para. 231).
3   "The holy mystery of love" (O'Donovan, 2021).

References

Aberbach, D. (1987). Grief and mysticism. *International Review of Psycho-Analysis, 14,* 509–526.

Adams, W. (1995). Revelatory openness wedded with the clarity of unknowing: Psychoanalytic evenly-suspended attention, the phenomenological attitude, and meditative awareness. *Psychoanalysis and Contemporary Thought, 18*(4), 463–494.

Belser, A. (2019, June 1–2). A queer critique of the psychedelic "mystical experience". Conference presentation, Queering Psychedelics, Chacruna Institute, San Francisco, California. www.youtube.com/watch?v=Q78zlERKLTc

Benjamin, J. (2004). Beyond doer and done to: An intersubjective view of thirdness. *Psychoanalytic Quarterly, 73*(1), 5–46.

Bion, W. R. (1962). *Learning from experience*. Karnac.

Bion, W. R. (1967). Notes on memory and desire. *The Psychoanalytic Forum, 3*, 271–280.

Bion, W. R. (1970). *Attention and interpretation*. Karnac.

Bobrow, J. (2010). *Zen and psychotherapy: Partners in liberation*. Norton.

Bonder, S. (2004). *Healing the spirit/matter split*. Mt. Tam Empowerments, Inc.

Bourgault, C. (2020). *The eye of the heart: A spiritual journey into the imaginal realm*. Shambhala.

Carhart-Harris, R. L., Leech, R., Hellyer, P. J., Shanahan, M., Feilding, A., Tagliazucchi, E., Chialvo, D. R., & Nutt, D. (2014, February 3). The entropic brain: A theory of conscious states informed by neuroimaging research with psychedelic drugs. *Frontiers of Human Neuroscience*. https://doi.org/10.3389/fnhum.2014.00020

Corbett, L. (1996). *The Religious Function of the Psyche*. Routledge.

Davoine, F., & Gaudilliere, D. (2004). *History beyond trauma: Whereof one cannot speak, thereof one cannot stay silent*. Other Press.

Dillard, A. (1974). *Pilgrim at Tinker Creek*. Harper Perennial.

Dithrich, C. (2021). *Beta elements and the relational field*. Unpublished manuscript.

Dourley, J. (2007). Jung, some mystics, and the void. In P. Ashton (Ed.), *Evocations of absence: Multidisciplinary perspectives on void states, Ch. 3*. Spring Journal Books.

Eliade, M. (1959). *The sacred and the profane: The nature of religion*. Harcourt, Brace, Jovanovich.

Elliott, A., & Spezzano, C. (Eds.). (2000). *Psychoanalysis at its limits: Navigating the postmodern turn*. Free Association Books.

Eshel, O. (2019). *The emergence of analytic oneness: Into the heart of psychoanalysis*. Routledge.

Fiorella, K. (2020). *Thinking in a marrow bone*. Unpublished manuscript.

Freud, S. (1930). Civilization and its discontents. *The Standard Edition of the Complete Psychological Works of Sigmund Freud, 21*, 57–146.

Gonzales, F. (2020). Trump cards and Klein bottles: On the collective of the individual. *Psychoanalytic Dialogues, 30*(4), 383–398. https://doi.org/10.1080/10481885.2020.1774335

Griffiths, R., Richards, W., McCann, U. R., & Jesse, R. (2006). Psilocybin can occasion mystical-type experiences having substantial and sustained personal meaning and spiritual significance. *Psychopharmacology (Berl), 187*(3), 268–283.

Grof, S. (2008). *LSD psychotherapy*. Hunter House.

Grotstein, J. (2000). *Who is the dreamer who dreams the dream?* Analytic Press.

Grotstein, J. (2007). *A beam of intense darkness*. Karnac.

Guralnik, O., & Simeon, D. (2010). Depersonalization: Standing in the spaces between recognition and interpellation. *Psychoanalytic Dialogues, 20*(4), 400–416.

Hill, S. J. (2019). *Confrontation with the unconscious: Jungian depth psychology and psychedelic experience*. Aeon Books.

Hillman, J. (1975). *Re-visioning psychology*. Harper & Row.

Hixon, L. (1992). *Great swan: Meetings with Ramakrishna*. Shambhala.

Hopper, E. (2003). *The social unconscious: Speaking the unspeakable*. Jessica Kingsley Publishers.

James, W. (1902/1982). *The varieties of religious experience*. Penguin Classics.

Jung, C. G. (1954/1970). A psychological approach to the dogma of the trinity. In H. Read, M. Fordham, G. Adler, & W. McGuire (Eds.), *The collected works of C. G. Jung* (R. F. C. Hull, Trans.) (Vol. 11, pp. 107–200). Princeton University Press. (Original work published 1942).

Jung, C. G. (1973). *Conscious, unconscious and individuation: The archetypes and the collective unconscious* (2nd ed., pp. 275–289). Princeton University Press.

Kalsched, D. (1996). *The inner world of trauma: Archetypal defenses of the personal spirit*. Routledge.

Kalsched, D. (2013). *Trauma and the soul*. Routledge.

Kurtz, S. (1989). *The art of unknowing: Dimensions of openness in analytic therapy*. Aronson.

Layton, L., Hollander, N. C., & Gutwill, S. (2006). *Psychoanalysis, class and politics*. Routledge.

Letheby, C., & Gerrans, P. (2017). Self unbound: Ego dissolution in psychedelic experience. *Neuroscience of Consciousness, 2017*(1). https://doi.org/10.1093/nc/nix016

MacLean, K., Johnson, M., & Griffiths, R. (2013, November). Mystical experiences occasioned by the hallucinogen psilocybin lead to increases in the personality domain of openness. *Journal of Psychopharmacology, 25*(11), 1453–1461. https://doi.org/10.1177/0269881111420188

Mayer, E. L. (2007). *Extraordinary knowing: Science, skepticism, and the inexplicable powers of the human mind*. Bantam Books.

O'Donovan, L. (2021, January 20). Presidential inaugural invocation. Washington, DC.

Ogden, T. (1994). The analytic third: Working with intersubjective clinical facts. *International Journal of Psychoanalysis, 75*, 3–19.

Parsons, W. (1999). *The enigma of the oceanic feeling: Revisioning the psychoanalytic theory of mysticism*. Oxford University Press.

Pearson, W., & Marlo, H. (2021). *The spiritual psyche in psychotherapy: Mysticism, intersubjectivity and psychoanalysis*. Routledge.

Peoples, K. (2000). Why the self is, and is not, empty: Traumatic and transcendent forms of emptiness. In A. Elliott & C. Spezzano (Eds.), *Psychoanalysis at its limits: Navigating the postmodern turn*. Free Association Books.

Peoples, K. (2021a, July). *When our hair stands on end: Encounters with non-ordinary states*. Conference presentation, International Psychoanalytic Association Congress, online.

Peoples, K. (2021b, October). *When the analytic third includes a psychedelic*. Conference presentation, Oregon Psychoanalytic Center, online.

Pontalis, J. B. (2003). *Windows*. University of Nebraska Press.

Purrington, (2020, September 15). Carl Jung's letter to Betty Grover Eisner [on mescaline]. *Carl Jung Depth Psychology*. https://carljungdepthpsychologysite.blog/2020/09/15/carl-jungs-letter-to-betty-grover-eisner-on-mescaline-2/

Richards, W. A. (2016). *Sacred knowledge: Psychedelics and religious experiences*. Columbia University Press.

Rundel, M. (2020). *Psychoanalysis and psychedelics: Convergences and divergences*. Unpublished manuscript.

Safran, J. (2003). *Psychoanalysis and Buddhism: An unfolding dialogue*. Wisdom Publications.

Samuels, A. (1985). *Jung and the post-Jungians*. Routledge.

Samuels, A., Shorter, B., & Plaut, F. (1986). *A critical dictionary of Jungian analysis*. Routledge.

Schwartz, H. (2013). *The alchemy of wolves and sheep: A relational approach to internalized perpetration in complex trauma survivors*. Routledge.

Stauffer, C. (2021, July). *Psychoanalysis and psychedelic-assisted therapy: A fortuitous alliance*. Conference presentation, International Psychoanalytic Association Congress, online.

Stauffer, C., Anderson, B., Ortigo, K., & Woolley, J. (2020, October). Psilocybin-assisted group therapy and attachment: Observed reduction in attachment anxiety and influences of attachment insecurity on the psilocybin experience. *ACS Pharmacology and Translation Science*. https://dx.doi.org/10.1021/acsptsci.0c00169

Stern, D. B. (2013). Field theory in psychoanalysis, Part 2: Bionian field theory and contemporary interpersonal/relational psychoanalysis. *Psychoanalytic Dialogues, 23*(6), 630–645.

Strassman, R. (2001). *DMT: The spirit molecule*. Park Street Press.

Suchet, M. (2016). Surrender, transformation, and transcendence. *Psychoanalytic Dialogues, 26*, 747–760.

Sullivan, B. S. (2010). *The mystery of analytical work: Weavings from Jung and Bion*. Routledge.

Tart, C. (1972). *Altered states of consciousness*. Doubleday.

Van der Kolk, B. (2015). *The body keeps the score: Brain, mind, and body in the healing of trauma*. IDreamBooks.

Vermote, R. (2021). The infantile mind. Conference presentation, International Psychoanalytic Association Congress, online.

White, J. (Ed.). (2012). *The highest state of consciousness*. White Crow Books.

Wilber, K. (1995). *Sex, ecology, spirituality: The spirit of evolution*. Shambhala.

Williams, S. (2019). *When trauma is a portal to the numinous: A Jungian perspective on numinous experience and psychedelic-enhanced psychotherapy*. Unpublished manuscript.

Yaden, D., Nguyen, K., Kern, M., Belser, A., Eichstaedt, J., Iwry, J., Smith, M., Wintering, N., Hood, R., & Newberg, A. (2017). Of roots and fruits: A comparison of psychedelic and non-psychedelic mystical experiences. *Journal of Humanistic Psychology, 57*(4), 338–353.

Chapter 10

Invoking the Numinous

Ritual, Medicine, and Magic in Psychedelic Psychotherapy

Camara Rajabari and Shanna Butler

Introduction

As authors of this chapter, we come together from both common and disparate standpoints, identities, and social locations to explore the concept of ritual. This exploration is informed by our lived experiences and our clinical work. Together, we have brought forward a multiplicity of ways to consider ritual within the context of psychedelic therapy. In Part 1 of this chapter, Butler describes some ways to define and contextualize ritual, moves on to consider cultural appropriation and the harms that result from members of dominant cultures reifying colonizer dynamics in the name of spirituality, and concludes with exploration and examples of ritual that center social justice values. The second half of the chapter brings a first-person narrative from Rajabari, in which she explores the concept of ritual and ceremony and the influential foundations of the Black Church and African traditional religions (ATRs) in her understanding of ritual and ceremony, and concludes with a descriptive reflection of her journey toward becoming a psychedelic psychotherapist.

Part 1

Seeking the Mysteries Through Ritual

The urge to seek the truth in one's suffering is as ancient as human existence. Seeded by the fundamental quality of curiosity, the human drive toward meaning is inevitable (Jung, 1977). The seekers and healers of all time, those who have gone before us and walked the labyrinth, treaded their path toward both the knowable and unknowable and sought the mysteries of the self, knew the importance of ritual as a means toward individuation (Chrzescijansk, 2017; Jung, 1972). Ritual is a container in which meaning is sought. Ritual is where mysteries unfold, where the universe whispers ancient secrets, where life-shaping patterns unabashedly show themselves, and where ecstasy soars and sorrow weeps. Ritual is the place where the deities arrive and commune with their human counterparts. Sacred wisdom springs forth in ritual, and grief has a place to shed another layer of its pain. Ritual

DOI: 10.4324/9781003167976-10

holds us, nurtures the soul outward, shines light into dark corners, and envelops brightness in the rich cloak of darkness. Ritual is where magic happens.

Ritual is both intention and surrender. It is directed hope. Ritual can be a sturdy foundation upon which a spiritual life, a noble quest, or a meaningful existence is built. To engage in ritual is to make sacred space from ordinary space. Ritual is as old as humans, with practices found across time and culture (Campbell, 1988; Jung, 1970). In a mythological sense, ritual helps us traverse the underworld by providing guidance, structure, and meaning even or especially in the midst of suffering. Persephone's consumption of the pomegranate seeds (Downing, 1994), Inanna's surrender of her royal protections (Wolkstein, 1983), and brokenhearted Orpheus' (Ovid, 2005) long walk back home were rituals that deepened painful events into meaningful experiences. It is the trail of breadcrumbs, a tether from our ordinary existence to the presence of divinity, to the numinous. Ritual offers instructions for moving between the realms of the self and the realms of the collective.

For many, ritual brings to mind images of sacred rites, well preserved mysteries, secret spells, and moonlit gatherings in the wild. While these images may be some of what ritual contains, it is not limited to ineffable acts nor reserved for use by the most seasoned of healers. Ritual belongs to all of us. While sacred indeed, the art of ritual is not restricted for those with certain skills or experience but rather is a purposefully constructed container that when imbued with desire and intention becomes an enigmatic third being: alive, active, generative, with limitless potential, and accessible by all.

For many cultures across time, ritual was the cornerstone upon which societies were built (Campbell, 1988), a shared space where healing, reverence, gratitude, and connection could occur. For cultures both historic and contemporary, ritual also includes the use of sacred plant medicine (Fotiou, 2020). From the use of peyote by Indigenous people of the American southwest and Mexico, iboga by West African communities, to psilocybin by Indigenous peoples in Mexico, the use of plant medicines in ritual space facilitates transcendence and serves as a vital cultural touchstone and a central support woven into the fabric of every day.

Colonization and Cultural Theft

Many cultures have, over time, cultivated and practiced unique rituals aimed toward enhancement of particular lived experiences and meaning making. There has also been a massive disruption of cultural practices and sacred ritual due to the violence of white body supremacy[1] and the heinous acts of colonization carried out by white Western people. For centuries, colonizers, imbued with lust for greed and power, have oppressed Indigenous peoples across the globe. Their aim at disrupting access to cultural practices and suppressing the wisdom of a particular culture served to instill hierarchy and domination through the traumatization of the social order; systematic dismantling of local structures; and, perhaps most poignantly, through stripping access to spiritual practices that form the backbone of social order and cultural meaning (Fotiou, 2020; George et al., 2020). Borrowing or non-reciprocal taking from other cultures is a direct result of white supremacy and the social privileges afforded to white individuals as a result of racist systems of domination. Taking what one wants without regard and acknowledgment and without permission or reciprocation is the heart of a colonizing psychological mindset that perpetuates oppression. The impact of colonization holds different meaning for each group affected; however, common themes of oppression include diminishment of vital resources, stolen land, forced relocation, conversion attempts away from Indigenous spiritual practices, erasure of native languages, criminalization of ritual practices, and the stripping of access to sacred plant medicines (George et al., 2020; Noel, 1987).

The story of Maria Sabina offers sharp insight into the impact of white Western intrusion and appropriation of the psilocybin mushroom ceremonies. Maria Sabina, born in 1894, was a Mazatec *curandera*, or healer who lived in a small village in Oaxaca, Mexico. She was revered for her healing abilities through the channeling of the wisdom of the psilocybin mushroom (Allen, 1997; Noel, 1987). Having encountered the *ninos santos* or saint children (psilocybin mushrooms) at a young age, Sabina cultivated her healing abilities in spiritual relationship to the psilocybin mushroom over the course of her life. In 1955, Gordon and Valentina Wasson, mycological researchers, visited Sabina's village, studying both the psilocybin mushroom itself as well as observing and participating in healing ceremonies facilitated by Sabina. Wasson's experience became "the first documented instance of outsiders being invited to participate in the Mazatec mushroom velada" (Stephen, 2020). Wasson recorded and published Sabina's ceremonial practices, "initially obscuring the location of the rite, and granting Sabina the alias of 'Eva Mendez'" (Stephen, 2020). After publishing his account in *Life* magazine, without Maria Sabina's consent, he shared her name and the name of her village, profoundly disrupting her life.

What followed was massive tourism from white Western people. These tourists were seeking enlightenment and implored Sabina to engage them in ritual with psilocybin. This type of tourism brought sharp criticism toward Sabina from her neighbors as well as the state government. Sabina found herself the subject of threats, violence, and further impoverishment, and was even jailed for a time (Allen, 1997). Her religious practice was raided by Mexican authorities, her home burned down, and her son murdered. She eventually died in destitute in 1985 (Stephen, 2020). Despite these harrowing challenges, Sabina continued offering her potent healing ceremonies facilitated by the psilocybin mushroom, frequently not charging for her work.

Sabina's story is not uncommon. The white gaze of the colonizer has long sought to consume the spiritual teachings of Indigenous cultures without centering the well-being of both the culture and the people from whom they seek the healing. The participation of white Western people in cultural practices not their own has frequently resulted in exploitation and significant lasting harm (Allen, 1997; Noel, 1987; Trichter, 2010).

White Supremacy Culture and Cultural Appropriation

Cultural appropriation and the history of white Western healers acquiring and commodifying spiritual practices from other cultures have caused tremendous, and in some instances, irreparable destruction toward the originating culture from whom the sacred teachings and rituals were taken (Mosley & Biernat, 2020; Taylor, 1997). The illness that is white supremacy has frequently separated white Western people from their innate connection to their spiritual self. The Christian church holds some responsibility in this division through its historical efforts to divide white Europeans from their ancestral connection to nature-based spirituality, which allowed direct access to the numinous. The massive hunting and killing of women who practiced herbalism and midwifery and were believed to be witches is a primary example of this separation through oppression (Ehrenreich, 2010).

Christian values uphold a system of religion that includes the necessity of an intermediary between humans and the divine, a role typically held by a priest or minister. While debatable as to the meaning and purpose of this practice, the outcome is often an overreliance on an external source to fulfill one's spiritual connection. If a satisfying spirituality is dependent on the approval of a human proxy, it makes access to this divine source tenuous at best. The result is a massive inner void that seeks fulfillment through material substances via capitalism (Barton, 2020). The ethos of entitlement and consumption of others' cultural practices is an attempt to assuage a vacuous emptiness that is unique to white identity and forged from the dredges of Christian values, supremacy, and racism. White supremacy teaches white people that anything and anyone is there for one's own purpose, satisfaction, and eventual disposal. Equity, respect, and boundaries are not part of the equation (Cushman, 1995; DiAngelo, 2012; Herzberg & Butler, 2019).

Whether we are considering the legacy of Maria Sabina and the unintentional sacrifices she made in introducing psilocybin to the white Western people or looking at the contemporary practices of spiritual tourism and those seeking the healing benefits of Ayahuasca in the South American jungles, it is vital that an ethical frame of cultural engagement be enacted. If our rituals are rooted in conscious or unconscious harm, it cannot be called healing. If efforts to liberate oneself oppress another, it cannot be true liberation.

Ritual as Social Justice

Creating ritual free of cultural appropriation centers an ethic that goes beyond the personal and extends toward collective care and liberation. If what is being sought is a psychological and/or spiritual experience rooted in integrity, it is imperative we think through all aspects of our actions and work to decolonize our practices. For those who hold white privilege, that means doing the work every day to understand the ways we have been conditioned to take, to harm, and to exercise dominance. This type of reflective accountability to dismantling inner and outer oppressive structures can also be a sacred ritual.

Some questions to consider when engaging in ritual, whether it be in the context of psychedelics or otherwise, are the following: *Where does this practice originate from? How did I learn to do what I am doing? Do I understand my full intention in this practice? Who benefits and who is harmed by my engagement with this practice? Does this practice hail from my own lineage? Can I connect more deeply with my own cultural traditions? If I feel disconnected from my cultural lineage, why is that? Is there reciprocity with the culture's traditions that I am engaging? If a ritualized practice is being shared freely with me from another culture, how am I giving back, uplifting and centering the needs of that group?*

Psychedelic Therapy and Ritual

A ritual is an intentional act. Knowing why we wish to engage in ritual allows for ample freedom, spontaneity, and creativity. Some rituals might include a great deal of planning, whereas others arrive in the moment and ask to be lived out spontaneously. Rituals appreciate a container whether spontaneous or planned.

Psychedelic therapy offers a significant opportunity to amplify the healing power of the therapy space by consciously enhancing the process of inner exploration. In the context of psychedelic therapy, ritual can be uniquely tailored to the person as they are in that moment in time. It can be playful, ruckus, joyous, silent, or grief filled. As psychedelic therapists, we have the opportunity to support our patients in building a sturdy container, in which we wait to see what or who arrives, where we can greet the unknowable.

Ritual can be found in the act of playing music, singing a song, lighting a candle, using divination cards, burning herbs, reciting poetry, dancing, silence, meditation, guided imagery, letter writing, anointing the body, bodywork, or somatic touch. Ritual makes space for the ancestral and imaginal realms to join participants in their efforts to heal. The invisible supports that lie just beyond our edges of conscious awareness wait patiently for an opportunity to arrive and mingle. Many a ritual becomes imbued with ancestors and elders, animal friends, guides, angels, deities, and beings beyond description. When the container is set, the arrival of help and support is limitless.

Reclaiming Ritual

Reclaiming the act of making ritual is important as the field of psychedelic therapy continues to unfold. By maintaining the lineages of sacred reverence for psychedelic use, we offer a veneration of the history of psychedelic medicines across time and space. Both contemporary Western practitioners working in the underground for decades as well as the long and vast lineages of people that have engaged with an expansive array of psychedelic medicines as part of ritual, ceremony, and cultural rites of passage for centuries know that it is not only the substance but the context, the set and setting, that supports curative potential. Furthermore, to adhere to an inclusion of ritual making supports psychedelic therapy in retaining its sacred form as safeguard against the over-medicalization of these medicines as legalization is ongoingly achieved.

For someone who is new to ritual making, whether it be the client or the psychotherapist, there are many ways to begin to introduce this practice. Investigating one's own lineage is a good place to start. When possible, delving into one's personal cultural connections can offer a rich opportunity for increased awareness and integration of past and present. For some, looking at personal cultural backgrounds is not possible due to lack of access, familial traumas, or unknown legacies. In these instances, when personal cultural lineages are unknown or a source of distress, we can turn toward the present moment and the natural world to harvest creativity and inspiration. In fact, this type of attunement is available to all of us regardless of personal cultural connection.

Turning toward the natural world is a universally accessible way of constructing ritual and begins with dually observing our dynamic outer environments and the landscapes of our inner world. There, we begin to see the images, the shapes, the metaphors, the colors, and the inner and outer symbols that thread each of us together. Nature performs rituals all day every day, such as the mighty oak outside my window that sheds its leaves each fall in a courageous act of letting go, or the vulture that swoops the air, which knows the alchemical ritual of putrefaction to purification as it consumes rotted carnage and then spreads its wings to drip the digested and transmuted substance from its body back to the earth to become vibrant compost. The ocean can tell countless tales of the way in which life ebbs and flows like waves.

As humans, we too can relate. We are the serpent that finds the stillness to shed our skin, or the chrysalis still in liquid form, no longer a caterpillar not quite a butterfly. We are the bear emerging from hibernation, hungry for nourishment, ready to introduce our newly born to the world. We are the moon, rising and setting, moving phase by phase from complete darkness to our full light. Harvesting these images as foundation for a ritual magnifies our personal work to include the collective rhythms that surround us all. We do not need to reach beyond what is present to us to find meaning and connection.

Examples of Ritual in Psychedelic Therapy

It would be remiss to not concretize the ethereal. The following therefore outlines how to initiate, construct, and carry out a ritual during psychedelic therapy sessions.

The preparation session is an excellent place to begin eliciting your client's vision for their journey ahead. We can then explore our client's relationship to ritual or constructing an intentional container. *What are their associations to the concept of ritual? What language are they most comfortable using to describe a purposeful container for their journey? What is their intention for engaging in the work? Are there images, symbols, archetypes, or metaphors that they are aware of in relation to this experience?* By collecting these thoughts, images, and emotions, both client and therapist are gathering vital ingredients to support the unfolding of desire and its symbolic representations as it relates to the client's forthcoming medicine session.

An altar or designated special location is often a helpful inclusion in ritual space and can be a supportive way to ground the intention into a physical manifestation. During the medicine session, the altar can be a place to return, to connect with meaning, find comfort, and access inspiration. If an altar is desired, the preparation session is an important time to invite imagination into the objects and items that will be included. In addition to altar items, it is helpful to think concretely about other supplies needed for the medicine session. Does the client wish to play special music, have access to art supplies, or read poetry? By giving solid consideration to details during preparation sessions, both therapist and client can arrive at the medicine session with a sense of direction and freedom. The following offers brief clinical examples of how ritual can be both planned and spontaneous, a sacred container for the numinous to enter.

Case Example (A)

A client whose intention was to work with her body and particularly her chest, which had endured trauma, created a ritual, in which she told the story of her trauma while focusing on her chest and upper torso. During periods of inward silence, she focused her energy on that part of her body and, as planned in the preparation session, periodically asked for physical contact on that body part from her therapist. To close the session, she found gentle movement with her chest and upper torso while sharing insight gleaned from the journey.

Case Example (B)

Another client had endured a devastating death of a loved one and felt partially responsible for the loss. His intention was to explore and challenge the part of himself that continued to feel at fault. During the preparation session, he explored the image of compost and the delightful feeling evoked when imagining his pain transforming into something fertile. He wanted to be supported by trees as he entered a compost state. On the day of the medicine session, he brought in leaves and branches from his yard to adorn the altar. While spending time inward, he allowed himself to release the bound-up pain and offer it as future soil. He also was able to connect with an image of the deceased loved one and experience shared space, in which the pain of this death could be mutually attended to. He emerged from his journey with a sense of renewal and readiness to embody the sturdiness of trees.

Clinical Example (C)

A final clinical example comes from a patient whose intention was to understand their dissociated body states. They had a sense that dissociation was connected to a very lost young part of themselves. For the medicine session, they brought in childhood photos and spent some time sharing about the photos and the young person in them. As a singer, they wanted to find a way to bring ritual sound to the experience, so they also brought in some special music that they associated with their young self. As they spent time inward, they found themselves in conversation with this young part, who expressed feeling unwanted and unloved. As this client emerged from their inward space, they played the music that they had brought and sang to their younger self. What resulted was a newfound intertwinement with this young part, where previously there had just been silence.

By making space for ritual in psychedelic therapy sessions, we have the opportunity to amplify the clinical work by concretizing the spiritual into the material through symbolic acts. As exemplified, ritual enlivens and deepens intentions and gives shape and guidance to medicine sessions. Ritual offers a lasting practice for our clients, one that supports immediate access to the inner work accomplished simply by connecting back to parts of the unique ritual container co-created in the psychedelic session.

We now turn to Rajabari, who explores from a first-person narration the way ritual, ceremony, and culture have forged a spirituality grounded in her lived experience as well as the incorporation of new and old traditions that have resulted in her current offerings as a psychedelic psychotherapist.

Part 2

The Human Life Cycle, Ritual, and Culture

In many cultures, there are a series of rituals that follow us throughout the life cycle of conception, birth, aging, death, and rebirth. I imagine that the first ritual space that we occupy is in the womb. Regardless of how conception took place, we are all sparked into existence, seeded, and shaped while in utero. Ritual guides our connection to the earth, creation, our people, our world view, and our understanding of Self. It helps us root into an awareness that much of life is a mystery—we cannot see or claim to know much of what we come into contact with. Ritual gives us a container in which to cultivate our connection with the unknown.

The Southern Black Church and Ritual

Forced to convert to Christianity, early enslaved Africans wove their traditional cosmologies into the religion of the colonizers. As the Bible was taught and remained in the forefront of Christian worship, enslaved Africans found ways to integrate ritual and ceremony that held the wisdom of their African ancestors. The early Black Church became a powerful repository of ritual and also served as a safe space for meaning making, community, and political organizing. Barnes (2005, pp. 969–970) proposed that rituals, songs, sayings, sacred meetings, and biblical stories helped Black congregations interpret events, focus efforts, and provide organizational vision.

Growing up in the southern Black Baptist and African Methodist Church, I was taught that the entity called God is unknowable. I grew up hearing, "God acts in mysterious ways," which reinforced the idea of a powerful entity that existed outside the bounds of human understanding. The Southern Black Church was considered a safe and secure container for self-expression in the Black community. Services included prayer, meditation, hymns, dedications, sermons, and devotional songs. Sacred ritual space was cultivated for the "calling in" of the "Holy Ghost," who was always invited and oftentimes invoked by a good sermon or even a powerful song. Depending on the church community, the Holy Ghost was the force of Spirit (God) and allowed for the transmission of emotional expression.

Growing up in the church, I knew how to recognize the energy of the Holy Ghost in the sensations of my embodying the energy of the congregation. I could feel the temperature change as the environment became warmer, and there was a certain pitch from the orator or singer that sent out an energetic beacon. When the Holy Ghost arrived, it sometimes occurred through "possession," in which a congregant served as a vehicle for the expression of God. Other practitioners helped those possessed by the Holy Ghost to stay safe in their expression. They fanned them and held them in comfort until the Holy Ghost left their body. It was considered a powerful and sacred moment to be possessed by the Spirit of the Holy Ghost. It meant you had surrendered to the ritual space and received the gift of God within.

Although I have shifted my spiritual practice away from the Christian religion, I credit the Southern Black Church and community with helping me to understand the role of ritual in relation to altered states of consciousness. The Southern Black Church community also modeled how to nurture and care for people in altered states. You allowed them to move, express, and emote while supporting them in staying safe in their body. The space was contained, so people could not run out of the church or engage in dangerous behavior. As the person returned to their ordinary state, no one shamed, questioned, or pathologized them or their experience. It was understood that they were experiencing a state beyond the community's current reality, and that they were being healed.

African Traditional Religion and Ritual

When I began to reconnect with ATRs, such as the West African Yoruba, Vodun, and Akan traditions, I immediately recognized passed down rituals, symbols, prayer styles, and movement practices that survived the Transatlantic Slave Trade and the traumatic oppression of chattel slavery. My ancestors kept their traditional practices alive by secretly integrating them into the Christian belief system. For example, in the Yoruba religion, deities were often syncretized with Catholic saints, like Saint Barbara for Shango or the Virgin Mary for Yemaya (Udo, 2020, p. 31). These practices assisted enslaved Africans in retaining a connection to their spirituality while adhering to strict laws that forbade the practice of African religion.

At the first Akan ritual ceremony I attended, I witnessed the possession of Spirit in an initiated practitioner. The Spirit then danced among the community, eating ritual foods and offering consultation to attendees. ATR ceremonies include significant preparation for ritual, which is often an all-day affair. Prayers and divination may take place to make sure the ritual space has the approval of the deities.

West African shaman Malidoma Somé of Burkina Faso observed that in the West, ceremony is often interchanged with ritual. Somé (1999, p. 143) explained that ceremonies are predictable—everyone knows what to expect, and the process and the outcome are clear—while ritual is "spontaneous and unpredictable." Somé (1999, p. 189) further observed that, particularly in the West, pre-existing assumptions, the need for control, and fear of the unknown can get in the way of opening to the spontaneous arisings that can come from ritual practices. For Somé, "reverence" and "trust" are essential first steps to rendering the ritual space sacred and safe enough to "embrace the possibilities for healing." "Ritual is like a journey," he states, "Before you begin, you own the journey; once the ritual begins, the journey owns you" (Somé, 1999, p. 190). African traditions hold that the unknown element of the ritual space is what allows the power of divine wisdom to express itself and facilitate healing.

My Journey With Sacred Medicine

My personal journey with substances begins with my father. My dad was a dynamic and charismatic personality; people loved him. He grew up in the southern United States during the Jim Crow era and told me countless stories about being Black in the South and of the traumas my family endured. Like many young adults during his time, my dad participated in the Great Migration of African Americans from the South to the Northern and Western United States. He had dreams of moving to California to live a life that was "free" of racism and filled with opportunities—experiences he never realized. He struggled with substance use most of his adult life and died in the early 1990s from an overdose.

Having grown up with a parent who struggled with substance use disorder and mental health issues, I went through my own complex feelings about substances. Parts of me felt like "drugs" had ruined my father's life and deeply impacted my early childhood, while other parts of me wondered whether substances also served as a resource for my father, helping to dull the pain of trauma, intergenerational wounding, and historical harms.

Years ago, in a religious ceremony, I felt the power of plant medicine and its ability to open me up to intergenerational healing. I understood in the tender moments of the ritualized ceremony what my African elders of the Akan traditions would say: "we stand on the shoulders of our Ancestors"—meaning we get our strength and knowledge from those who came before us. In the Adinkra language, this process is called Sankofa, which means to "retrace one's steps, return to one's roots." Experiencing the deep connection of my ancestral bloodline through ritual left me with a powerful image of sitting at the feet of Divine Mother with all my ancestors known and unknown. Ritual helped me to connect to my lineage's creation story, in which there was no beginning and no end.

Becoming a Psychedelic-Assisted Therapist

I identify as a spiritualist and an artist. I believe in the psychospiritual power of art and healing. I was introduced to the field of psychedelic-assisted therapy in a class on psychopharmacology and was immediately drawn to this area of study. In many ways, it naturally made sense to me that psychedelics could assist us in healing through NOSC. After I graduated, I trained with Sage Institute (sageinst. org) and MAPS. The decision to pursue training in psychedelic-assisted therapy has deepened my inquiry into the potential to heal intergenerational trauma through arts-based ancestral veneration and ritual.

The Potential of Ritual in Psychedelic-Assisted Therapy

I have come to imagine an energetic thread that connects the many spiritual teachings and psychological theories I embrace as a clinician. In my early training with MAPS, I was struck by the teaching of allowing the client to access and trust their "inner healing intelligence," supported by the non-directive presence of the clinician (Mithoefer, 2016, p. 8). This philosophy resonated with the humanistic psychological view of the client as the expert of their own experience and the therapist as an empathetic collaborator. MAPS also encouraged embracing the Eastern philosophical concept of the "beginner's mind" as a way of staying open to whatever arises in session with a client. I connect this with Somé's observation that Westerners' tendency to grasp for control is "antithetical to ritual" (1999, p. 190), and instead we must remain open and humble to what emerges from the client's experience.

As a therapist who seeks to integrate ancestral wisdom, creative arts, and Western psychotherapy, I find myself wanting to bridge my culture and relationship to ritual with my therapeutic approach as well as my client's experiences. For example, I was trained by Western institutions to evaluate and diagnose using evidence-based tools; yet, my social, cultural, and political beliefs hold diagnosis with more complexity. I consider the impact of generational wounds, historical harms, and systemic oppression on mental health. The ritual space I hold in psychedelic-assisted therapy is trauma informed, client centered, and imaginal. I hold intentional space for whatever needs to be embodied and expressed—grief, joy, anger, and the unknown.

I began to visualize a ritualized creative process, in which I imagined a psychedelic-assisted journey between a therapist and a client as a circle within a circle. Leaning into Somé's thoughts on ceremony, the outer circle symbolizes the preparation and the clinical environment—the *container* for the session. As the therapist, I would create the "ceremony" of tending to the "set and setting" through preparation: a predictable process that includes such considerations as cultivating emotional safety, discussing consent for the use of touch, being a resource for the client by attending to their needs, and making agreements around when and how to initiate communication after the client has taken the medicine as well as what steps to take in an emergency.

The inner circle represented by a dotted line is the "ritual" aspect of the session, where there is space to trust the divine inner wisdom of the client and the medicine by inviting in the fluidity of intention and trusting the imagery, visions, and psychic content that spontaneously emerge as material in service of healing. The dotted circle is permeable. It makes space for the process of ritual, where the client can bring in dreams from the night before the session and synchronistic experiences that point to their transition into ritual space. I have witnessed "ritual guides" show up as crow cawing outside, the imagery of a beloved ancestor, or a smell that reminds the client of childhood. In these moments, I encourage curiosity around the appearance of these guides. What message do they bring regarding the client's healing process? Can the client use their own divine inner wisdom to connect to the entirety of their medicine experience? Somé (1999) described ritual as "not stepping into the same river twice" and further explained, "the Indigenous belief is that a ritual happens only once and is never repeated again (p. 191)." It is important that the clinician recognize that the ritual space of the psychedelic session is dynamic. The therapist cannot be a passive participant with a clinical gaze but instead must seek to balance the tension between the outer circle of safe, secure containment and the inner dotted circle, offering careful clinical holding alongside spaciousness for spontaneous arising.

Ancestral Work and Appropriation Within Psychedelic-Assisted Therapy

I was introduced to ancestral healing work through a teacher of the Sangoma tradition of South Africa. I was taught to work with elements of the earth and to utilize my intuitive knowledge as a tool to access the Spirit realm. I also was taught about the reciprocal nature of divine relationship with Spirit and our ancestors. In many ATRs, there are protocols for how and when we communicate with Spirit and ancestors. A large majority of African and Indigenous traditions are closed— not accessible to people outside of family and community bloodlines. Breaking these "rules" or guidelines could result in unforeseen circumstances or catastrophic events. For years, people in the West have extracted spiritual practices of Black and Brown cultures without permission or understanding of the context of such practices. This is why great care and respect are essential when engaging in spiritual practices that involve a culture other than your own.

Ancestor work, ritual, and ceremony differ across cultures and communities. A practice that is open to everyone in one community may be completely closed in another. The act of "calling in" ancestors, using certain ceremonial herbs/plants/roots, prayers, symbols/images, and certain instruments/songs, could be very offensive if you are not initiated and/or have no traditional lineage connections or personal relationship with the practices or spiritual tools you are using.

I consider myself an ancestral psychotherapist and find ancestral work to be a powerful component of ritual practice when held in a good way. In a clinical setting, ancestral work invites in the exploration of intergenerational resilience and healing. I have experienced clients seeking to work with ancestral healing who have no formal connection to ancestral work. I spend time speaking with them about their desire for ancestral healing. I offer the guidance of my own teachers, which suggests that we only invite in the energy of those ancestors who are evolved and are ready/willing to work with the client. I support them in bringing in familial objects, photos, and/or symbols that connect them with their healed ancestors. I also offer the idea that they could begin by simply setting an intention to know their ancestors better.

Integrating Ritual Respectfully

As a clinician, I make myself available to support clients in developing a relationship with the unknown. I center the client in setting up the "ritual" space by inviting in their cultural and community practices. I ask what they would like my role to be in any ritual or spiritual work they wish to introduce to their session. I also let it be known that I do not need any role, and it could be possible that they may need privacy before the session or afterward to open and close their ritual space. If they have specific concerns about spiritual practices, I work with them to find a safe way to respect the sacredness of their work while understanding my role as a clinician, and personal Spiritual practices could be intrusive if not held in a good way. A primary example of this is time. The earliest and most powerful lesson I learned reconnecting with my cultural traditional practices was that "spirit has its own time," meaning we cannot put an end time on ritual. I have been in numerous traditional ritual spaces, where ritual went all night into the next day; yet, in Western clinical spaces, the psychedelic space is contained by time. I cannot say I agree with this, because the ritual does not fit neatly into hourly slots of time. I often remind my clients that the medicine journey may begin before our set time for the session and may continue long after the session ends. I communicate that I will do my best to work with their medicine experience while acknowledging the parameters of time. It is important that clinicians are not so rigid with time that they fail to observe that the client is still activated by the medicine and their ritual experience.

Ritual space in psychedelic-assisted therapy will differ from client to client. Some clients will desire an altar, candle, incense, photos, special objects, or other spiritual tools—it is best to leave that up to the client. Sometimes, ritual elements can simply be imaginal. Ritual could look like trusting the client's divine inner wisdom in the medicine session, or helping them remember their thoughts and dream imagery through note taking. Many clients connect with the idea of setting an intention, which in and of itself is very powerful. The client gets to explore the question of intention with curiosity and from a place of inquiry, trusting that their inner wisdom can provide an answer. I may ask the client if they need support creating an intention or if the process might be facilitated by journaling, creating art, or engaging with another practice.

Depending on the space, a ritual lighting of a candle to start the session and the extinguishing of it at the end of the session can be powerful. Reading of poetry or picking a tarot or oracle card at the start and/or end of the session can provide a bridge into or out of ritual space. The client may want to bring in nature elements that represent water, fire, earth, and air to create a simple altar or focal point.

Conclusion

As a clinician, I do not create ritual. Instead, I am a steward and a witness. I understand that my duty is to do my own work regarding the complexities of cross-cultural psychotherapy and the intersections of identity, culture, and community. I have grown up knowing grand, expansive, and transformational ritual processes and ceremonial spaces. I have also learned the value of simple intention setting as a highly transmutative process. Ultimately, my role is to provide a safe space for honoring the *unknown*, a powerful and essential offering in psychedelic-assisted therapy sessions.

Note

1   White body supremacy is defined as individual and institutional attitudes, practices, and policies that elevate the white body as the standard against which all other persons' worth is measured (Menakem, 2017).

References

Allen, J. W. (1997). María Sabina: Saint mother of the sacred mushrooms. *Ethnomycological Journals, 1*. Psilly Publications.

Barnes, S. (2005). Black church culture and community action: Purdue University; the University of North Carolina Press. *Social Forces, 84*(2), 969–970.

Barton, C. (2020, June, 22). The violence of the void. *Medium*. https://xamillearton.medium.com/the-violence-of-the-void-f1f97c202043

Campbell, J. (1988). *The power of myth*. Double Day.

Chrzescijanska, M. (2017). The sacrifice ritual and process of individuation: Analysis of a model. *International Journal of Jungian Studies, 9*(2), 97–107.

Cushman, P. (1995). *Constructing the self, constructing America: A cultural history of psychotherapy*. De Capo Press.

DiAngelo, R. (2012). *What does it mean to be white: Developing white racial literacy*. Peter Lang.

Downing, C. (1994). *The long journey home: Re-visioning the myth of Demeter and Persephone for our time*. Shambhala.

Ehrenreich, B., & English, D. (2010). *Witches, midwives, and nurses: A history of women healers*. Feminist Press.

Fotiou, E. (2020). The role of Indigenous knowledges in psychedelic science. *Journal of Psychedelic Studies, 4*(1).

George, J., Michaels, T., Sevelius, J., & Williams, M. (2020). The psychedelic renaissance and the limitations of a White-dominant medical framework: A call for indigenous and ethnic minority inclusion. *Journal of Psychedelic Studies*, *4*(1).

Herzberg, G., & Butler, J. (2019). Blinded by the White: Addressing power and privilege in psychedelic medicine. *Chacruna*.

Jung, C. G. (1970). *Collected works of C. G. Jung, volume 11: Psychology and religion: West and east*. Princeton University Press.

Jung, C. G. (1972). *Collected works of C. G. Jung, volume 7: Two essays in analytical psychology*. Princeton University Press.

Jung, C. G. (1977). *Collected works of C. G. Jung, volume 18: The symbolic life: Miscellaneous writings*. Princeton University Press.

Menakem, R. (2017). *My grandmother's hand: Racialized trauma and the pathway to mending our hearts and bodies*. Central Recovery Press.

Mithoefer, M. (2016). *Multidisciplinary Association for Psychedelic Studies (MAPS), manual for MDMA-assisted psychotherapy in treatment of posttraumatic stress disorder* (p. 8). Santa Cruz.

Mosley, A. J., & Biernat, M. (2020). The new identity theft: Perceptions of cultural appropriation in intergroup contexts. *Journal of Personality and Social Psychology*.

Noel, D. C. (1987). Shamanic ritual as poetic model: The case of María Sabina and Anne Waldman. *Journal of Ritual Studies*, *1*(1), 57–71.

Ovid, A. D. (2005). *Metamorphoses* (C. Martin, Trans.). W.W. Norton & Co.

Somé, M. (1999). *The healing wisdom of Africa: Finding life purpose through nature, ritual, and community*. Penguin Putnam.

Stephen, J. (2020, November 10). R. Gordon Wasson & Maria Sabina: First contact with magic mushrooms. *Truffle Report*. https://truffle.report/maria-sabina-and-r-gordon-wasson-psychedelic-first-contact-warning/

Taylor, B. (1997). Earthen spirituality or cultural genocide?: Radical environmentalism's appropriation of Native American spirituality. *Religion*, *27*, 183–215. doi: 10.1006/reli.1996.0042

Trichter, S. (2010). Ayahuasca beyond the Amazon: The benefits and risks of a spreading tradition. *Journal of Transpersonal Psychology*, *42*(2), 131–148.

Udo, E. (2020). The vitality of Yoruba culture in the Americas. *Ufahamu*, *41*(2), 31.

Wolkstein, D. (1983). *Inanna, queen of heaven and earth: Her stories and hymns from Sumer*. Harper & Row.

Chapter 11

Psychedelic-Assisted Internal Family Systems Therapy

Robert M. Grant

Introduction

Psychedelic medicine is a promising approach for the treatment of anxiety, depression, and trauma, as well as couples' therapy, transforming use of substances, building community, and fostering attunement with the environment. Internal Family Systems (IFS) is a model for psychotherapy, which "plays well" with psychedelics, and has its own capacity to foster healing experiences through NOSC.

The Internal Family Systems Model

Richard Schwartz pioneered the development of IFS in the 1980s. He reports that he was using his training in family systems therapy for the treatment of a young client with bulimia who had been cutting herself (Schwartz & Sweezy, 2020). As was still common practice, he obtained a safety contract and felt confident that he and the client had made an agreement in good faith. The following week, he was devastated to find that his client had cut herself again—this time more severely than before and on her face. As he explored what happened, the client told him she had a part who had agreed to their safety contract, but she later felt overwhelmed by another part filled with anger who vehemently objected to their agreement. Dr. Schwartz thus began to formulate a model of the psyche that accounted for people having a multiplicity of parts. The notion that the mind is not monolithic is deeply embedded in psychotherapeutic and cultural traditions, most notably Jungian, Gestalt, and psychodynamic theories. The deep cultural antecedents of the multiplicity of the mind are discussed in detail in the book titled *Many Minds, One Self* (Schwartz & Falconer, 2017).

The name Internal Family Systems originally came from Dr. Schwartz's training in family systems therapy. The name may be a misnomer, as family members are not usually included in IFS therapy sessions. I sometimes explain to clients that internal families of parts are like external families—they live together and do not always get along; sometimes they fight, sometimes they ignore each other, and sometimes one part colludes with another against a third. An internal family of parts can do just about anything that a family of people does.

DOI: 10.4324/9781003167976-11

The multiplicity of the mind manifests in many common experiences—people experience ambivalence in most important realms of their lives. Consider a person assessing whether to stay in a marriage or leave. They may have strong desires to stay for the children, for financial security, for appearances among friends and co-workers, to avoid conflict or to avoid disappointment. Yet, there may be equally strong desires to leave, motivated by aspirations for greater independence, safety, or adventure. These conflicting desires can lead to erratic, paralyzed, or self-destructive behavior. A part that is afraid of disappointing others may insist on staying in an unsafe relationship. Another part may lash out with violence against the partner or oneself. Yet, another part may try to relieve suffering by drinking excessively. We can come to understand why these behaviors occur and find more satisfying ways forward by getting to know the various parts at play.

There are less-extreme examples of ambivalence in daily life. What to order at a restaurant may bring up parts who have different tastes (sweet or savory) or concerns about weight, fitness, or what others at the table may think. Shopping for groceries, choosing a show to watch, or deciding what shirt to wear may all be informed by a spectrum of parts. Thoughts and emotions can also be expressions of parts. Certain parts may consistently dominate the internal conversation (as with intrusive thoughts), while other parts sit in silence out of view, feeling sad, wounded, or overwhelmed.

Different people perceive parts in different ways or differently over time. Some people "see" images of their parts as distinct people within themselves—for example, by visualizing an inner child. Others perceive their parts as animals or mythic creatures. Still others sense their parts without any visual image, instead experiencing them in their bodies as sensations or internal voices.

The IFS model of the mind is inherently non-pathologizing. According to IFS, all people have parts—which consist of *protectors* (including *managers* and *firefighters*) and *exiles*—as well as a *Self*. Everyone's parts sometimes become polarized with one another; some parts are exiled and carry burdens imposed on them during traumatic experiences, and people suffer as a consequence. There is a diversity of forms and degrees that suffering can take.

Protective Parts (Managers and Firefighters)

Protective parts serve to protect a person from pain, anxiety, shame, or other forms of distress. There are two types of protective parts: managers and firefighters. Protective parts are said to be "managers" if they prevent suffering in peaceful ways. Examples of managers include timekeeping parts (who keep people on time), diplomatic parts (who try to keep other people minimally satisfied), caregiving parts (who take care of other people or parts), and work-oriented parts (who seek validation through professional accomplishments). Managers carry out "ego functions" that manage the stresses of inner and external challenges. Managers are often charged with being rational, sometimes conceived as being internally consistent, or explaining beliefs and behaviors.

Destructive parts are called "firefighters" based on the metaphor that a firefighter will sometimes destroy a structure to put out a fire. (Anecdotally, I have trained with firefighter professionals who object to this characterization, pointing out that actual firefighters spend most of their time preventing fires and helping people and animals survive.) The concept of parts who seek to relieve suffering in destructive ways has been helpful for understanding behavior. In this model, destructive behavior can be understood as driven by an imperative, perceived by a part with limited perspective, to spare the internal family system from pain, anxiety, suffering, or shame. A firefighter's destructive behavior might include cutting and other self-harming behaviors, drinking to the point of personal and social harm, and even suicide. IFS is unique in that it regards firefighters as protectors because their intentions are to protect the internal family system from overwhelming pain. Befriending firefighters, learning their intentions, and listening for what they would rather do are the first steps in helping them become less extreme.

Exiles

According to the IFS model, traumatic experiences, especially in childhood, can lead to the development of parts called "exiles," which are often subconscious or exiled from consciousness. Exiles hold the most distressing and overwhelming aspects of a traumatic experience, which are called "burdens" in the IFS model and can include unbearable beliefs, memories, and emotions, such as shame, grief, and fear. These parts and the burdens they carry are exiled to keep their overwhelming pain, suffering, and affect from consciousness. Burdens may come into consciousness as intrusive thoughts, obsessions, or ruminations, causing distress, depression, or anxiety. Protector parts work hard to keep exiles and their distressing burdens out of conscious awareness by behaving in ways characterized by the stage of childhood when the trauma occurred. An exile may have one or more manager parts who keep the exile and its distressing burdens at bay. Managers may be backed up by firefighters who will use more extreme means, like violence or inebriation, to push the part back into exile if the manager fails to contain it.

The Self

The Self is a core aspect of each of us that is able to observe and witness our experiences and parts with curiosity and compassion; it has the quality of being able to witness trauma without itself being traumatized. Some communities experienced with psychedelics may refer to this as "spirit," "soul," "consciousness," or the "inner healing intelligence." One premise of the IFS model is that everyone has a Self, no matter how traumatized they are; however, access to the Self may be limited in those who suffer from severe emotional dysregulation or extreme substance use. The qualities of Self include the eight C's: clarity, courage, confidence, creativity, connection, compassion, curiosity, and calmness, and five P's: playfulness, patience, presence, perspective, and persistence. The IFS view of health and actualization involves Self-leadership—a state of mind in which emotions, thoughts, and behaviors are led by Self and thus reflect Self qualities, as opposed to states influenced by the leadership of parts, who may be driven by an imperative to suppress painful memories, emotions, and thoughts.

Transformation Through IFS Therapy

IFS therapy is intended to create new experiences and durable changes in how one's parts relate to Self energy. IFS sessions often involve working with managers, who have important functions in daily life but may interfere with a deeper healing process if they are not led by Self qualities. An effective session will typically start by identifying and befriending any managers present and coming to understand their underlying function, fears, and needs. Managers may be serving to monitor safety; keep track of time; establish expectations for social behavior; or perform duties that fulfill perceived expectations as a client, spouse, parent, or other social role. Managers may fear, for example, that if they stop performing their role, an exile will overwhelm the Self with feelings. Managers may also fear that the therapist will have a negative reaction to exiled parts, or that they would be rejected from the system if their role is no longer needed. Correspondingly, managers may thus need reassurance that the Self can make contact with exiles without being overwhelmed, or that the therapist will help them identify a new role that is more fitting if theirs were to become obsolete. This process is called "unblending" in that distance is created between the Self and the manager parts, such that the managers can be better seen, can come to appreciate the existence of the Self, and can trust that their needs will be tended to.

A primary goal of developing this relationship between the client's Self and manager parts is to get permission to work with exiled parts, typically granted as the manager agrees to step aside, to step back, or to rest. Such permission is granted only when the manager's fears are assuaged, and they perceive respectful, compassionate, and friendly regard from the Self, as well as from the therapist. Firefighters may also need attention, and the approach is similar, although firefighters are more reactive and more likely to benefit from direct conversation with the therapist's Self through a process that is called "direct access." A protective part who experiences the healing power of connection with Self energy and rests in that—even for a moment—can often return to that state later when needed to stay in calm confidence.

More durable transformation occurs when the IFS process comes to completion. If the beginning of the session succeeds in befriending the protectors, they may be willing to "rest" or temporarily step to the side so that attention can be given to exiled parts carrying burdens. From a state of Self-leadership, the client is guided in finding and befriending an exile, listening to its story, and holding compassion for its pain. The part may be willing to describe in detail its experience of prior trauma and express any related emotions they are carrying. Calmly witnessing this process is essential. Curiosity about what more had occurred is also important, if the protective parts are willing to have the complete story told.

When the exiled part feels the client's Self has heard the whole story, they can be asked if they are willing to leave the traumatic environment, a process that is called "retrieval" in the IFS system. If willing, the part can be invited to imagine a place they would rather be—for example, a peaceful place in nature (pastures and beaches are popular) or in the client's home. The client is then invited to help the previously exiled part to move to the desired place. Once there, the exiled part is invited to consider whether there are any burdens it has been carrying that do not belong to it and are no longer necessary now that they have left the traumatizing situation. If they are willing, they are invited to let go of their burdens (e.g., fear, sadness, shame, or maladaptive beliefs about themselves), typically to light, wind, fire, earth, or water, although any massive element can work. Once unburdened, the part is invited to call in qualities that are desired to take the place previously occupied by burdens. Recently unburdened exiles will often invite in qualities of Self, especially compassion, confidence, courage, calm, clarity, and playfulness.

The final step is to establish a ritual to maintain the relationship between the Self and the previously exiled part. The recently unburdened part is asked to suggest a ritual with the prompt, "How does that part want to stay in connection with you?" The ritual is best if it is specific and feasibly performed at least twice a week for a month. Examples include viewing a photo; performing a gesture; looking at the sky; or including the part in a yoga routine, meditation, or prayer. People who are able to experience all of these stages in the IFS process typically feel permanently transformed by the experience, never returning to the exact same patterns of emotion, thought, or behavior. Of course, other issues may arise, but these same dynamics are often durably shifted.

The details of this process of retrieval and unburdening matter. The properly trained IFS therapist learns to facilitate the process of retrieval and unburdening over the course of hundreds of hours of supervised practice in certification courses offered by the IFS institute. While IFS can be used safely by any mental health professional to "unblend" from protectors, work with exiles requires supervised practical training, because exiles are exquisitely vulnerable and can be retraumatized by parts in the client or the therapist who have an agenda for them, however well intentioned.

IFS and Psychedelic Therapy

IFS combines well with psychedelic therapy and shares several common premises and values, including the following IFS principles.

Embracing Multiplicity of the Mind

People having psychedelic experiences are frequently aware of complex and sometimes contradictory images and memories. They may perceive joy and dread during their journey, sometimes in the same moment. People also often perceive distinct parts of themselves during psychedelic journeys. Models of psychedelic therapy tend to encourage normalization of the multiplicity of the mind. The IFS view that different experiences and parts can and do co-exist simultaneously in each of us helps provide perspective to these complexities, which may otherwise seem chaotic or contradictory.

All Parts Are Welcome: Reconnecting With Dissociated Experiences

A core premise of IFS is that all parts are welcome, including those that cause suffering, such as exiles and firefighters. Working with these parts through the practices described earlier allows them to contribute to the person's welfare in a new way going forward. Similarly, some psychedelic traditions embrace "shadow work," aiming to understand and integrate that which has been split off from conscious awareness. In fact, psychedelics are known to facilitate greater access to previously dissociated feelings, memories, and parts of the self. Through the process of working with dissociated material in psychedelic therapy, compassion and creativity are fostered by delving into traumatic memories and cultivating expression and acceptance of feelings, desires, and fears that may have previously been experienced as taboo or shameful.

Therapists as "Hope Merchants"

Both IFS and psychedelic therapists are trained to hold space for hope, an essential motivator for traveling along the healing path. Hope also encourages protective parts to rest so that a more durable solution can be found in moments of distress.

Hope can also lead to unrealistic expectations and ensuing disappointment. While transformative healing and change are sought, the psychedelic-assisted IFS therapist does well to avoid promising any particular results. The path toward healing can be long and nonlinear with some setbacks for every advance. Furthermore, relapse can occur. Typically, relapses happen when exiles are left behind, the whole story of the trauma was not shared, or promises made to stay in contact with exiles are not kept. Furthermore, people with severe or repeated trauma histories may have groups of exiles that can only be engaged over time or as a group. As the relationships among the internal family of parts become less burdened by past trauma, the person may engage more fruitfully with people in their external family and community. This work will take time. Hope for healing is therefore essential for IFS to work, but false promises about the road being easy or rapid are not useful.

Similarly, the lure of new, effective, and efficient medicines brings new hopes and challenges. How psychedelic therapists can be hope merchants without becoming "snake oil salesmen" is an ongoing challenge and topic for discussion in medical ethics. False and baseless claims of immediate efficacy made in psychedelic medicine advertisements and the media are unethical, especially given that the therapy is expensive and takes time. It is important to remember that both therapists and clients want to avoid unrealistic expectations and resulting disappointment, especially when resources are limited.

The IFS model suggests ways to foster hope without deviating from what is truly possible, based on the notion of Self-leadership. Therapists can engage clients in a discussion of the possibilities for lasting psychological transformation. Therapists may introduce the idea that such change comes from within, guided by the person's inner healing intelligence, or Self, rather than from a medicine or other external source. In IFS, and in some psychedelic therapy frameworks, the person's Self is given the credit for healing.

An illustrative example often used to describe the inner source of healing is a situation in which someone has a deep cut in their skin and goes to an emergency room for stitches. The stitches hold the skin edges together but do not cause the healing. Rather, the healing occurs through the body's own process of secreting extracellular fluids into the wound, allowing migration of cells that produce fibrotic connections, followed by rebuilding the skin architecture. The psyche can be said to heal in a similar way: when held in a safe therapeutic space, neuronal pathways in the brain begin to shift; parts of the brain holding traumatic memories reconnect with parts of the brain that perceive the safety of the current situation; and the psyche builds new ways of processing emotions, sensations, and traumatic experiences.

Seeking Consent at Every Step

IFS therapists are taught to seek consent from the client's parts at every stage of the treatment. This is important because parts who are pushed aside by a manager, perhaps in collusion with a part of the therapist who wants to see more healthy behavior, will often retaliate with more extreme behavior and emotions. An IFS therapist returns to a common question at every step, "Is it okay if we pay attention to that part?" If a protector does not consent, the client and the therapist can direct curiosity (a quality of Self) to the question of why paying attention to that part is not acceptable. If such curiosity is not welcome, attention turns to what is acceptable at that time.

Given the vulnerable states that psychedelics induce, frequently obtaining consent throughout psychedelic therapy is essential. The IFS approach to protectors is well suited as a model for discussing consent in psychedelic therapy. The goal is to focus, befriend, show compassion and curiosity, seek consent often, and build trust and confidence. Someone participating in psychedelic therapy is well served if they feel safe with their provider; feel seen; and trust they will not be manipulated, coerced, or forced into anything.

Working With Expanded States of Consciousness

The root of the word *psychedelic* is "soul and mind manifesting." A psychedelic experience may involve mystical experiences characterized by visions, images, visitations by spirits, amplified bodily sensations, a sense of unity and beauty, and deep insight. Such experiences can occur in IFS sessions as well. IFS therapy is psychedelic—a mind manifestor—whether or not a psychedelic medicine is used. In my experience offering non-medicine IFS therapy, I have witnessed mystical experiences arising in moments when protector parts were able to rest, allowing access to exiles and the Self. I recall clients experiencing "domes of healing light" being lowered over entire cities, rifts in the earth opening and swallowing up predators, and detailed personal conversations with ancestors who had died many years before—experiences which have a common resonance with reports from psychedelic sessions.

Reaffirming these experiences—whether they occur in IFS therapy or a psychedelic session—is helpful for sustaining the benefits of the therapy. Some clients will question or dismiss these experiences as they return to a regular state of consciousness. A key role of both the IFS and the psychedelic therapist is to help the client trust the significance of their experience and help them make meaning of it. Experiencing such visions in the context of IFS helps both therapist and client understand that psychedelic experiences arise from a mind that has been untethered from managing parts who keep track of time, space, relationships, sensations, and emotions.

An experienced IFS therapist becomes accustomed to these expanded states of consciousness and learns to stay present with them. At the end of IFS sessions, there is always a closing process, in which managers are asked to come back in and comment on what they perceived. This is similar to the process of integration after a psychedelic session, in which people are asked to describe what they experienced as they return to ordinary states of consciousness, helping the client's analytical mind to make sense of and integrate expanded states into their sense of self.

How Does Psychedelic Medicine Facilitate IFS?

Psychedelic medicine can facilitate IFS in several ways. First, it can increase access to the Self. For example, ketamine experiences are often characterized by clarity, creativity, connection, and playfulness—all qualities of Self. In some ketamine sessions, protector parts are able to rest. People tend to enjoy the temporary cessation of ruminations and intrusive thoughts (like self-judgment) coming from protective parts. Sometimes, people with strong self-defeating core beliefs will find they have some space from them toward the end of the session. Other ketamine sessions may bring protective parts into focus, so that they can engage in a Self-led conversation with other parts. For example, a patient may become very aware of an inner critic, initially prompting turmoil, which can evolve into an inner conversation about what the inner critic is afraid would happen if it stopped being so critical and what it would rather do if it did not feel compelled to be self-critical. These sometimes tumultuous conversations with protectors can be quite healing, provided the client and the therapist are able to maintain a sense of safety and confidence. While ketamine often brings out Self-qualities of clarity and calmness, other psychedelic medicines may increase access to other Self-qualities. For example, MDMA typically floods the person with compassion for self and others.

Ketamine-Assisted IFS

Ketamine is a psychedelic medicine that is highly effective for treatment of depression and suicidality and is used for these and other conditions. Ketamine therapy is provided in a wide range of settings and doses by a growing number of practitioners. At low doses, ketamine has subjective effects of calming, mood elevation, and heart opening, similar to MDMA. At higher doses, ketamine can be similar to classical psychedelics, affording visual imagery and potentially ego dissolution. At still higher doses, ketamine is a dissociative anesthetic. Low and medium doses are used for treatment of mental health conditions by a growing number of practitioners.

Ketamine has offered me a rich ground for developing the craft of psychedelic-assisted IFS therapy. My experience with ketamine-assisted IFS therapy provides some helpful examples, which I will describe in the remainder of this chapter. Lessons learned at my clinic, Healing Realms Psychotherapy, as well as in other environments, inform the following suggestions for practice. All of these suggestions should be regarded as provisional, available to be adapted to different practices and clients.

Preparation

The preparation phase of a psychedelic treatment is essential for establishing safety, which in turn allows surrender to the deeper psychological and spiritual explorations conducive to healing. IFS offers a comprehensive approach to consent. While any ketamine practice will seek written informed consent to treatment, the IFS therapist is aware that such consent is typically signed by a manager part. Such managers may push aside concerns of other protectors and exiles. Proceeding with treatment based only on the written informed consent document risks a backlash by parts who were pushed aside.

From an IFS framework, a post-treatment surge of anxiety can be understood as a backlash from parts who were pushed aside during treatment or during the informed consent process. Attention to all the parts can help to avoid this backlash. Frank Anderson (n.d.), a psychiatrist and senior trainer in the IFS system, asserts that no psychoactive medicine should be given until "all parts agree." While Anderson is referring primarily to antidepressants and mood stabilizers, I believe the same principle applies to psychedelics. Perhaps more so.

During each preparation visit, I always ask if there are any questions or concerns that have come up. This conventional question will elicit common concerns around safety, efficacy, legality, format of the treatment, costs, my experience as a clinician, and information about outcomes. This is just the beginning. After achieving a more substantive level of connection with the client, I will deepen the question by reminding the client that their questions and concerns do not have to make sense, and they need not explain why they are asking. I promise them not to take anything personally. Only with this preface will I hear about the concerns of other parts—namely firefighters and exiles. It is essential to give these concerns adequate attention. Some concerns commonly expressed by these parts include:

- "I have a part that is afraid that you will touch me sexually."
- "I may experience psychosis and never come back."
- "I will do something or talk about something that will make me feel ashamed."
- "You will do something or talk about something that will make me feel ashamed."
- "I might not get better despite your best efforts, and you will be disappointed."
- "I might get better and then have to face more frightening problems."

An experienced clinician will appreciate that any of these concerns can open fruitful exploration of related memories, feelings, or other concerns. The introduction of psychedelic medicine is best delayed until these concerns are fully addressed to the satisfaction of all the parts. It may help to remind the concerned part that ketamine experiences are typically brief—lasting 60 to 90 minutes depending on dose, that the initial dose will be low enough to allow movement and speech, and that the concerned part will be invited to come fully back into consciousness before the session is over.

Exceptions to proceeding with ketamine therapy when some parts disagree are few. One exception may be with people who suffer from active suicidal ideation, given that ketamine has known rapid efficacy, and there is some urgency to ameliorate a life-threatening situation (Burger et al., 2016; Hu et al., 2016).

Given that spiritual experiences are common during ketamine sessions, we also discuss spirituality during preparation sessions. I ask the client to describe their religious background, if any, and their current spiritual beliefs, including whether they experience ancestral spirits. I ask them to identify any religious trauma, which may be related to punishment, gender, or sexuality. Some will say that they have no spiritual beliefs or experiences. If so, I express curiosity about whether they lament this lack of experience. (Some do; others do not.) I also describe my spiritual journey from being raised as an Episcopalian to an academic interest in the history of religions, to agnosticism, to atheism, and then to "radical empiricism" described by William James. Radical empiricism embraces spiritual experiences without needing to explain them and is a helpful concept to prepare for psychedelic experiences.

Medicine Session

Ketamine-assisted IFS sessions are best if they are three to four hours in duration. The first phase of the session is spent getting into Self, often involving catching up on recent events and feeling into current emotion all aimed to cultivate the qualities of curiosity and confidence. Accessing curiosity and confidence is facilitated by allowing the client to speak for any parts that have concerns or distress, and addressing these concerns with calm, curiosity, and clarity (all Self qualities). Ketamine dosing should be delayed until the client has some access to Self, either in themselves or through connection to the therapist, who may need to provide curiosity, confidence, and courage for both themselves and the client. In some cases, the IFS therapist will need to find ways to keep themselves calm and curious even when the client cannot. Staying calm is a skill that both psychedelic guides and IFS therapists should keep well honed. A phrase that helps, if heartfelt, is "I feel your distress, and you are safe here with me in this place right now. I am curious if you can feel safe here now?" The goal is not to achieve unblending (separation or equanimity) from *all* active protectors prior to ketamine administration. Rather, the goal is to achieve *some* unblending and some access to Self, manifested by some calmness and curiosity about where the journey may lead and confidence that the therapist and the space will keep the client safe. If there has been a preparation session in the prior few days, this pre-dosing period may be as short as 20 to 30 minutes.

Prior to administering the ketamine, I specifically verify that the client agrees to the following boundaries: 1) the client will stay in the office until we all agree that it is safe for them to leave, 2) there will not be any sexual contact with the therapist (although the client is welcome to express or bring up sexual themes), and 3) the client will not hit or physically harm the therapist or anyone else in the room. Under ketamine, these boundaries are rarely transgressed but are still important to name explicitly.

I emphasize that there will be a clear differentiation of roles, and everyone in the room will be participating in the journey in different ways. I note that the therapist's role is to keep the client safe, hold space for their experience to unfold, and offer compassionate witnessing. I let the client know that all of their parts are welcome, and invite them to be open to, focus on, and speak for any parts that call for attention. The therapist also stays open to their own parts and provides any attention they require, either during the session or afterward, seeking out consultation if needed. The therapist generally does not speak for their own parts during the session, unless needed to serve the client's process.

Ritual prior to ketamine dosing can support access to Self. We use rituals that invoke sound and scent, as these sensations are intimately connected to emotional memory and may serve to activate neural pathways that store traumatic memories. These rituals should be customized to each client and therapist/client dyad. For further discussion of client-centered ritual, see Chapter 10. The ritual I use typically involves the following elements, adapted to the individual needs and desires of each client:

1. Starting the session with a chime serves to convey that the situation is shifting from an external focus to an internal focus. With the chime, I say that, "I invite in the spirit of ketamine and the person's inner healing powers so that they may collaborate in ways that we barely understand." References to "spirit" may be altered if the client has expressed aversion to spirituality during preparation sessions. (Such aversion is best to fully explore before psychedelics are given.) The basic message is that the effects of ketamine therapy are not fully elucidated, and the guide does not have the answers—nor needs to have answers—for healing to

occur. This invites the client to have confidence in their own healing capacities and the "rational" or "explaining" parts to rest, knowing that healing can happen even if we do not understand exactly how.

2. I burn fragrant plant or resin and use a fan composed of feathers from local bird species to bathe the client in the scent. This practice should be discussed prior to the session; it is best if the selected plant is derived from the client or the therapist's own cultural tradition—it is important to avoid cultural appropriation through this practice. The scent should be pleasant to the client.

3. I use a rattle to go around the room pointing to all four corners and walls. This use of a rattle invokes a sense of spaciousness that is characteristic of many ketamine journeys. The rattle may also ease people into a more calm or meditative state.

4. I then use a meditation that specifically invokes the directions in terms of Self-qualities defined by IFS. I draw attention to the east, direction of sunrise, new beginnings, creativity, and innocence. The south is used to invoke playfulness, nourishment, and warmth. The west is used to invoke an oceanic sense of home and belonging (appropriate to my practice located on the West Coast of California). I use the north to invoke qualities of courage and clarity. I focus on the ceiling to invoke a sense of spaciousness. I then focus at length on gravity and the ground as a metaphor for unconditional love, stating that gravity holds us to the ground, whether or not we believe we deserve to be held, whether or not we understand gravity. (Indeed, gravity remains one of the unsolved puzzles in physics; yet, everyone counts on it.) I name that the room is part of a building that is nestled securely into the soil of the earth. Bedrock lying below the soil is so massive and strong that it holds all things effortlessly, and the waters that flow below the rock connect us with everything that is. The qualities of confidence and connection evoked here also invite Self. I then turn attention back to the room, and note, "How gently the air touches our skin, so gently that we are free to move, to grow and to change." I then focus on the inner direction by asking us to breathe the air in deeply, and feel the nourishment of the oxygen that is picked up by our blood and circulated to bathe every cell of the body. I ask the client to imagine that with every breath out, that same air carries from their bodies that which they no longer need. I end by remarking that the process of nourishment and cleansing is as easy as breathing in and out. This is intended to build confidence and invite any performative parts to rest.

5. After this meditation, I ask everyone in the room to express an intention. People in the room include the client and the therapist and may also include a co-therapist, a student, or a family member—or in a group therapy setting, all group members. I prepare any co-therapist, student, or family member who will be present to know the question is coming. Typically, the client goes first. The therapist's intentions may include to keep the client safe (our designated practical role) as well as whatever else is invoked in the therapist. Having everyone express interrelated intentions helps cultivate connection, curiosity, and compassion, all Self qualities that foster healing.

6. Finally, I ask if the client is ready to proceed with the ketamine administration. While nearly all of my clients have peacefully and enthusiastically affirmed their intention and consent for ketamine treatment, a few have balked. These situations have led to fruitful explorations of parts that have objections and wait until the last minute to express them.

In this method, the 60 to 90 minutes after ketamine dosing is best reserved for quiet inward contemplation. A few clients, typically those receiving a low dose, may want to talk. I accommodate that if I have a sense that the desire for talk is Self-led. Alternatively, a part that insists on talking during the ketamine peak may seem defensive or a "chatterbox." For example, I recall a client who spoke incessantly after dosing, rattling off a stream of consciousness, and finally saying, "I am afraid that if I stop talking, I will cease to exist." I suggested that they try that, and they did, with much greater success in their inner exploration.

During the peak of an appropriately dosed ketamine experience, people are lightly sedated, defined as verbally responsive to verbal prompts in a normal voice. Without prompts, they will typically lie still and breathe deeply in a cyclic manner. When the ketamine dose is high enough, a pattern of deep and cyclic breathing often spontaneously occurs, reminiscent of Holotropic Breathwork (Grof & Grof, 2010). I have wondered how much of the ketamine hallucinogenic experience is due to the direct effects of the medicine alone and how much is due to the deep cyclic breathing stimulated by the effects of the ketamine. Research on this topic would be appropriate.

As clients start coming out of their ketamine experience, they will usually begin moving their arms or legs in a purposeful way or roll over on their side and will respond to verbal prompts with more complete sentences. As this happens, I typically offer an open-ended prompt used in Eye Movement Desensitization and Reprocessing therapy: "What are you noticing now?" (Shapiro, 2017). If the response is brief, I will respond, "Go with that," and wait for several minutes. At first, attention will often shift every time the question is asked, highlighting how ketamine can interfere with focus—an important prerequisite for working with parts. When the person begins noticing consistent themes or parts over time and is more awake and interactive, we can transition into IFS work.

Immediate Post-Ketamine IFS

Once the client has emerged from the ketamine experience, interaction with the therapist may allow for more focused work with parts. I encourage the client to focus on an image, a sensation, a body part, or a memory that came up during the journey. These often represent parts. In ketamine journeys, parts may not manifest as "personas" or little people as they typically do in IFS alone. Rather, parts may appear as harp strings, crickets, goats, or lampposts, for example. These symbolic representations of parts may well respond to questions that are asked of parts, such as, "How old are you?" This may set in motion a conversation about the part's experience, past memories, concerns, and burdens. The part may be willing to be retrieved and can then unburden and bring in desired qualities. I have noticed that post-ketamine IFS sessions, which include retrieval and unburdening, are often significantly transformative. In such instances, clients typically remark that their experience of their depression or anxiety is durably altered.

It is important not to rush parts into retrieval or unburdening; pressuring parts is more likely to occur during psychedelic therapy and can lead to backlash after the treatment. The circumstances of psychedelic therapy, or a therapist who is blended with an achieving part, may lead to an agenda to achieve results quickly. This is not helpful. In addition, some psychedelic therapists have a part that wants to be a hero, bringing relief when others could not. I am familiar with my heroic part, and I have learned through experience that this part is better invited to rest during psychedelic sessions. Under the influence of ketamine, people may cooperate with an overly directive approach. However, this is not expected to produce durable healing and may leave the client with less confidence and heightened feelings of dependence on the medicine or the therapist.

The best way to facilitate healing—including retrieval and unburdening—is through adequate preparation and remaining in Self, creating the conditions in which both the client and the therapist can access the qualities of curiosity, compassion, and confidence. People with complex PTSD and those who have protectors that are skilled managers may take longer to achieve these important phases of the work. The therapist is well advised to let the process happen in its own time and not to take anything personally, whether or not the session goes in the direction they had hoped.

As the client emerges from deeper interactions with exiles, it is important to ask whether protectors who stepped aside at the beginning of the session were able to see what happened during the session. They have often witnessed the journey and are softer and more Self-led by the end of the session. Congratulating them and inviting them to celebrate with the other parts can be helpful. Sometimes, after a medicine-assisted IFS session, protector parts may surface and be quite suspicious. A rational part may believe that the entire experience was a hallucination, and that none of it mattered. That part may collude with a fatalistic part who believes the client cannot get better or does not deserve to get better. Addressing these parts' concerns at the end of the session will help avoid an otherwise rough landing.

For example, when a protector insists that the traumatic events did not "really" happen, it can be helpful to remind the client that the experience that just occurred is real and important, regardless of what "really" happened many years ago. Also, clients with strong materialist protective parts may doubt any direct experience with ancestral spirits and spirit guides; asking those materialist parts to rest for a moment to allow the full experience to be appreciated is often helpful. It may also be important to engage with these protectors, allowing them to express their concerns and treating them with curiosity and compassion. Important information may surface regarding ways protectors felt their needs were not tended to prior to entering into the ketamine experience, which can then be used to inform future ketamine sessions.

At the end of every ketamine session, I remind the client that whatever arose came from their own psyche. Ketamine is a simple molecule serving only to open the door to the healing power of the psyche. I say that I am grateful for the opportunity to witness their process, and that my role was limited to keeping them safe. "Everything that was healing in this session came from you." This helps to evoke a sense of the client's power at the end of the session. People coming out of a psychedelic experience often feel reverence for or dependent on the medicine or the therapist. This may be appealing to parts in the therapist who enjoy the appreciation and other parts that enjoy the business income. Yet, these dependencies can also be disempowering, or even addictive, possibly for both the therapist and the client. Appropriate insight and skill in managing the transference and countertransference are essential. I always take steps to ensure that the client feels empowered and grateful for their own inner healing powers after an IFS or psychedelic experience.

Integration

Integration of psychedelic sessions is important for sustaining the healing process. IFS begins the integration process toward the end of the session, whether the treatment involves medicine or not.

If exiles have been contacted—whether or not they were retrieved or unburdened—I ask how the exile would like to stay in connection with the client's Self. I encourage the client to wait for the answer rather than let a manager respond with what the exile should want. The goal is to find some thought or behavior that would help maintain a connection between the Self and the part—something that is feasibly done at least two or three times a week for the next month. Requests I have witnessed from exiles include, "Look up at the sky for a few moments in the morning" or "Make the gesture that I made just now before going to sleep at night." Relapse may occur if the promise is broken; however, exiled parts will often settle for just a bit of contact, which is better than the years of abandonment they had experienced previously.

Other causes of relapse include an exile finding that another exile was left behind. As discussed previously, it is common for those with complex PTSD to have multiple exiles sheltering together in a traumatic memory. With these clients, it is important to ask exiles who surface to identify any other exiles stuck in the same setting before suggesting retrieval. IFS can be used during integration sessions to explore this possibility.

I find it important to schedule an integration session or a phone call with the client on the day after a medicine session. This provides an opportunity to check in with protectors who may have stepped aside or rested during the session. For example, a materialist part may disbelieve in any experience that seems "spiritual" or "woo-woo." Asking that part to consider the symbolic meaning of these experiences may be helpful. In one circumstance, I worked with an orthodox Jewish person in March. He had asked that we incorporate some of his traditional practices into our ketamine process, which I welcomed. The ketamine session went well and resulted in an elevation in mood (which is typical of ketamine sessions at the end of the day). The client reported images of burdensome fluids draining out from a deep place. The following day, a protective part was present, who felt his depression had returned, and the client was discouraged. I reminded him that Passover was coming and wondered whether that had significance for his ketamine experience. He became animated and retold the story of hardship and seas (fluids) parting to allow exodus to a better place. We talked about letting go of past maladaptive beliefs, and the client became enthused about his prayers for the coming Passover. The protective part was allayed through developing a deeper understanding of what had happened in the ketamine session, and the client was able to incorporate his process of letting go of depression into his Passover celebrations. He later told me that the ketamine session was pivotal in his healing; while he continued to experience sadness at times, his suicidality had dissipated.

It is important to check in after a ketamine session to ensure protective parts are functioning to support the client's safety, given that protectors are often essential for resilience, especially in hazardous situations. Protective parts may continue to "rest" after a psychedelic experience, including timekeepers, mood stabilizers, people pleasers, financial managers, and sexual managers. While some respite can be healing, returning to normal social and occupational demands requires that these protectors function, hopefully in more Self-led ways.

An integration session or call the day after a medicine session provides an opportunity to highlight important events from the day before; reinforce sensations associated with confidence and unity; and link the symbolic process with the client's thoughts, bodily experiences, social life, environment, and spiritual practice. I will also remind the client of the importance of keeping promises to exiles. I am always pleased when clients decide to "tidy up," call an old friend, play in the dirt, or paint after a journey. While these activities may seem trivial, they bridge the symbolic and material realms. This integration session or call is also convenient for checking on sleep, self-care, and side effects.

How IFS Fits in a Social Justice Framework

IFS offers insight into how psychedelic medicine could engage more openly with challenges of social justice and inclusion, including our legacies of racism, sexism, heterosexism, individualism, and materialism. In the IFS model, these "isms" are regarded as legacy burdens inherited from ancestors and social context. Like individual burdens arising from personal traumatic experiences, these collective burdens can lead parts into extreme behavior and subsequent exile from consciousness. Exiles carrying legacy burdens driven by the traumatic experiences of ancestors can be understood, retrieved, and unburdened through a process resembling the method discussed previously for working with exiles burdened by personal trauma. The management of legacy burdens requires additional skill and techniques; however, these are described in the second edition of IFS therapy (Schwartz & Sweezy, 2020) and taught in level 2 IFS certification courses. How psychedelic medicine practices confront these legacies could make the difference between transformative healing and temporary escape by a privileged few from toxic systems.

By eschewing presumption and staying in curiosity, the IFS approach encourages each person to lead their own process, rather than being led by a guide who claims to know what path to take. The concept of a guide in psychedelic therapy is fraught. There can be an assumption that the guide has traveled farther down the path of healing than the client. This notion presumes that the guide and the client are on the same path. This can lead some therapists to claim to have more experience and knowledge than they have, and some clients to become dependent on their therapist. In the IFS model, the therapist is not regarded to be wiser, more mature, or more evolved than the client; rather, the therapist is available to witness—in a curious and Self-led manner—the client's process of healing, and help the client develop relationships between the Self and their parts.

Differences in ethnic background, race, gender, and trauma history highlight how different people have different paths. Even those with similar identity markers often have very different life journeys. A basic premise of IFS is that each person has a unique family of parts, and each internal family system is different—even when there are superficial similarities that tempt stereotyping. Each person's internal family system lives within a cultural system that has its own unique history and dynamics. The invitation from IFS is to stay curious about these dynamics, presume nothing, ask questions, show compassion, have courage to see plainly what happened, and invite next steps toward retrieval and unburdening. The respectful approach of IFS to the multiplicity and diversity of the psyche can be broadened out to encourage respect for the multiplicity and diversity of our culture at large.

The IFS model has been taken up by a wide range of people of different cultures, identities, and backgrounds. For example, the open approach of IFS has been readily adapted for use in China, where the name of the model was changed to Inner Peace Coaching. This renaming highlights the Self-quality of calm and the non-pathologizing intentions of the practice. The IFS model has been embraced by a burgeoning number of Black, Indigenous, and People of Color and sexual and gender minorities. Furthermore, licensed professionals and non-professionals are welcome into IFS trainings, and the certification process is the same, although non-licensed persons use the title "IFS certified practitioner," while licensed persons use the title "IFS certified therapist."

Conclusion

IFS and psychedelic practice fit well together by sharing a theoretical foundation that highlights the multiplicity of the psyche, welcoming of all parts of the psyche, non-pathologizing intent, seeking consent at every step, a non-directive approach, respect for non-ordinary and mystical states of consciousness, and optimism about healing. IFS provides a useful framework for the preparation, treatment, and integration of psychedelic experiences. Ketamine and MDMA, in particular, can facilitate the IFS process by increasing access to the Self and allowing protectors to rest. IFS has been adopted by diverse cultures and peoples, and it reflects the core values of curiosity, creativity, and Self-leadership.

IFS is an antidote for an emerging epidemic of misconception that psychedelic medicines are required for healing experiences to occur. Yet, for some people, IFS therapy leads to impasse, burdened by their personal history and legacies of racism, sexism, heterosexism, materialism, and individualism. Psychedelic medicine can facilitate a way through impasse and foster a strong connection between the therapist and the client, and more importantly, between the client's Self and their family of parts. Family systems operate on internal, external, communal, and global levels. Hope for durable healing through communion among family systems is the common promise shared by the best of psychedelic and IFS initiatives. May we keep this promise.

References

Anderson, F. (n.d.). *The internal family systems approach to psychopharmacology.* www.psychotherapynetworker.org/blog/details/592/the-internal-family-systems-approach-to-psychopharmacology

Burger, J., Capobianco, M., Lovern, R., Boche, B., Ross, E., Darracq, M. A., & McLay, R. (2016). A double-blinded, randomized, placebo-controlled sub-dissociative dose ketamine pilot study in the treatment of acute depression and suicidality in a military emergency department setting. *Military Medicine, 181,* 1195–1199.

Grof, S., & Grof, C. (2010). *Holotropic Breathwork.* State University of New York. www.dipsu.dk/Holotropic%20Breathwork%20by%20Stanislav%20Grof,%20MD.pdf

Hu, Y. D., Xiang, Y. T., Fang, J. X., Zu, S., Sha, S., Shi, H., & Ungvari, G. S. (2016). Single i.v. ketamine augmentation of newly initiated escitalopram for major depression: Results from a randomized, placebo-controlled 4-week study. *Psychological Medicine, 46,* 623–635.

Schwartz, R. C., & Falconer, R. (2017). *Many minds, one self.* Center for Self Leadership.

Schwartz, R. C., & Sweezy, M. (2020). *Internal family systems therapy* (2nd ed.). Guilford Publications.

Shapiro, F. (2017). *Eye movement desensitization and reprocessing (EMDR) therapy. Third Edition: Basic principles, protocols, and procedures.* Guilford Publications.

Chapter 12

Dimensions of Attunement

Music Listening, Resonance, and the Vibrational Field in Relational Psychedelic Therapy

Eric Sienknecht

> Reason gets in the way of so much, doesn't it?
> Let the imagination take over
> And lead you far from that small, worn platform,
> Out along those strange currents
> That flow from the mouths of Muses
> Into the Wilderness Beyond . . .

Most of us have heard in one way or another of the remarkable synergy between music and psychedelics and ways in which this particular alchemical combination has been the source of inspiration for creative endeavors and facilitated healing processes for people throughout time. Music has been an indelible component of sacred plant ceremonies in Indigenous societies for thousands of years. In Western societies, arguably some of our greatest works of art have sprouted from the rich soil of music- and drug-induced reveries. Since the 1950s in the U.S.A., music and psychedelic medicines have been used together in psychotherapy for the treatment of mental health conditions. This combination has been shown to potentiate thera-peutic outcomes (Kaelen et al., 2018) and has become a consistent component of psychedelic therapy treatments.

In this chapter, I will describe the importance of using music in psychedelic ther-apy sessions and illustrate the various roles and functions it serves in expediting therapeutic progress. I will then explore in detail, based on my clinical experiences with ketamine- and MDMA-assisted therapy, ways of thinking about and using music in sessions, with particular emphasis on the impact of music on the relational and vibrational fields. Finally, I will share a clinical case example to illustrate one way of thinking about and working with music in a psychedelic session.

Clinical Use of Music and Deep Listening

Although it is a matter of some debate, I will make my position clear at the outset that I believe music to be an essential ingredient of good psychedelic therapy. I propose that we think about music as a fundamental component of the psyche-delic therapy setting, rather than a modification or adaptation. As melody plays

DOI: 10.4324/9781003167976-12

an integral role in bringing harmony to musical compositions, so music creates a cohesive environment for the psychedelic session and enhances therapeutic effects.

Some psychotherapists may be suspicious or reluctant to introduce such a potentially powerful influence as music into the space of the therapeutic relationship. While one might argue that music imposes a kind of scaffolding that could foreclose potential directions of the therapeutic process, this concern does not actually bear out in clinical practice. Rather, in most cases, the client's process is guided primarily by their inner healing intelligence and catalyzed by the medicine; the musical scaffolding simply deepens or enhances a process that is already unfolding. Stan Grof (1980, p. 142) made similar observations in his work with LSD in the 1970s:

> The danger of programming associated with specific music is not as serious as it might seem. The potential for manipulating and controlling the experience is rather limited . . . although a certain general atmosphere or emotional tone will be suggested from the outside [by the music], the subject will elaborate it very specifically. The resultant sequences will still be manifestations of the individual's own unconscious, reflect the content of his or her memory banks, and represent a meaningful self-revealing gestalt . . . [music] does not seem to reduce the therapeutic significance of the psychedelic experience that it triggers or modifies.

The question I aim to explore in this chapter is not whether to use music, but rather how to think about the use of music in psychedelic therapy sessions, as well as how to talk with our clients about it so that they orient to and make use of the music in a generative way.

Listening Into Music

It is important for psychedelic therapists to be open to the power of music's subjective influence. By virtue of the often unspoken or ineffable nature of one's experience of music, it is often unknowable how the client is experiencing the music played in sessions. However, the experience of music can be shared through the act of listening and through emotional and somatosensory resonance with the music; in this way, the therapist can connect more directly with the client's experience.

The client will experience the music in a psychedelic session in different ways, depending on how they are primed to engage with it. To create conditions for deepening the client's relationship with and use of music in sessions, the process of music listening itself should be explicitly addressed in the initial phases of treatment (intake and preparatory sessions). We might distinguish between two different ways of listening to music: 1) listening *to* music and 2) listening *into* music—or deep listening—in which the listener enters *into* the musical field and allows themselves to *feel* it. In the first mode, the listener's subjectivity is largely still online and operational, filtering the experience of the music through their preferences and judgments and discerning such things as whether they like the music or not, or whether the music is consonant or dissonant. In the second mode, the listener enters a more open and receptive state of mind, immersing in and merging with the somatosensory, vibrational surround of the musical field. Depending on the client's familiarity or lack thereof with this way of listening, the therapist may choose to invite the client to practice listening to a few tracks in this way as part of preparation.

To clarify further the conditions for optimizing this way of listening, we introduce to the client the concept of "beginner's mind" (Suzuki & Dixon, 2010) to point to a particular orientation, in which one remains curious about their process and allows it to unfold organically, without attachment to a specific outcome or agenda (Mithoefer, 2017, p. 9). When listening in this way, music can be a place to rest one's attention, and, by doing so, one can enter into a more receptive state and into the present moment. When introducing this way of listening, we prime clients with questions like, "What is the story the music is telling?" and "What is it calling you to feel?" With this orientation, the music acts as a substitute for thought and mental activity, offering a more direct way of attuning to the present-moment experience.

One of the more challenging aspects of a psychedelic session can be the initial phase after taking the medicine, as the effects start to be perceived. During this phase—as well as in other phases—music can serve to support the client in staying present with whatever is arising: "[Music] provides a meaningful structure for the experience and creates a continuous carrier wave that helps patients to overcome difficult parts of the sessions and move through impasses" (Grof, 1980, p. 141). As fears, sadness, and other previously unconscious and unprocessed "shadow" (Jung, 1963) material arise, music can help clients stay present and not retreat or distract in typical ways. We can think about this as a practice—welcoming all that arises, even when connecting with shadow material; learning to stay curious about it; and trusting that it is coming up for a reason. As one learns they can navigate the storms and feel, tolerate, and survive that which they have been avoiding, repressing, or dissociating from, their sense of inner space expands, and they find safe harbor in their own minds.

Functions of Music in Psychedelic Sessions

Early psychedelic researchers delineated several functions that music serves in psychedelic experiences. In their work with LSD psychotherapy, Bonny and Pahnke (1972) describe music as a tool for facilitating the surrender of ego functions, catalyzing the release of emotionality, facilitating peak experiences, helping to promote a sense of timelessness, and directing and structuring the experience. Grof describes the specific roles of music similarly: music evokes emotion, facilitates deepening of process, provides structure, supports letting go of defenses and surrendering to the experience, facilitates movement through impasses, and provides a sense of continuity while navigating through NOSC (Grof, 1980). More recently, Mendel Kaelen, a contemporary psychedelic researcher and neuroscientist, specified four functions of music based on his research, which corroborates these earlier conclusions: accessing emotional release, facilitating peak experiences, evoking autobiographical processing and mental imagery, and providing care and reassurance (Kaelen, 2021). In this section, I will briefly examine each of the four functions delineated by Kaelen.

Accessing Emotion and Facilitating Release

Why is music so important to us, and how can it say so much without saying anything at all? Studies in the psychology of music hint at an answer: the primary motive people report for listening to music is to connect with emotions (Juslin & Laukka, 2008). It is well known that music is processed by the limbic system, the brain region responsible for processing emotion (Blood & Zatorre, 2001). "Music can be an effective stimulus in helping to bring out affectively charged memories" (Chandler & Hartman, 1960). Listening to music also has been shown to decrease activation in the prefrontal cortex (Ferreri et al., 2013). By facilitating connection with our emotions, music offers a doorway into memory that is unmediated by logical thinking.

With regard to psychedelic therapy specifically, well-curated and culturally attuned music selections afford clients a powerful container for emotional expression, without pressure to formulate and express verbally. As Kroeker (2019) notes,

> Musical expression has the ability to carry the same fluid potency as the verbal exchange but without taking us out of the open symbolic *right brain* realm and the emotion-oriented amygdala system. Our feelings tend to stay *online* during the musical exchange, whereas the verbal exchange can quickly take us into our intellectualized logos orientation.
>
> (p. 5)

Indeed, it could be argued that the greatest therapeutic potential of music in psychedelic sessions lies in its capacity to enhance and deepen emotional awareness and expressiveness (Kaelen et al., 2018). We see this powerful cathartic process illustrated in psychedelic sessions—as well as in Holotropic Breathwork sessions[1]—in which clients connect with previously repressed emotionality that is then expressed and released, often quite dramatically. These types of cathartic releases have been shown to correlate with positive therapy outcomes (Belser et al., 2017).

The phenomenon of *frisson* provides an interesting example of how music can bypass the analytical mind, help us to access emotions, and engage a complementary physiological response. It is not uncommon for clients in psychedelic sessions to report somatic sensations of tingling, buzzing, and even prolonged shaking accompanying emotional release. Although in some cases this may be a feature of trauma processing—an instinctive discharging of stress described by Peter Levine and Frederick (1997) in his Somatic Experiencing work—it may alternatively be a feature of deep aesthetic appreciation. Frisson is also referred to as "aesthetic chills" or "goosebumps" and can occur when one is moved by an evocative piece of music, an exquisite piece of art, or an epic cinematic storyline and score. This appreciation of beauty triggers the release of dopamine, activating the autonomic nervous system and increasing muscle tension, skin resistance, and depth of breathing, while causing hair follicles to stand erect on the skin. Frisson can also be experienced as waves of energy or shivers moving along the spine that typically involve transient euphoria. In various esoteric and spiritual traditions, frisson has been associated with the sequential activation of higher energy centers or chakras, the rising of Kundalini energy, and an expansion of conscious awareness, which can be cultivated and sustained for longer periods of time through certain types of yoga and meditation (Feuerstein, 1998).

Facilitating NOSC and Peak Experiences

Music and psychedelics serve as guides for accessing inner resources not readily available in ordinary states of consciousness. The poet William Blake wrote, "In the universe, there are things that are known, and things that are unknown, and in between, there are doors" (1794). Music opens these doors and guides us on a pathway through the mysterious territory. Music in psychedelic sessions provides a "sense of continuity and connection in the course of various unusual states of consciousness" (Grof, 1980, p. 141).

To this end, some research has investigated specific types of music that more effectively support NOSC and mystical experiences (Barrett et al., 2017). Qualitative analysis of musical selections recommended by expert guides for use during the peak period of psilocybin experiences revealed a preference for New Age, world music, and classical music (often orchestral or choral pieces). Additionally, common qualitative features (e.g., predictable phrase structure, consistent and homogenous instrumentation, slow tempo, simple meter, continuous movement that builds, and culturally non-European) and quantitative features (low perceptual brightness and high perceptual fullness) of "peak period stimuli" were found.

Furthermore, music has been used for centuries in ceremonies and rituals to induce trance states for the purpose of healing. Ludwig (1966) delineates common features among trance states: "alterations in thinking, change in sense of time and body image, loss of control, change in emotional expression, perceptual distortion, change in meaning and significance, a sense of ineffability, feelings of rejuvenation, and hypersuggestibility" (pp. 225–234). For the sake of our purposes here, we can define the trance state as an NOSC distinct from the "normal" waking state of consciousness, in which the subject has let go of any expectations or attachments to outcome and is open to what is unfolding in their present experience. In this state, the subject's consciousness is not obscured or reduced; yet, awareness of normal limits, such as time, space, body, and ego, is deprioritized and instead immersion in the inner world and imagination becomes the focus.

The key elements of trance induction are rhythm and melody (Pilch, 2006, p. 38). Certain kinds of music have been used in many cultures to essentially hypnotize the thinking mind into a more receptive, lower-frequency state of consciousness. In his study of the trance phenomenon, Winkelman (1986) describes the ancient practice of *auditory driving*: a universal component of shamanic healing traditions that involves repetitive drumming, singing, and chanting to induce trance states. In these states, "the cortex is easily set into oscillation at the alpha frequency, and that a wide-variety of percussion procedures produce or enhance this state of dominance of slow-wave frequencies" (p. 178). This is corroborated by EEG studies of subjects in trance states, which reveal increases in theta and alpha frequencies in frontal brain regions (Fachner, 2011, pp. 273–274). Winkelman further specifies that trance states share psychophysiological similarities: parasympathetic dominance, slowed brain wave patterns, and heightened limbic system activity (Winkelman, 1986, p. 174). Interestingly, other practices, such as meditation and dance, also involve increases in lower brain wave frequencies (Kohlmetz et al., 2003).

Regardless of the intention, dose, and music used, the possibility of entering into trance and accessing NOSC should be made explicit in the preparation phase of treatment. The therapist should provide specific examples of the range of NOSC that one may experience (e.g., out of body, near death, ego dissolution, and mystical experiences) and describe qualities of each, from the potential fear, terror, and liberation of ego dissolution to the expansiveness, awe, and sense of unity of the mystical experience.

Accessing the Imagination, Evoking Mental Imagery, and Processing Memories

Music can open the doorway to imagination, autobiographical memories, and visionary capacity. Music listening in psychedelic sessions has been shown to modulate neural circuitry responsible for mental imagery and autobiographical memory, enhancing the vividness of these phenomena (Kaelen et al., 2016).

The guiding and structuring aspect of music in the visionary space has been observed and described by cultural anthropologists partaking in sacred plant medicine ceremonies as participant observers. In many of these ceremonies, "Music and visualization seem causally linked, with music serving as a kind of software that instructs the course of the visual programing of the experience (Dobkin De Rios, 2006, p. 98). In iboga ceremonies with the Mitsogho people in Gabon, Uwe Maas and Suster Strubelt described music as acting as a "safety rope reaching from this life to the hereafter," serving as "a means of locomotion in the visionary space" and "facilitating remarkably spiritual communication and improving mental and physical well-being" (Maas & Strubelt, 2006, pp. 106–107). Marlene Dobkin del Rios and Fred Katz transcribed recordings from ayahuasca ceremonies with the Chama and Cashinahua people of Peru and described music functioning as a "jungle gym for the person's consciousness during the drug state" and "providing a series of pathways and banisters through which the drug user negotiates his way" (Dobkin De Rios, 2006, p. 99). They further explain:

> Rattles, singing, chanting and vocal productions in general may be a very important part of the hallucinogenic experience in that the "jungle gym" is built up, torn down, and rearranged in a sort of "block-building" of consciousness to serve specific cultural goals.
>
> (Ibid., p. 99)

They note that, "Healers were adamant about the importance of music in the healing session and the role that melody played in programming the actual content of the vision in their 'icaros,' or chants." (Ibid., p. 98)

Many of those in Western culture—therapists as well as clients—suffer from a kind of imaginal atrophy as the capacity and practice of envisioning are undervalued. Providing a safe space and right music provides an opportunity for clients to reconnect with their imagination and, perhaps, to other dimensions of consciousness and reality. Rediscovering our capacity to go within and have meaningful and profound experiences with ourselves and our inner worlds can deepen a sense of intimacy with the self and repair the wounds of self-abandonment and self-neglect. We are helping clients rediscover a home within.

Providing Support, Reassurance, and Soothing

Music is a source of support in the psychedelic experience; it can reduce stress, soothe autonomic nervous system activation, and lower cortisol levels (De Witte et al., 2022). Moreover, music has been historically used in shamanic ceremonies to counteract stress and reduce muscle tension, heart rate, and blood pressure (Winkelman, 2000, pp. 196–197).

Research has found that the use of music in psychedelic therapy can promote "calm and a sense of safety" (Kaelen et al., 2018, p. 1). Music therapists, such as Summer (2010), have advocated for careful selection of supportive music (i.e., music with minimal dissonance and dynamic changes) to help clients "access positive internal resources before moving on to more challenging material" (Battles, 2018, p. 4). Supportive or "soothing" music should be used alternately with "deepening" music to calm and activate the nervous system throughout the session (Kaelen, 2021, p. 370). Soothing music "does not strongly demand attention, and it allows the listener to explore various aspects of him- or herself and the experience freely" (Ibid., p. 370). Supportive music is best used in opening and closing phases of the experience, but it can also be used at various periods of the more dynamic phases of the session when indicated by the client's process, such as after the completion of processing intense emotion or to help regulate nervous system activation.

Preparing Music for Sessions

To design effective playlists for a psychedelic session, the therapist should have a good-enough understanding of the client's relationship with music. In the preparation session(s), it is important to inquire into the client's musical tastes and preferences. Many clients will make general statements, such as, "I like everything except Country." It is important to ask them to further describe what music they like, even asking about specific songs or albums that they have enjoyed listening to. The goal here is not to collect specific tracks for the playlist, but rather it is to get a sense of the genres and styles of music they prefer. It is also important to ask whether there is any music or sounds that they find off-putting or triggering. For example, if a client has been sexually abused by a priest, sounds of church bells or possibly even chimes should not be included, unless there is explicit consent from the client to use these sounds to revisit past traumatic experiences.

The following components should be incorporated to prepare a good psychedelic playlist: flow, variety (in cultural influences and emotional tones), mirroring of the medicine effects, and support and connection with higher vibrations. The playlist should make sense and move seamlessly from one song to the next. Similar to a good story, the playlist should take the client on a journey, and tracks should be arranged in a way that follows and builds upon previous tracks.

Each track should be appropriate to the specific phase of the journey: opening, building, peak, descent, and closing (Kaelen, 2021, p. 370). The opening phase should include slow, spacious, and soothing sounds. The building phase should include slightly higher tempo tracks that introduce elements of rhythm and beat while alternating between soothing and deepening tracks. In the peak phase, the music should continue alternating between soothing and deepening tracks but emphasize higher-tempo, more kinetic rhythms. The descent phase includes deeper, emotional, cinematic, and heart-opening tracks with continued alteration between soothing and deepening tracks. The closing phase should include meditative, spiritually themed, and largely soothing tracks.

Tracks should be arranged in a way that matches and supports the arc of the effects of the specific medicine being used. The therapist should know the dose–response curve of the medicine they are working with and select and arrange tracks that support each phase of the arc. The intensity of the tracks in each phase should mirror the anticipated intensity of the medicine effects. For example, with ketamine sessions, the duration of effects is much shorter than classical psychedelics, and the shorter arc of the medicine effects should be accounted for: peak effects come on relatively quickly after taking the medicine (within 5–30 minutes, depending on route of administration and individual sensitivity factors), tail effects last about twice as long as the ascent to the peak, and intensity of effects slowly lessen in the return to baseline. With MDMA, psilocybin, or LSD, the dose–response curve is much longer, with peak effects generally occurring one and a half to three hours after taking the medicine.

Furthermore, the style of music used in the playlist should enhance the effects of the medicine. For example, with ketamine, lower tempo (ranging from 60 to 120 BPM), ambient, and richly textured atmospheric tracks, including ambient sounds of waves crashing, bird calls, or children laughing, are generally more conducive to accentuating the spacious states of mind that people typically encounter. With MDMA, in contrast, higher-tempo tracks (ranging from 110 to 160 BPM), particularly during building and peak phases, provide greater enhancement of the effects.

Generally, it is best to use music that is unfamiliar to the client to optimize the novelty of the experience and avoid material to which the client may have associated memories. To this end, contemporary artists, like East Forest and Jon Hopkins, have created entirely new, instrumental soundscapes, albums, and mixes specifically designed to support clients in psychedelic sessions. Several of my colleagues, myself included, have used platforms, like Ableton and Audacity, to curate unique mixes for sessions.

Additionally, songs with lyrics, particularly in the listener's native tongue, can be distracting during the onset and peak of the medicine. It is typically better to reserve vocal tracks for the end of the journey to invite the client back into their body and to evoke a heart-centered experience.

The playlist should include a variety of tracks that are expected to evoke a range of emotions, as rich and varied as the human experience. Darker tracks and dissonant sounds can be important in evoking challenging emotions and memories and working toward acceptance and integration of repressed material. However, darker tracks should be used in moderation, and the ultimate goal of the playlist should be to uplift the client and aid them in accessing higher vibrations.

It is also important for the therapist to be able to hear the music the client is hearing. If the client will be using headphones, a simple device called a "headphone splitter" allows music to be played through a speaker and headphones simultaneously. This facilitates the therapist's connection to the client's process through the music and enables "therapists to empathize with the patient's current state, as well as observe how they were responding to a particular piece of music" (Kaelen et al., 2018, p. 507).

Dislike of and Resistance to Music

In the preparation session, it should be discussed how any dislike or resistance to the music will be handled. The client should understand that there may be times during the journey when they have challenging reactions or feel resistance to the music. In these moments, they can let the therapist know what is coming up for them. The concept of the inner healing intelligence can be used to prime the client to be open to and curious about whatever is arising, including agitation, fear, sadness, or any other uncomfortable emotions. If the discomfort is due to a lack of resonance with their inner process, it may be appropriate to change the track to support their process. However, if the distress is due to the client's dislike of the music or resistance to the nature of the material the music is evoking, then the client should generally be encouraged to stay with the material and try to move through it (Kaelen et al., 2018). In these cases, the therapist should first explore the client's distress and identify its source. They can then either encourage the client to stay with their process or change the music as needed. It is important that the client understands this method explicitly (from conversations in preparation phase), so they can fully surrender to their experience and know that there is a clear procedure in place for managing music-related distress.

Dimensions of Attunement

How can the psychedelic therapist optimize their presence and attunement with the lived experience of the client, as well as the sensory/vibrational tone of the session, so that they are best available to support the client? How does the therapist sensitize themselves to the subtleties of their own felt sense and their inner healing intelligence? Here, I will describe three dimensions of attunement that are important in this process: attunement to self (of the therapist), attunement to the relational field, and attunement to the vibrational field.

To further explore attunement, two essential principles of psychedelic therapy must be explained: non-directive/inner-directed psychotherapy and inner healing intelligence. These principles were originally delineated by Grof in his work in Holotropic Breathwork and later adapted for use in the MAPS MDMA-assisted psychotherapy treatment protocol. In the Manual for MDMA-Assisted Psychotherapy, the non-directive approach is described as,

> A general sense of permission, allowance, and receptivity, so that the locus of movement or therapeutic action is coming from within the participant rather than the therapists. Therapists become curious, asking questions or prompting awareness of an internal process. Participants are not so much "directed" inward as they are invited inward, encouraged through gentle suggestion from the therapists.
>
> (Mithoefer et al., 2017, pp. 10–11)

The goal of this approach is to support the client's innate capacity to connect with their inner healing intelligence and to allow it to lead them to process specific psychic material, memories, or experiences in order to heal. Mithoefer et al. (2017) describe inner healing intelligence with the following analogy:

> The body knows how to heal itself. If someone goes to the emergency room with a laceration, a doctor can remove obstacles to healing (e.g., remove foreign bodies, infection, etc.) and can help create favorable conditions for healing (e.g., sew the edges of the wound close together), but the doctor does not direct or cause the healing that ensues. The body initiates a remarkably complex and sophisticated healing process and always spontaneously attempts to move toward healing. The psyche too exhibits an innate healing intelligence and capacity.
>
> (p. 11)

With the help of the psychedelic and the music, the inner healing intelligence acts as a radar of sorts to navigate through NOSC and hone in on deeper psychic material—typically obscured by the conditioned mind—that needs attention and understanding.

Attunement to Self of the Therapist

In non-directive psychotherapy, the therapist also seeks to connect with their own inner healing intelligence. Just as the client is instructed to enter into a receptive state of mindfulness in the beginning of the session, using their breath and the music, the therapist also shifts into a more receptive space, allowing the surround of the room to impact them and noticing the details of their sensory experience— quality of breathing, posture, sounds, smells, etc. The work here is to breathe into one's present-moment experience and connect with the observing self, or witness consciousness. The therapist may even momentarily enter into a light trance state; this may signify an important syncing up with and deepening into a shared experience of consciousness.

Attunement to the Client and the Relational Field

Once connected with their self-experience, the therapist seeks to attune to the client's experience. Throughout the medicine session, clients are invited to direct their attention inward, with the option of listening to the playlist, and using headphones and eye shades to block out external stimuli. However, the therapist is also available for verbal processing when desired by the client. During these periods of inward attention, the music, which has been referred to as "the hidden therapist" (Kaelen et al., 2018, p. 505), becomes a primary support for the client. In these sessions, the aim is to let the client's inner healing intelligence guide the process; the therapist seeks to be non-directive and follow the client's lead. As such, the therapist must often rely on non-verbal perceptive and intuitive capacities rather than dialectical engagements, such as interpretation or meaning making.

Music is also a source of support for the therapist in the psychedelic therapy session. To the extent that both the therapist and the client are open to allowing the music to move them, a sharing of vibrational frequencies is possible, helping the therapist to stay attuned and in sync with the client's process. It is helpful to stay open to ways in which the beat, the melody, and the rhythm of the music are tuning and calibrating the corporeal instruments of the psyche–soma of both the therapist and the client.

In music theory, the term *resonance* describes the phenomenon of the sharing of vibrational frequencies between two separate bodies. For example, when two guitars are placed in close proximity to each other and a note is played only on one of them, the other will resonate, humming in the same note. Similarly, empathic attunement is facilitated by mirror neurons in resonance with the other:

> New developments in neurophysiology show that exposure to language develops mirror motor neurons when an active sound is perceived. . . . It is possible for us to know what is happening in the other person, as intersubjectivity, when we resonate with them.
>
> (Aldridge & Fachner, 2006, p. 11)

Resonating is a non-verbal dimension of relating and of empathizing, which holds the capacity to change the frequency of the other.

It might be helpful to consider each psychedelic therapy session as a meeting of two subjects attempting to make music together. As in music, so in therapy—attention to emergent qualities of the session, such as call and response, timing, tone, intonation, and rhythm, is needed to effectively attune, resonate, and harmonize. Shapiro et al. (2017) describe the here-and-now, improvisational, and bottom-up aspects of the art of attunement in psychotherapy: "The rhythm of back-and-forth relational flow, call and response, utterances punctuated by silences, synchronized rhythms of affective and autonomic responsiveness will be unique to each dyad and each moment" (p. 236).

The psychedelic therapist takes an interest and stays curious about the subtleties of their client's experience, noticing shifts in the client's behavior—breathing, movement, and other non-verbal aspects of their experience. What might be happening for them and how might they be expressing aspects of their process? Are they holding their breath, or is there a deepening of breath or a sigh? What unspoken meanings or feelings are being expressed through tone or intonation of the voice? What might they be sensing, feeling, seeing, and dreaming?

In attuning to the relational field, the therapist and the client are resonating, syncing their vibrational tones, frequencies, and rhythms. How does the client's engagement with the shared space (physical, psychic, and energetic) influence the therapist's experience? What is the quality of the shared sensory experience? Is it harmonic? Dissonant? Use of the voice by the therapist should be harmonious as opposed to disruptive: considerations of *how* (e.g., soft or loud) and *when* (in prep phase or at height of peak experience) to speak should be informed by the therapist's attunement to the flow of the session and the client's process.

Rigidity of personality and cognitive/emotional inflexibility can be sequelae of trauma, abuse, and neglect and are often rooted in early attachment wounds and patterns of interpersonal misattunement. Clients will often consciously or unconsciously seek to repeat these patterns in psychotherapy through reenactments in the interpersonal domain, "replaying a mournful, affective melody in the keys of hurt, sadness, fear, anger, and shame" (ibid., p. 233). The therapeutic encounter can be thought of as a "relational duet," where the therapist and the client acknowledge moments of dissonance and misattunement, enter a more harmonious and coherent relational flow, and ideally achieve synchronous togetherness. In this way, we are attuning, mirroring, resonating, and attending to help clients facilitate emotional expression, revise patterns they feel compelled to repeat, and reestablish a "coherent life narrative" (Siegel, 2007). See Chapter 5 for a further elaboration of tending to the relational field and working with enactments.

Attunement to the Shared Vibrational Field

Finally, we can attune to the vibrational field, which is inherently shared and connecting. Music is a tool for synchronization of two or more bodies and is highly efficient in synchronizing movement (Repp, 2005), emotions (Juslin & Laukka,

2008), and even physiological responses such as heart rate and blood pressure (Czepiel et al., 2021). The rhythm of the listener's heartbeat actually entrains to the rhythm of the music, almost as if the body is being calibrated and tuned to the frequency of the vibrational field.

The potential for the therapist and the client to merge through shared awareness of sensory phenomena, such as music—what psychoanalyst Peter Goldberg refers to as "sensory symbiosis"—can be overlooked in psychotherapy. As Goldberg (2012) explains, "In the act of jointly perceiving an object, one is rendered experientially indistinguishable from the other" (p. 796). He uses the example of gazing with a client upon various items in his office, together noticing the details and patterns within them, and making contact through curiosity and appreciation of sensory data, without having to make sense of it together through language. The sense of connection, in this case, was not created through meaning making but more primarily through "a shared location of attention." This form of seeking connection through the sensory field is not a regressive trait, as has been traditionally thought, but rather a progressive one; it is a seeking to transcend individual ego consciousness to be "free of the demand to relate to the other as object" (p. 796), to merge self with the world, and to arrive in the domain of pre-symbolic and trans-egoic Being—the undifferentiated realm of "at-one-ment" (Winnicott, 1960). This drive toward sensory symbiosis should be recognized and met by the therapist, as it may represent a wish to connect at a deeper, less formulated level and to share in a new experience of the world together.

Cultural Factors of Music Selection

While musical taste is highly individual and subjective, musical structure and meaning are also socially constructed. Musical perception, like psychedelic experience, is dependent on context. As Fachner (2011) explains, "Drug effects are necessarily situated and involve complex interactions between their pharmacological components and their psychological and physiological setting within a specific aesthetic context that frames the production, perception, and cognition of music" (p. 267). The perception of and meaning evoked by a particular song are informed by cultural as well as personal context.

When inducing trance states through music in various cultural practices, the selected music is a "context-dependent phenomenon relating to the cultural meaning of symbols and action during ceremonies" (Fachner, 2006, p. 20). Likewise, in psychedelic therapy, the therapist spends time in the preparation phase exploring and understanding the client's musical tastes in the context of their sociocultural matrix and influences. It is recommended that selection of particular types of music and inclusion of specific instruments and sounds be informed by the cultural values systems, in which the client is embedded as well as the client's cultural identity. Williams et al. (2020) suggest that,

> Music conducive to psychedelic healing for White Americans may be inadequate for those from other cultural backgrounds . . . it is important to consider

potential alterations, supportive measures, or alternatives to the typical Western playlist (e.g., new age music, space music, folk, post rock, etc.) that will better suit the individual needs of each patient based on their preferences, safety needs, age, and rich cultural background and heritage.

(pp. 44–45)

Although music has the power to open us up to unforeseen depths and heights, a misattuned musical selection can result in distractedness, resistance to the process, feeling unmet or misunderstood, and alienation from the therapist (Kaelen et al., 2018). Aligning music selection with the client's preferences, intention for the medicine session, and cultural background is a central aim in constructing effective playlists.

Case Example

Sam is a middle-aged, white, straight, cisgender man who is highly accomplished in his work but tormented by a prevalent sense of anxiety and depression related to his high-stress work life, which was also affecting his relationships. He complained of lack of joy, persistent worrying, and underlying "existential dread" related to a sense of meaninglessness. We did two series of six KAP sessions over the course of nine months with a three-month break between the series. During these sessions, he was able to access his observing self, or witness consciousness, which allowed him to gain perspective on the roots of his anxiety. His use of and insights into his relationship with music were essential in this process.

Sam grew up in a family where great emphasis was placed on productivity and achievement, and emotions were seen as an impediment to overcome. Not surprisingly, his parents were emotionally unavailable and dismissive of his emotional experience. He once explained, "Some of my most basic existential questions, my parents failed to answer. They didn't celebrate or embrace curiosity. I always had to be optimizing something; I never could let go and just be." He became adept at suppressing his emotional needs to please those around him and excelled in his school and work life. However, he described frequent feelings of overwhelm, being consumed by a "frantic" state of mind, and periodic depressive episodes.

Another detail of note is that he began playing piano at a young age, and performing well became yet another way to measure his achievement. It was not until he entered his teenage years that he discovered music as a resource. He explained that listening to music while bike riding or spending time alone in his room was perhaps the only thing that helped him feel and process his emotions, including sadness, anger, hurt, awe, and joy. He had found a way to begin making sense of his emotional landscape. He once mused, "There's a mapping of emotions through music."

As we prepared for his sixth KAP session, Sam expressed his intention to gain insight into his fear of expressing his needs. After receiving the intramuscular ketamine injection and as the effects were coming on, he connected with a sense of deep contentment and peace. He described having "arrived" and being in touch with "a calm, steady state of existence, a spacious, fluid, floaty space." He noted that this expansive space was shaped in time with the music: "Humming with the music. Resonance. Warm and energizing. Breathing with the music. Surfing." He felt increasingly "cozy" and "comfy." From this spacious state of mind, he gained insight into his fear of expressing his needs. He recalled an early fear of not being loved or accepted when having needs, and he connected this with his current fear of expressing his needs. He stated, "What I want isn't okay, so I don't express it."

As he continued to commune with the music, a visionary space opened. "There's a new expanse on the other side," he sighed. His hands moved gracefully in the air. He then began to notice a felt-sense experience that was *beyond* his anxiety. "The somatosensory experience is fascinating right now. The sensation. This music is a rebirth, a re-incantation of a thing I want to express. The one true melody. Being hard on myself doesn't exist in that place." As he explored further, he reflected, "This raw, connected felt sense gets contorted, suppressed, based on others' expectations. I was taught to appreciate and pursue the reward, not the journey, to care about the wrong thing!" Sam also explained that his constant attempts to control his environment were so deeply ingrained that he would not have known how to transcend them without psychedelics. He now saw how these attempts to control do not have to be so automatic, that he could access spaciousness and self-compassion instead.

In our integration session, we continued exploring this new experience of liberation from his conditioned mind and his increased access to self-compassion. Sam was able to name the anxiety as being related to a core invalidation of his emotional responses. He spoke of an urge to practice mindfulness, so that he could extend this more expansive state of awareness into his daily life: "I cannot let the anxiety take hold. Instead, I can practice being curious about it—a more gentle note, more fluid approach." He saw how when he succumbs to anxiety, he ignores his felt sense and underlying feelings, which contain valuable information. He committed to tuning into his felt sense more often and reaffirming his authority over his emotions.

In this session, Sam was able to access a felt sense of "okayness" and reclaim his relationship with his authentic self that transcended his conditioned anxiety about judgment and expectation from himself or others. He reconnected to his special relationship with music as a map of his emotions and guide to his inner world. In the integration sessions, he committed to using mindfulness and music listening as a practice to stay connected with himself in a more authentic way. As the therapist, I strove to stay attuned to Sam's process on multiple levels—narrative/cognitive, emotional, and somatosensory. The music was an essential aspect of the healing that occurred, facilitating access to emotions, providing support in navigating ego dissolution, and helping Sam connect with relevant memories as well as a deeply supportive sense of spaciousness and ease.

Conclusion

Music is a powerful tool and catalyst for psychedelic experience; these two complementary medicines have been combined for thousands of years to support healing and transformation. We are now rediscovering the healing potential of music and psychedelics and applying ancient techniques and practices in the modern clinical setting. We have reviewed some of the fundamentals of optimizing clients' experience with music, explored the nuances of listening and attunement, examined ways in which the therapist can use music to enhance their own attunement to and resonance with the client and their process, and considered ways in which music can allow for shared experiences that transcend verbal communication. As we move the field of relational psychedelic therapy forward, it will be crucial for therapists, clients, researchers, and musicians to continue to engage in interdisciplinary cross-fertilization and to collaborate in developing innovative ways of using music to deepen relational attunement, facilitate transformative and healing experiences, and optimize therapeutic outcomes.

Note

1   Holotropic Breathwork is a therapeutic modality developed by Stanislav and Christina Grof that combines a specific breathing method with evocative music to access and work with NOSC for healing. The term "holotropic" is derived from the Greek "holos" (whole) and "trepein" (to move toward), meaning "moving toward wholeness."

References

Aldridge, D., & Fachner, J. (2006). *Music and altered states: Consciousness, transcendence, therapy and addictions*. Jessica Kingsley Publishers.

Barrett, F. S., Robbins, H., Smooke, D., Brown, J., & Griffiths, R. (2017). Qualitative and quantitative features of music reported to support peak mystical experiences during psychedelic therapy sessions. *Frontiers in Psychology*, 8, 1238. https://doi.org/10.3389/fpsyg.2017.01238

Battles, P. (2018). Music as a catalyst for altered states of consciousness and peak experiences in the treatment of depression, anxiety, and PTSD. *Expressive Therapies Capstone Theses*, 89. https://digitalcommons.lesley.edu/expressive_theses/89

Belser, A., Agin-Liebes, G., Swift, T., Terrana, S., Devenot, N., Friedman, H., . . . Ross, S. (2017). Patient experiences of psilocybin-assisted psychotherapy: An interpretative phenomenological analysis. *Journal of Humanistic Psychology*, 57(4), 354–388. https://doi.org/10.1177/0022167817706884

Blake, W., Lessing, J., & Rosenwald Collection. (1794). *The marriage of heaven and hell*. Retrieved from the Library of Congress. www.loc.gov/item/50041675/

Blood, A., & Zatorre, R. (2001). Intensely pleasurable responses to music correlate with activity in brain regions implicated in reward and emotion. *Proceedings of the National Academy of Sciences of the United States of America*, 98(20), 11818–11823. https://doi.org/10.1073/pnas.191355898

Bonny, H., & Pahnke, W. (1972). The use of music in psychedelic (LSD) psychotherapy. *Journal of Music Therapy*, 9, 64–87.

Chandler, A., & Hartman, M. (1960). *Lysergic acid diethylamide (LSD-25) as a facilitating agent in psychotherapy*. A. M. A. Archives of General Psychiatry, 2. Box: 3, Folder: 1. Stanislav Grof papers, MSP 1, Series 3, Sub-Series 2, File 3, Item 23, Purdue University Archives and Special Collections. Retrieved July 3, 2022, from https://archives.lib.pur-due.edu/repositories/2/archival_objects/25032

Czepiel, A., Fink, L., Fink, L., et al. (2021). Synchrony in the periphery: Inter-subject correlation of physiological responses during live music concerts. *Scientific Reports, 11*, 22457. https://doi.org/10.1038/s41598-021-00492-3

De Witte, M., Da Silva Pinho, A., Stams, G., Moonen, X., Bos, A., & Van Hooren, S. (2022). Music therapy for stress reduction: A systematic review and meta-analysis. *Health Psychology Review, 16*(1), 134–159. doi: 10.1080/17437199.2020.1846580

Dobkin de Rios, M. (2006). The role of music in healing with hallucinogens. In D. Aldridge & J. Fachner (Eds.), *Music and altered states: Consciousness, transcendence, therapy and addictions* (pp. 97–100). Jessica Kingsley Publishers.

Fachner, J. (2006). Music and altered states of consciousness: An overview. In D. Aldridge & J. Fachner (Eds.), *Music and altered states: Consciousness, transcendence, therapy and addictions* (pp. 15–37). Jessica Kingsley Publishers.

Fachner, J. (2011). Drugs, altered states, and musical consciousness: Reframing time and space. In D. Clarke, & E. F. Clarke (Eds.), *Music and consciousness: Philosophical, psychological, and cultural perspectives* (pp. 263–280). Oxford University Press. http://dx.doi.org/10.1093/acprof:oso/9780199553792.003.0074

Ferreri, L., Aucouturier, J., Muthalib, M., Bigand, M., & Bugaiska, A. (2013). Music improves verbal memory encoding while decreasing prefrontal cortex activity: An fNIRS study. *Frontiers in Human Neuroscience, 7*, 1–9. www.frontiersin.org/articles/10.3389/fnhum.2013.00779

Feuerstein, G. (1998). *Tantra: The path of ecstasy*. Shambhala.

Goldberg, P. (2012). Active perception and the search for sensory symbiosis. *Journal of the American Psychoanalytic Association, 60*(4), 791–812. https://doi.org/10.1177/000306511245569

Grof, S. (1980). *LSD psychotherapy*. MAPS.

Jung, C. (1963). *Psychology and religion: West and East*. Pantheon Books.

Juslin, P., & Laukka, D. (2008). Emotional responses to music: The need to consider underlying mechanisms. *Behavioral and Brain Sciences, 31*, 559–75. doi: 10.1017/S0140525X08005293

Kaelen, M. (2021). The use of music in psychedelic therapy. In C. S. Grob & J. Grigsby (Eds.), *Handbook of medical hallucinogens* (pp. 363–376). The Guilford Press.

Kaelen, M., Giribaldi, B., Raine, J., Evans, L., Timmerman, C., Rodriguez, N., & Carhart-Harris, R. (2018). The hidden therapist: Evidence for a central role of music in psychedelic therapy. *Psychopharmacology, 235*(2), 505–519. https://doi.org/10.1007/s00213-017-4820-5

Kaelen, M., Roseman, L., Kahan, J., Santos-Ribeiro, A., Orban, C., Lorenz, R., . . . Carhart-Harris, R. (2016). LSD modulates music-induced imagery via changes in parahippocampal connectivity. *European Neuropsychopharmacology: The Journal of the European College of Neuropsychopharmacology, 26*(7), 1099–1109. https://doi.org/10.1016/j.euroneuro.2016.03.018

Kohlmetz, C., Kopiez, R., & Altenmüller, E. (2003). Stability of motor programs during a state of meditation: Electrocortical activity in a pianist playing "vexations" by Erik

Satie continuously for 28 hours. *Psychology of Music, 31*(2), 173–186. https://doi. org/10.1177/0305735603031002293

Kroeker, J. (2019). *Jungian music psychotherapy: When psyche sings* (1st ed.). Routledge. https://doi.org/10.4324/9780429459740

Levine, P. A., & Frederick, A. (1997). *Waking the tiger: Healing trauma: The innate capacity to transform overwhelming experiences*. North Atlantic Books.

Ludwig, A. M. (1966). Altered states of consciousness. *Archives General Psychiatry, 15*(3), 225–234.

Maas, U., & Strubelt, S. (2006). Polyrhythms supporting a pharmacotherapy: Music in the iboga initiation ceremony in gabon. In D. Aldridge & J. Fachner (Eds.), *Music and altered states: Consciousness, transcendence, therapy and addictions* (pp. 101–124). Jessica Kingsley Publishers.

Mithoefer, M. (2017). *A manual for MDMA-assisted psychotherapy in the treatment of posttraumatic stress disorder*. https://maps.org/research-archive/mdma/MDMA-Assisted-Psychotherapy-Treatment-Manual-Version7-19Aug15-FINAL.pdf

Pilch, J. (2006). Music and trance. In D. Aldridge & J. Fachner (Eds.), *Music and altered states: Consciousness, transcendence, therapy and addictions* (pp. 38–50). Jessica Kingsley Publishers.

Repp, B. (2005). Sensorimotor synchronization: A review of the tapping literature. *Psychonomic Bulletin & Review, 12*(6), 969–992. https://doi.org/10.3758/BF03206433

Shapiro, Y., Marks-Tarlow, T., & Fridman, J. (2017). Listening beneath the words: Parallel processes in music and psychotherapy. *American Journal of Play, 9*, 228–251.

Siegel, D. J. (2007). Mindfulness training and neural integration: Differentiation of distinct streams of awareness and the cultivation of well-being. *Social Cognitive and Affective Neuroscience, 2*(4), 259–263. https://doi.org/10.1093/scan/nsm034

Summer, L. (2010). Music therapy and depression: Uncovering resources in music and imagery. In A. Meadows (Ed.), *Developments in music therapy practice: Case study perspectives* (pp. 486–500). Barcelona Publishers.

Suzuki, S., & Dixon, T. (2010). *Zen mind, beginner's mind*. Shambhala.

Williams, M., Reed, S., & Aggarwal, R. (2020). Culturally informed research design issues in a study for MDMA-assisted psychotherapy for posttraumatic stress disorder. *Journal of Psychedelic Studies, 4*(1), 40–50. doi: 10.1556/2054.2019.016

Winkelman, M. (1986). Trance states: A theoretical model and cross-cultural analysis. *Ethos, 14*(2), 174–203.

Winkelman, M. (2000). *Shamanism: The neural ecology of consciousness and healing*. Bergin & Garvey.

Winnicott, D. (1960). The theory of the parent-infant relationship. *International Journal of Psychoanalysis, 41*, 585–595.

Chapter 13

Psychedelic-Assisted Group Therapy

Christopher Stauffer and Brian T. Anderson

I was seeing in a sacred manner the shapes of all things in the spirit, and the shape of all shapes as they must live together like one being. And I saw that the sacred hoop of my people was one of many hoops that made one circle.

~**Heȟáka Sápa** or "**Black Elk**" (1863–1950), *wičháša wakȟáŋ* of the Oglala Lakota people (Black Elk & DeMallie, 1986)

Systems are groups of interconnected elements that form a unified whole. Depending on the scope of our lens, we can define systemic boundaries around a single cell or an entire galaxy, both our internal and external family systems, our broader social networks, or any of the myriad ecosystems we share with other organisms. In this chapter, we focus on *psychedelic-assisted group therapy*. There is still so much we do not know about individual psychedelic-assisted therapy; introducing the topic of psychedelic-assisted *group* therapy ostensibly adds magnitudes more complexity.

Research has demonstrated that a primary therapeutic mechanism of psychedelic-assisted therapy is a profound firsthand experience of mystical unity (James et al., 2020), during which a participant transcends their limited default system of consciousness and can integrate information (and perhaps wisdom) from a broader perspective. "The interconnectedness of all things" is an inherently overpowering concept. Similarly, group dynamics can seem overwhelming for researchers, clinicians, and participants to navigate. However, according to chaos theory, within the apparent randomness of complex systems, patterns emerge. Subatomic particles, the DNA double helix, crystal formations, and the structure of solar systems are all examples of self-organizing fractal patterning that pervades our ever-expanding range of perceptual awareness and symbolizes the harmonious interwoven fabric of the universe. When people form a group with the intention of healing, as in group therapy, the gestalt can be utilized therapeutically. While some of the emergent patterns of a group therapy cohort may readily reach the conscious awareness of group participants, many aspects are enacted unconsciously. A systems perspective is foundational when inviting group participants to reflect on these patterns as they surface.

DOI: 10.4324/9781003167976-13

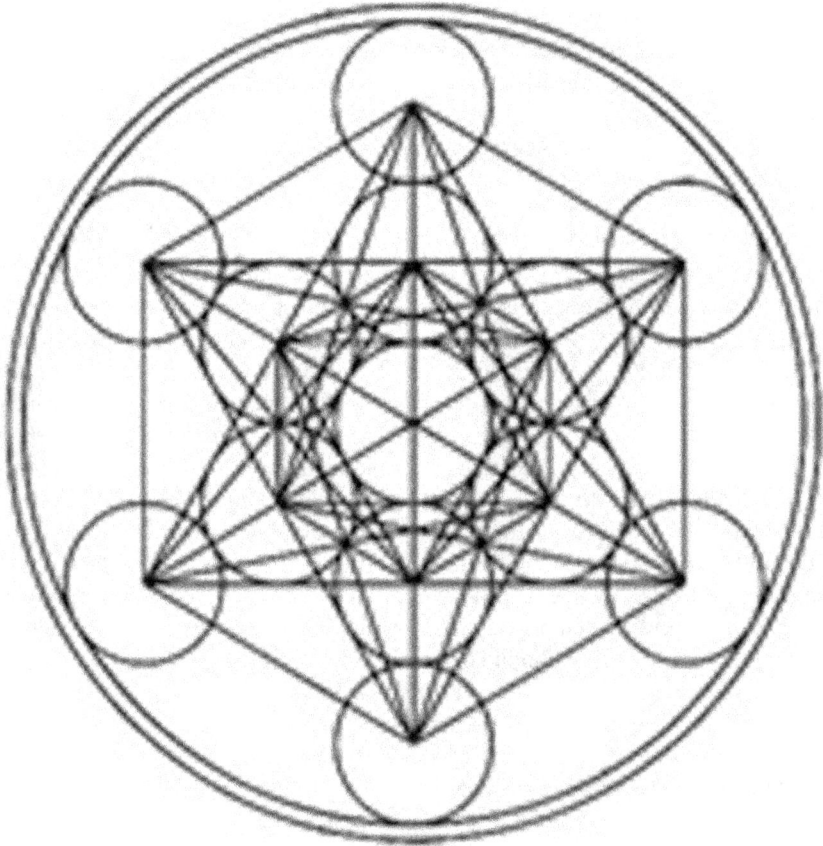

Figure 13.1 Image of Metatron's cube

Modern protocols for individual psychedelic-assisted therapy already comprise small groups of three: a participant and two co-facilitators. This moves the treatment beyond the traditional dyadic to what Bowen family systems theory refers to as a "triangle," the smallest basic unit of an emotional system and the central way through which emotional process is both transmitted and stabilized (Titelman, 2008). Group psychotherapy typically involves one to two facilitators and a cohort of four to nine participants. However, a group cohort of, say, two co-facilitators and six participants is not just six individual treatments. It represents a matrix of interlocking triangles created by eight foci as well as a superimposed layer representing *group cohesion* (G. M. Burlingame et al., 2018) or *cohesiveness* (Yalom & Leszcz, 2020). If navigated well enough, the emerging themes and emotional processes of a cohesive group can provide powerful and unique opportunities for healing both individual and collective wounds. We aim to reinforce the idea that psychedelic-assisted group therapy, while introducing complexity and additional risks that must be attuned to, has the potential for unique therapeutic benefit well beyond mere time- and cost-effectiveness to address scalability—features that are often touted as primary motivations for incorporating a group modality.

The process of gathering in small circles with a healing intention and ingesting substances that expand our sense of connection is nothing new. Indigenous communities in the Americas and beyond have carried and protected centuries-old traditions of psychedelic plant and fungi use in the context of communal rituals for individual and collective health; rites of passage; and for the pursuit of knowledge, power, and the harmonious stewardship of everyday relationships among community members (Furst, 1976; Schultes & Hofmann, 1992). The varied reasons why different traditional communities use psychedelics in group settings are manifold. There are many salubrious effects of traditional ceremonies that can also be found in group therapy, such as corrective attachment experiences, a sense of safety from being with others "like me" when going through an emotionally challenging process, and even the mere fact of not being in isolation. Nonetheless, traditional communal ceremonies and the Western model of group therapy are different processes, and cultural misappropriation should be avoided when incorporating psychedelic medicines into group therapy (e.g., using distinct practices and symbols from one cultural group without serious training and instruction in how to do so appropriately).

In the following sections, we will briefly summarize the first wave of psychedelic-assisted group therapy research from the mid-20th century, dissect our preliminary experiences merging psychedelic-assisted group therapy with modern scientific rigor, review the evidence base for group therapy in general, and recommend strategies for ongoing psychedelic-assisted group therapy research and eventual practice.

20th Century Psychedelic-Assisted Group Therapy Clinical Research

Early therapeutic research with classic psychedelics,[1] before becoming Schedule I substances[2] in the 1970s, often involved the study of group work (Trope et al., 2019). A number of publications have detailed clinical approaches to conducting psychedelic-assisted group therapy (Chwelos et al., 1959; Sessa & Fischer, 2015; Stolaroff, 2004). A recent systematic review of English- and Spanish-language publications on classic psychedelic-assisted group therapy clinical trials found that the most methodologically sound mid-20th century studies of these group therapies focused on treating "neuroses" (anxiety and mood syndromes) or "alcoholism" (Trope et al., 2019). The populations, methodologies, and outcome reporting of these early studies varied considerably, with many studies employing single-arm open-label designs, mostly of oral LSD with or without accompanying psychotherapy. Reporting of safety data was minimal.

One main conclusion we can draw from these publications is that the manuscripts did not report any serious adverse reactions to the treatments—inferring that no participants died, were hospitalized, or had a persisting major impairment in functioning due to the treatment. Also, in the case of the alcohol use treatment studies, better clinical outcomes were associated with intentionally combining the drug sessions with a group therapy approach that was specifically designed to support psychedelic experiences. Finally, the only trial that compared individual and group LSD dosing sessions for "neurotic patients" in an ongoing group therapy cohort found that patients had better outcomes when the LSD was administered in individual dosing sessions. This points to the potential benefits of inward-directed experiences while under the acute effects of certain psychedelics, even when using group settings to enhance social support in preparation and integration.

±3,4-Methyl enedioxy methamphetamine (MDMA) was introduced into psychotherapy in the 1970s by way of Ann and Alexander Shulgin (Shulgin & Shulgin, 1991). Early accounts of the therapeutic use of MDMA describe couples and group settings, although publications mainly reflect brief case studies or protocol outlines rather than clinical research (Adamson & Metzner, 1988; Gasser, 1994; Greer & Tolbert, 1986; Naranjo, 2001; Passie, 2018). Torsten Passie (2018) mentions that group work with MDMA quickly became a common approach among practicing therapists, noting "MDMA appears to have advantages [over classic psychedelics] for group settings because of its capacity to help people free themselves from interpersonal distrust and communication blocks without interfering with cognition" (p. 14). A typical weekend retreat with 12–16 group members involved a Friday night intention sharing session, a daylong MDMA session on Saturday, followed by a Sunday morning integration circle. It was not advised for someone to participate in an interactive group therapy experience who had not previously had a facilitated individual experience to first orient to the non-ordinary state and other aspects of the experience.

Ralph Metzner (1998) characterized two approaches to MDMA administration in a group context that emerged during the 1970s and early 1980s. One approach involved interaction among the participants during the session. Some groups practiced structured interaction, where the group sat or lay in a circle, and each participant had a turn with a "talking stick." An alternate version of an interactive therapy group, described by the Chilean psychiatrist Claudio Naranjo, involved non-directed unstructured interaction among groups of people who typically had ongoing relationships outside of therapy. Participants had the option to withdraw from group process at any point during the session, but Naranjo noted, "Again and again I have had the impression that as the result of the catalytic effects of MDMA upon the participants, the group becomes a spontaneously organizing system, for the good of all" (Naranjo, 2001, pp. 208–221). The second approach—endorsed by Leo Zeff, a psychotherapist who, during the late 1970s and 1980s, administered MDMA to some 4000 people and trained more than 150 facilitators—involved each person engaging with their own internal process and communicating only with facilitators if needed. Per Zeff, "Sometimes people like to get up and do some hugging and then we set them right back down" (Stolaroff, 2004, p. 81).

In the 1980s, rave culture saw the combination of MDMA, music, and movement in a large-scale naturalistic experiment in psychopharmacology, ritual, and *communitas*[3] (Turner, 2012). Although use of psychoactive substances in such unregulated contexts comes with heightened risk, many participants reported having had healing experiences in a rave context (Hutson, 1999). However, to regulatory bodies, rave culture appeared to resemble too closely the psychedelic-inspired counterculture of the 1960s and is often touted as the impetus behind the Drug Enforcement Administration categorizing MDMA as a Schedule I substance in 1985, despite its therapeutic potential at the time.

Lack of modern scientific rigor in earlier studies and the rescheduling of psychedelic medicines, which put considerable constraint on ongoing research, have left us without a stable evidence base for conducting psychedelic-assisted group therapy. The field is once again in a position to explore this modality, now with a stronger framework of general group therapy knowledge and revised research methodology.

21st Century Psychedelic-Assisted Group Therapy Clinical Research

While the combination of group therapy with psychedelic drug administration was a fairly common practice in psychedelic medicine in the mid-20th century, and this work continued in Europe in legal clinical treatment sessions in the late 20th century and into the 21st century (Gasser, 1994; Passie, 2012), there was a gap in protocolized clinical research in this area for several decades.

In 2018, we conducted the first psychedelic-assisted group therapy clinical trial of the 21st century (Anderson et al., 2020). This study was an open-label pilot safety and feasibility trial of psilocybin-assisted group therapy for demoralization in older, male, gay-identified, long-term AIDS survivors. Eighteen men with moderate-to-severe demoralization enrolled in the trial, representing three group therapy cohorts of six participants each. Each cohort underwent four group preparatory sessions of 90 minutes each, and then each participant had an *individual* psilocybin session in which they ingested a capsule with 0.3 mg/kg or 0.36 mg/kg synthetic psilocybin. This was followed by an individual integration session the day after the medicine session and then four to six group integration sessions of 90 minutes each. The group therapy in this trial was based on a process-oriented existential group therapy called supportive expressive group therapy that was initially developed for women with metastatic breast cancer. This trial found that with modern clinical trial methodologies, it can be feasible and safe to administer high-dose psilocybin to a chronically distressed patient population with complex medical and psychiatric histories while having the vast majority of non-medicine psychotherapy sessions offered in a group format. The clinical outcomes also suggest that this intervention has a strong potential to be efficacious in treating demoralization among marginalized patients with serious medical illness and significant trauma histories.

As of 2022, recruitment is open for two clinical trials of psilocybin therapy using group therapy elements for the treatment of depression in patients with cancer: one at an oncology clinic in Maryland (ClinicalTrials.gov NCT04593563) and the other at a cancer institute in Utah (NCT04522804). In Maryland, the preparation and integration sessions are to be conducted in group cohorts of four participants each, while the medication sessions occur as four simultaneous sessions in separate rooms. In Utah, cohorts include up to six participants, and medicine sessions occur with all participants in the same space with one therapist per participant. We have also designed a clinical trial of MDMA-assisted group therapy for veterans with PTSD, with plans to begin recruiting in 2023. In this protocol, participants will undergo two MDMA sessions three to five weeks apart, the first being an individual MDMA session with two co-facilitators and the second being a group MDMA session with six participants and a team of four co-facilitators present. Most of the preparation and integration will be conducted as group sessions led by two co-facilitators. Over the next several years, research on psychedelic therapy conducted in various group formats is likely to continue to unfold.

Evolution of Group Therapy Principles

Formal group therapy has undergone many academic iterations over the past several decades. In a cheeky reference to the paternalistic medical landscape while working on his doctoral dissertation, "The Social Dimensions of Personality: Group Structure and Process," Timothy Leary wrote, "In 1947, a medically trained psychiatrist considered group therapy as recklessly dangerous as requesting a group of patients to perform perilous surgical operations on each other" (Leary, 1982, p. 6). Several decades later, a comprehensive evidence base exists demonstrating that group therapy is a safe treatment option with efficacy at least equal to that of individual therapy for many mental health issues (G. Burlingame & Krogel, 2005; Burlingame et al., 2004).

Eric Berne, a contemporary of, and arguably influenced by, Timothy Leary, surmised in his 1966 book *Principles of Group Treatment* that "knowledge of group dynamics for a group leader is as essential as knowledge of physiology for a physician" (Berne, 1966, p. 138). Irvin Yalom, who first published *Theory and Practice of Group Psychotherapy* in 1970 (Yalom & Leszcz, 2020), refers to the therapy group as a microcosm of everyday reality for its members, who will recreate automatic attachment dynamics and behavioral patterns that are also evident for them outside of the group therapy setting. Therapeutic change then occurs via facilitated emotionally reparative experiences within the group setting, which Yalom calls *the corrective recapitulation of the primary family group*. This phenomenon counters well-worn maladaptive relational patterns rooted in early family dynamics that are, unfortunately, largely reinforced during uncontrolled interactions in real-world settings. Corrective recapitulation of the primary family group is one of 11 evidence-based therapeutic factors of group therapy that Yalom and his colleagues have identified. The others include:

- Instillation of hope
- Universality
- Imparting information
- Altruism
- Development of socialization techniques
- Imitative behavior
- Interpersonal learning
- Group cohesiveness
- Catharsis
- Existential factors

To expand on a few more of these factors, *universality* allows individuals with similar experiences and issues to know that they are not alone, and group therapy *instills hope* by allowing group members to see others at different stages in the treatment process. *Group cohesiveness*, the group therapy analogue to *therapeutic alliance* in individual therapy, results in members of a group cohort gaining a sense of belonging and acceptance as they unite over a common treatment goal.

In sum, group therapy is effective for a wide range of mental health issues, and unique therapeutic factors of group therapy have been identified through decades of research.

Psychedelic-Assisted Group Therapy Design

Generally, not explicitly modifying a treatment manual from individual therapy for group settings has been shown to lower group therapy effectiveness (G. M. Burlingame et al., 2004). Michael Mithoefer et al.'s (2017) "A Manual for MDMA-Assisted Psychotherapy in the Treatment of Posttraumatic Stress Disorder," published by the Multidisciplinary Association for Psychedelic Studies (MAPS) and publicly available online (Mithoefer, 2017), is an evidence-based foundational resource for individual psychedelic-assisted therapy. The approach described in the manual is based on distilled knowledge from early psychedelic therapy research, including Grof's work with LSD and Holotropic Breathwork. MAPS trains facilitators on an "inner-directed" approach to therapy based on empathic presence and trust in the participant's inner healing intelligence—a person's innate capacity and drive to be the source of their own healing. The manual also describes the process of orienting a participant to working therapeutically with NOSC, the creation of an appropriate set and setting, the safe and therapeutic use of touch, and the essential process of integration. This manual provides a solid approach to individual psychedelic-assisted therapy; however, factors pertaining to the group container and navigation of group process should be incorporated to adapt the manual for psychedelic-assisted group therapy.

There are a variety of resources available to support the adaptation of individual treatment models to a group context. Yalom's *The Theory and Practice of Group Psychotherapy* is a comprehensive guide for understanding and implementing psychodynamic group therapy (Yalom & Leszcz, 2020). Motivational interviewing, a client-centered descendant of Rogerian therapy with a humanistic orientation, emphasizes that people are naturally inclined to pursue wellness and growth (a notion that is akin to the "inner healing intelligence") and outlines many practical techniques and a broad spirit compatible with the MAPS model. Wagner and Ingersoll's *Motivational Interviewing in Groups* is another helpful resource for adapting an existing individual approach into a group format (Wagner & Ingersoll, 2013). Aspects of other group manuals can be incorporated, for example acceptance and commitment therapy (Westrup & Wright, 2017) or cognitive processing therapy (Chard et al., 2009), depending on the clinical population and intention of the group.

Group therapy can take on many different formats. Throughout this chapter, we are primarily referring to "closed," "time-limited" group therapy, which is different in structure and intention from psychoeducational or support groups, which are often drop-in groups with open-ended formats. A closed group, which starts and ends with the same cohort of pre-selected participants, allows for a greater sense of trust and safety to develop among the group cohort. Ideally, the structural role and administration of any psychoeducational components during group sessions are shared by two co-facilitators, while the group process is co-created among co-facilitators and participants. While group cohesion has been shown to explain positive outcomes regardless of the treatment length, this is strongest when a group lasts more than 12 sessions (Burlingame et al., 2011). Many of these aspects distinguish group therapy from a "weekend retreat" model, an important distinction as psychedelic work continues to expand.

Recruitment and screening are much more challenging for group interventions compared to individual. Several potential participants must be recruited, screened, and considered for enrollment within a limited time frame in order for the group to have enough eligible participants for a single cohort. At the most basic level, an experienced and detail-oriented coordinator is required to harmonize the schedules of group participants, co-facilitators, and support staff. Eligibility criteria will vary, but at the very least all participants must have adequate flexibility in their schedules. Group composition might also take into account the preferred level of heterogeneity of demographic, diagnostic, and personality characteristics among participants, which will differ depending on the framework and intention of specific groups. The American Group Psychotherapy Association has developed clinical practice guidelines for assembling a group (Burlingame et al., 2006).

There are many additional design elements to consider with psychedelic-assisted group therapy. Should group sessions be reserved solely for preparation and integration? Or should psychedelic sessions be conducted in a group setting? If group psychedelic sessions are deemed appropriate, should the dosing regimen be the same as in individual sessions? Should an individual psychedelic session be required for each group member prior to participation in a group psychedelic session? This may be a particularly pertinent question for psychedelic-naïve participants or participants with more severe psychopathology, in which case it may be important to introduce the participant to psychedelic experiences and assess their capacity to navigate them prior to entering these realms in a group setting. How many individual preparatory or integration sessions, if any, should be incorporated into a group protocol? With the current standard of care for individual psychedelic work being a two-is-to-one facilitator-to-participant ratio, what is an ideal ratio for group work? Many open questions remain that are pertinent to the safe and responsible conduct of psychedelic-assisted group therapy. Despite a limited evidence base, we begin to address some of these questions here.

Psychedelic-Assisted Group Therapy Arc

Group Preparation

During the preparation phase, group co-facilitators must juggle the tasks of orienting group members to NOSC, creating an apt set and setting, establishing group guidelines and norms, and beginning to build group cohesion. Participants may be more or less familiar with a group therapy setting or engaging in a "here-and-now" approach (focusing on what is arising in the moment rather than on past events), which is encouraged in most group therapy manuals. This may inform the number of group preparatory sessions included in the protocol. Techniques typically taught to prepare a participant for a psychedelic session, such as diaphragmatic breathing, mindfulness, and other forms of grounding, can be used to open and close each group preparatory session.

Preparation for psychedelic-assisted therapy involves intention setting. Co-facilitators must navigate each group participant's personal intention as well as the intention of the group as a whole. Individual preparation time may be needed for personal intention setting, deepening rapport with providers, discussing specific personal symptoms and historical information, and establishing individual safety. Participants are encouraged to approach psychedelic sessions with "beginner's mind," remaining open to whatever emerges, and to understand that the process of healing is nonlinear. It is vital for participants to understand that there is no "typical" psychedelic experience in preparation for the variety of experiences group members may have.

Therapeutic concepts, such as inner healing intelligence or honoring resistance, can be applied at both the individual and group levels. Just as an individual's own drive and capacity to heal will unfold in the right set and setting, we urge participants to trust that the group's healing intelligence will manifest. Co-facilitators can watch for and respect any resistance from group members, meeting any apparent opposition to group process with curiosity and obtaining permission from all participants before moving into deeper emotional intimacy as a group. Finally, group leaders should assess whether some group therapy members may need additional individual preparation sessions prior to a psychedelic session. Flexibility in scheduling, in the name of safety, should always be a consideration.

Psychedelic Administration in Group Work

When psychedelic sessions are conducted with each group member individually after group preparation, keep in mind that scheduling several individual psychedelic and integration sessions within a relatively short amount of time will require a high level of coordination. If too much time elapses between the first participant's individual psychedelic session and the last participant's individual psychedelic session, group cohesion might be sacrificed. This must also be balanced with potential facilitator exhaustion from conducting multiple individual sessions in a short time frame.

Creating the set and setting for a group psychedelic session require extra attention compared to individual sessions. Participants can collectively contribute to the creation of an altar or some other symbolic "transitional object" that can serve as a grounding reference during the psychedelic experience. Music playlists will need to have an arc that is likely to work for all participants during the session, or the technology setup might allow for multiple sets of noise-canceling headphones with individual volume control, different music track options, or an option for silence. There must be adequate space for all group members to lie flat and for co-facilitators to access each participant with ease during the session. It is helpful for each participant to have a mat that demarcates their personal space, where, depending on the protocol, they may be asked to remain for most of the session. It is helpful to have plenty of blankets on hand and other items to address the individual comfort needs of each participant. From Leary's *Changing My Mind*,

One suggestion is to place the heads of the beds together to form a star pattern. Perhaps one may want to place a few beds together and keep one or two some distance apart for anyone who wishes to remain aside for some time. The availability of an extra room is desirable for someone who wishes to be in seclusion.

(Leary, 1982, p. 115)

There is no quality evidence base yet to determine the optimal ratio of facilitators to participants. Multiple participants might require individual attention at the same time. With a group psychedelic session, it is typically predetermined by the co-facilitators when the group's focus will be external (e.g., the opening and closing of the session) and when the group members' focus is to be on their own inner process.

The group can begin and end with a collective ritual that is already familiar to group members from preparatory sessions. Some psychedelic group spaces involve specific cultural or ceremonial practices that may not be appropriate when working with a variety of individuals in a professional therapeutic context. When establishing components of the opening and closing ceremonies of the group session, facilitators should take care to avoid rituals or practices that may alienate any given member. Nonetheless, ritual is important. Knowledge of each participant's culture and spiritual practice as well as history of previous harm from participation in religious, spiritual, or healing practices will help facilitators create an inclusive ritual and overall set and setting. Specific practices may be co-created during the preparatory phase, with all participants' input and explicit consent on an ongoing basis.

There is not a definitive way to conduct a group psychedelic session. If parallel inner work is preferred, "the group" can be established as a secure base from which to start individual explorations and to return to whenever participants need additional support from facilitators. It is important to keep in mind that a group process is occurring even when all participants are focused inward. Conversely, intentional group process through interaction of group members during a psychedelic session may be facilitated or allowed to occur organically. Facilitators might want to coordinate roles so that there is always at least one facilitator monitoring the group as a whole and assuring that any individual requests for assistance are attended to immediately. Intentionally bringing the group back together at the end of the session, either from inner work or various group interactions, can be beneficial for supporting group cohesion and creates space for a closing ritual.

Group Integration

In a group setting, psychedelic-assisted therapy can have a Gestalt quality, with each individual experience tied to the collective and vice versa. Systems theory tells us that when one part of a system changes, the other parts will initially resist the change to maintain homeostasis. As a group matures, individuals can embody different roles for the group, which may or may not be a role they are familiar with in their regular lives. Recognizing and normalizing emerging dynamics in group therapy are not dissimilar from how we approach multiplicity in individual psychedelic-assisted therapy. For example, when a group member takes on a scapegoat role, it is important to witness and assist in delicately integrating the experience into the larger group, just as it is important to witness and integrate exiled parts in an IFS framework (see Chapter 11). Transmuting conflict and resistance among members into compassion, curiosity, and other components of "Self energy," as defined in IFS, can aid both group and individual integration, ultimately manifesting as improved social functioning outside of the group. Just as individual psychedelic-assisted therapy involves helping intimate others outside of the therapy adjust to the major therapeutic changes their loved one experiences over the often relatively brief treatment course, with a group therapy cohort we must consider each participant's outside support system in addition to the system of the therapy group.

We have found that it can be particularly challenging for participants to stay with their own process during group integration. Despite preparing participants for the uniqueness of every psychedelic experience, participants will still compare and contrast their experience during a psychedelic session with those of others in the group. This may present a particular challenge for participants dealing with rejection trauma, shame, or harsh inner critics. Nonetheless, this can bring up valuable grist for the integration mill but only with adequate facilitation. Co-facilitators can pay particular attention to groupthink when it comes to applying positive or negative valence to specific qualities of the psychedelic experience, such as mystical-type experiences, among a group cohort. Beginner's mind, nonlinearity of healing, and ongoing unfolding of the process are handy concepts to reemphasize during group integration sessions. It may be appropriate to include individual integration sessions in the protocol, especially if each participant has their own individual psychedelic session, or make individual integration optionally available if needed.

Psychedelic-Assisted Group Therapy and Communal Healing

Cost and demand on trained psychedelic providers may limit a course of psychedelic treatment to the realm of a short-term or adjunctive service vs. long-term treatment, with a minimal number of medicine and integration sessions being offered. One factor that differentiates the use of psychedelics in traditional settings from psychedelic use in the context of psychotherapy is the stark contrast in how integration is approached. Among traditional communities with established cultures of psychedelic use, it is common for many community members to have had psychedelic experiences. In these settings, integration can happen through day-to-day interactions with the wider community. When psychedelics are used in the context of medical treatment in North America and Europe, the opportunity for deep integration may end once participants leave the clinic or laboratory where the therapy occurred. Providers might consider referring participants to an ongoing integration group when available to provide ongoing community support and integration.

Within society, our personal safety and power, or lack thereof, are either diminished or amplified by our alliances with different social groups and our identity within those groups. For example, certain members of a family or society are consistently oppressed or scapegoated, forcing them to choose between cycles of perpetration–victimization and isolation. Psychedelic-assisted group therapy offers an opportunity to bring together individuals with shared traumatic experiences or other forms of suffering to engage in communal healing. This can be particularly relevant when facilitators do not have an obvious relationship to the participant's lived experience (e.g., mismatch in race, gender identity, or sexual orientation) or when a participant does not have a strong sense of social support or community outside of the treatment setting. Healing that is intended to alleviate societal harms (e.g., racism, transphobia, homophobia, etc.) might benefit from focusing beyond the individual participant and looking outward at oppressive systems and their impact on individuals and communities.

As an emerging field, we must strive for inclusion and accessibility for communities with a disproportionately high prevalence of psychiatric diagnosis and underrepresentation in research and treatment utilization (e.g., Black, Indigenous, and People of Color and LGBTQI+). Of note, it can be helpful to avoid using traditional psychiatric diagnoses to determine eligibility for group cohorts, particularly cohorts composed of individuals from socially marginalized populations. Psychiatric diagnoses can be further stigmatizing, whereas reconceptualizing symptoms as a result of (possibly ongoing) systemic oppression can foster a safer and more therapeutic environment. Group psychedelic work has the capacity to uncover the resilience within a community rather than discretely address the "pathological symptoms" of individuals already isolated by systemic injustices.

Whether psychedelic-assisted therapy consists of a small group of two co-facilitators attending to the set, setting, and social support of one individual or a group cohort of multiple participants, we are certain that healing requires a communal approach. As we near regulatory decisions to approve psychedelic-assisted therapy, scalability is a significant consideration; however, until we collect and analyze the data, there is no guarantee that psychedelic-assisted group therapy will be a more cost- or time-efficient model, or that it will measure up to the efficacy of individual psychedelic-assisted therapy. There are many questions yet to be answered, and standards of care for psychedelic-assisted group therapy will continue to develop as more research is conducted.

Human evolution beyond kin-related altruism is a core component of civilization. Our ability to collaborate on activities that sustain and protect our perceived in-group has led to a relatively rapid evolution from tribes to kingdoms to nations to international alliances aimed at sharing and preserving the limited resources of our Earth. In the shadow of teamwork, the adversary emerges. Conflict between nations, religious sects, and political parties has resulted in trauma that has rippled through our impressively adaptive gene pool for generations. Combining group therapy with psychedelic medicine has the potential to offer unique insights into communal healing. Like honey bees observing a waggle dance[4] and being alerted to danger or the location of life-sustaining nectar (Riley et al., 2005), we, too, stand to benefit from holding space for the hive mind to witness the wisdom of our shared shadow and resulting resilience. Much like the geometric fractal patterns that make up the universe, psychedelics can serve as a bridge between science and art, ordinary and mystical, the individual and the collective.

Notes

1   Classic psychedelics include lysergic acid diethylamide (LSD), mescaline, N,N-dimethyltryptamine (DMT), and psilocybin. Classic psychedelics are all serotonin 2A receptor (5-HT2AR) agonists.
2   Schedule I substances are defined by the Drug Enforcement Administration as drugs with no currently accepted medical use, a high potential for abuse, and are typically allowed only in highly regulated research settings.
3   A profound experience of communal connection and equality that transcends typical social norms.
4   By performing a waggle dance, successful honeybee foragers can share information with other members of the colony about the direction and distance to patches of flowers yielding nectar and pollen, water sources, new nest-site locations, or attacks by rivals or predators.

References

Adamson, S., & Metzner, R. (1988). The nature of the MDMA experience and its role in healing, psychotherapy, and spiritual practice. *ReVision: A Journal of Consciousness and Transformation, 10*, 59–72.

Anderson, B. T., Danforth, A., Daroff, P. R., Stauffer, C., Ekman, E., Agin-Liebes, G., Trope, A., Boden, M. T., Dilley, P. J., Mitchell, J., & Woolley, J. (2020). Psilocybin-assisted group therapy for demoralized older long-term AIDS survivor men: An open-label safety and feasibility pilot study. *EClinicalMedicine, 27*, 100538. https://dx.doi.org/10.1016/j.eclinm.2020.100538

Berne, E. (1966). *Principles of group treatment*. Oxford University Press.

Black Elk, & DeMallie, R. J. (1986). *The sixth grandfather: Black Elk's teachings given to John G. Neihardt*. Bison Books.

Burlingame, G., & Krogel, J. (2005). Relative efficacy of individual versus group psychotherapy. *International Journal of Group Psychotherapy, 55*, 607–611. https://doi.org/10.1521/ijgp.2005.55.4.607

Burlingame, G. M., MacKenzie, K. R., & Strauss, B. (2004). Small group treatment: Evidence for effectiveness and mechanisms of change. In M. J. Lambert (Ed.), *Bergin & Garfield's handbook of psychotherapy and behavior change*. Wiley.

Burlingame, G. M., McClendon, D. T., & Alonso, J. (2011). Cohesion in group therapy. *Psychotherapy, 48*(1), 33.

Burlingame, G. M., McClendon, D. T., & Yang, C. (2018). Cohesion in group therapy: A meta-analysis. *Psychotherapy, 55*(4), 384–398. https://doi.org/10.1037/pst0000173

Burlingame, G. M., Strauss, B., Joyce, A., MacNairSemands, R., MacKenzie, K. R., Ogrodniczuk, J., & Taylor, S. M. (2006). *CORE battery*. An Assessment Tool Kit for Promoting Optimal Group.

Chard, K. M., Resick, P. A., Monson, C. M., & Kattar, K. A. (2009). *Cognitive processing therapy therapist group manual: Veteran/military version*. Department of Veterans' Affairs.

Chwelos, N., Blowett, D. B., Smith, C. M., & Hoffer, A. (1959). Use of d-lysergic acid diethylamide in the treatment of alcoholism. *Quarterly Journal of Studies on Alcohol, 20*, 577–590.

Furst, P. T. (1976). *Hallucinogens and culture*. Sharp Publishers.

Gasser, P. (1994). Psycholytic therapy with MDMA and LSD in Switzerland. *Newsletter Multidisciplinary Association for Psychedelic Studies, 5*(3), 3–7.

Greer, G., & Tolbert, R. (1986). Subjective reports of the effects of MDMA in a clinical setting. *Journal of Psychoactive Drugs*, 319–327.

Hutson, S. R. (1999). Technoshamanism: Spiritual healing in the rave subculture. *Popular Music and Society, 23*(3), 53–77. https://doi.org/10.1080/03007769908591745

James, E., Robertshaw, T. L., Hoskins, M., & Sessa, B. (2020). Psilocybin occasioned mystical-type experiences. *Human Psychopharmacology, 35*(5), 2742. https://doi.org/10.1002/hup.2742

Leary, T. (1982). *Changing my mind, among others: Lifetime writings*. Prentice-Hall.

Metzner, R. (1998). *The unfolding self: Varieties of transformative experience*. Origin Press.

Mithoefer, M. (2017). A manual for MDMA-assisted psychotherapy in the treatment of posttraumatic stress disorder [Review of a manual for MDMA-assisted psychotherapy in the treatment of posttraumatic stress disorder]. *Multidisciplinary Association of Psychedelic*

Studies, 8(1). https://s3-us-west-1.amazonaws.com/mapscontent/research-archive/mdma/TreatmentManual_MDMAAssistedPsychotherapyVersion+8.1_22+Aug2017.pdf

Naranjo, C. (2001). Experience with the interpersonal psychedelics. In J. Holland (Ed.), *Ecstasy: The complete guide* (pp. 208–221). Park Street Press.

Passie, T. (2012). *Healing with entactogens: Therapist and patient perspectives on MDMA-assisted group psychotherapy.* Multidisciplinary Association for Psychedelic Studies (MAPS).

Passie, T. (2018). The early use of MDMA ("Ecstasy") in psychotherapy (1977–1985). *Drug Science, Policy and Law.* https://doi.org/10.1177/2050324518767442

Riley, J. R., Greggers, U., Smith, A. D., Reynolds, D. R., & Menzel, R. (2005). The flight paths of honeybees recruited by the waggle dance. *Nature, 435*(7039), 205–207. https://doi.org/10.1038/nature03526

Schultes, R. E., & Hofmann, A. (1992). *Plants of the gods: Their sacred, healing, and hallucinogenic powers.* Healing Arts Press.

Sessa, B., & Fischer, F. M. (2015). Underground MDMA-, LSD-and 2-CB-assisted individual and group psychotherapy in Zurich: Outcomes, implications and commentary. *Drug Science, Policy and Law, 2*, 2050324515578080.

Shulgin, A. T., & Shulgin, A. (1991). *PIHKAL: A chemical love story.* Transform Press.

Stolaroff, M. (2004). *The secret chief revealed.* MAPS.

Titelman, P. (2008). The concept of the triangle in Bowen theory: An overview. In P. Titelman (Ed.), *Triangles: Bowen family systems theory perspectives* (pp. 3–61). The Haworth Press/Taylor and Francis Group.

Trope, A., Anderson, B. T., Hooker, A. R., Glick, G., Stauffer, C., & Woolley, J. D. (2019). Psychedelic-assisted group therapy: A systematic review. *Journal of Psychoactive Drugs, 51*(2), 174–188. https://dx.doi.org/10.1080/02791072.2019.1593559

Turner, E. (2012). *Communitas: The anthropology of joy.* Palgrave Macmillan.

Wagner, C. C., & Ingersoll, K. S. (2013). *Motivational interviewing in groups.* The Guilford Press.

Westrup, D., & Wright, M. J. (2017). *Learning ACT for group treatment: An acceptance and commitment therapy skills training manual for therapists.* Context Press.

Yalom, I. D., & Leszcz, M. (2020). *The theory and practice of group psychotherapy.* Hachette UK.

Chapter 14

The Upside of Coming Down

The Opportunities and Challenges of Psychedelic Integration

Jessica Katzman and Harvey Schwartz

Introduction

This chapter will present a history and overview of psychedelic integration, including the value of intentional practices and the most common obstacles to successful outcomes. In the *spirit* of integration, this effort also represents a collaborative conversation between the authors, who each co-founded separate KAP practices in San Francisco. We hope to model how working in cooperative community and supporting each other's growth allow for cross-pollination so vital to this novel and evolving field. In contrast with the increasingly prescriptive and reductive manualized approaches to mental health treatment, we offer our ongoing dialogue with each other, between our various disciplines, and with *you*, the reader.

Weaving Wholeness

From the Latin *integrare* (to make whole and to begin again; the act of bringing together the parts of a whole), the term *integration* signifies creating wholeness out of separateness. Integration of peak experiences involves identifying the vestigial threads in the tapestry of the altered state, then weaving these ephemeral filaments into the warp and weft of one's daily life and usual sense of self.

Successful integration incorporates the psychological, somatic, relational, transpersonal/spiritual, and practical realms of our experiences. Stabilizing and synthesizing new experiences and insights from non-ordinary states of consciousness (NOSC) encourage more durable changes, sustaining the benefits accrued from psychedelic sessions. Unpacking these momentary revelations for practical applications helps foster greater flexibility and resilience in the human psyche.

From Altered States to Altered Traits

One of the previous century's major missteps in clinical use of psychedelics manifested as the tendency to over-idealize the seductively powerful altered states of consciousness in themselves, as many of our pioneering predecessors overlooked how the return to everyday stress and tedium can gradually close a recently opened

DOI: 10.4324/9781003167976-14

heart and mind. The visceral, dazzling insights vividly comprehended in yesterday's NOSC infamously become ephemeral in today's ordinary consciousness; transient new understandings may dissolve into vague impressions or diffuse into oblivion. Significant others may unintentionally express concerns about the change process that contributes to the evaporation of seemingly credible perspectives.

The *problem of generalizability* implies the difficulty of transferring singular experiences into lasting changes. Roger Walsh (2012) describes the challenge of moving *from state to trait*,

> For those people who are graced with mystical experience—whether spontaneous, contemplative or chemical—the crucial question is: what to do with it? It can be ignored, be allowed to fade, or even dismissed, or perhaps clung to as a psychological/spiritual trophy.
>
> (2002, p. 80)

Religion scholar Houston Smith also noted the difficulty of transforming flashes of illumination into abiding light (1992). Jamie Wheal, co-author of *Stealing Fire*, was recently interviewed about the struggle to apply flow/mystical experiences into quotidian life, "There's only a fraction of [peak breakthrough experience] that we can bring back into our [ordinary] state of consciousness, and into our lives . . . [so] we're going to the waterfall with thimbles" (Kotler & Wheal, 2019, p. 42).

Transformational, expanded states may indeed induce enduring shifts by giving us glimpses of a broader worldview and/or a more openhearted way of being, providing a source of inspiration and guidance for beneficial life direction. However, there is no guarantee that brief forays into these moments of unity consciousness will result in lasting, sustainable change without ongoing practice. Walsh advocates for synergizing the chemical with the contemplative, strengthening the human container through discipline so that these phenomena may eventually endure. Thus, altered states may lead to altered practices, values, orientations, commitments, and relationships with others/the community/the world.

Clinical History

The term *integration* was initially identified in Jungian/archetypal psychology as well as in treatment of trauma/dissociative disorders. These traditions emerged independently and predate contemporary psychedelic therapy; yet, all share common philosophical underpinnings: interpreting symbols, working with all parts of a psychic system, and—perhaps most importantly—honoring the transcendent inner healing and guidance systems, which inherently move us toward wholeness.

In the dissociative disorders field, this term is used to reflect the primary objective of unifying split-off aspects of the personality, which were developed and compartmentalized to survive intense traumatic conditions. Recovery from PTSD or dissociative identity disorder involves opening new communication channels between separated/sequestered aspects of one's identity, enhancing internal coherence, boosting self-compassion, and strengthening the ability to face distressing memories without becoming overwhelmed or overly identified with the material.

Integration is also central to the individuation process in Carl Jung's depth psychology, which is the underlying purposeful direction of human development that guides one toward the person one is meant to be (Miller, 2004). Jung stressed the role that integration plays in human development by bringing "activated unconscious and symbolic material into a constructive and synthetic relationship with the conscious mind" through interaction, association, and active imagination (Hill, 2013/2019; Jung, 1969).

Few traditionally trained psychotherapists are fluent in both psychedelic-assisted therapy and mainstream psychology; this may be due to their own limited experience and/or fears around liability and legality. On the other side of the coin is the emerging psychedelic integration subspecialty, an uncharted zone where almost anyone can hang out a shingle and call themselves an "integration specialist" or "integration coach," with little-to-zero experience in psychotherapy or clinical training. The unique vulnerability of altered states calls for the highest level of expertise and trustworthiness, as mismanagement of post-journey experiences can lead to re-traumatization or even, in severe cases, escalate into psychiatric crises.

Literature Review

Psychedelic-assisted therapy has only recently gained a prominent role in psychiatry and psychology, reemerging after decades of suspended research and practice. The previous body of clinical knowledge accrued during the 1950s–1960s (predominantly with LSD-based treatments) was unfortunately truncated by governmental restrictions on clinical research, based on the criminalization of private citizens' experimentation, promulgated as the morally virtuous War on Drugs. One of the many terrible legacies of this era is our professional developmental delay, manifesting in the current dearth of academic literature on the subject of psychedelic integration.

Today's major psychedelic-assisted research and therapy protocols using MDMA, psilocybin, and ketamine all include strategies for integration, often stressing its value as potentially greater than the medicine sessions on their own. Recent and evolving perspectives appear on blogs, online forums, book chapters in edited volumes on psychedelic therapy, workbooks/guidebooks for post-journey integration, and online magazines. The most comprehensive models of psychedelic integration thus far have been outlined by House (2007), Marsden and Lukoff (2007), and Coder (2017). Marsden and Lukoff (2007) focus on meaning making, transitioning back into everyday life and community, taking responsibility for one's own life and destiny, and the value of giving and receiving feedback immediately after the experience. House (2007) developed a five-stage process as a container for altered states, from intention to psychological purification and release to cognitive/emotional/behavioral implementation. He advocates for dedicated therapeutic processing over time to rebalance ruptured psychic frameworks; sustain mental spaciousness; and metabolize all content evoked by such potentially confusing, powerful, and metaphorical experiences.

In her companion guide for integration following visionary plant medicine ceremonies, Coder (2017) has elaborated one of the most cohesive, inclusive, and far-reaching approaches. She cautions journeyers and healers alike about the dangers of being abandoned by shamanic leaders to process on their own after ceremonies without a systematic way to integrate the experience, which can be disorganizing and overwhelming. She is particularly concerned about the tendency many have to seek further peak experiences (i.e., more ceremony), rather than digest prior content. As an ardent advocate of intensive integration, she offers a user-friendly manual to guide participants through a post-ceremony process that maximizes safety and beneficial effects. She outlines ten key recommendations: expert guidance, trauma release, spiritual discipline/practices, reflection/inner listening/creativity, meaning making, spaciousness and time, nature and grounding, adequate physical care (diet, rest, exercise, and movement), cultivating virtues, and returning to the world.

In reviewing the aforementioned contributors, we noted the commonly occurring themes of *safety*, *durability*, *relationship*, and *consolidation*, with overlapping goals such as:

- Smooth the return to ordinary life (safety and stabilization)
- Reflect on original intentions
- Debrief disturbing, overwhelming, and/or transcendent experiences
- Encourage participants to share feedback with therapists/sitters
- Identify coping strategies for regression/relapse prevention; prevent premature termination of treatment
- Enhance self-monitoring and observing ego functions
- Navigate interpersonal challenges and intimacy
- Revise limiting or pathogenic beliefs; address conflicts between parts of the self
- Boost self-compassion and self-forgiveness
- Protect against making major life changes or decisions immediately following peak experiences
- Witness, review, and capture the journey narratives, images, feelings, body sensations, encounters, perceptions, and revelations (with writing, drawing, recording, etc.)
- Provide ongoing safety and self-care recommendations
- Clarify values; commit to practical applications for newfound wisdom and support for behavioral changes
- Identify coping strategies for potential changes in identity and worldview
- Incorporate strategies for meaning making and symbolization on multiple levels (ego, metaphoric, somatic, transgenerational, and transpersonal)
- Sustain mindfulness
- Avoid spiritual bypass

A Bridge to Community

It is essential to recognize the Indigenous origins of integration dynamics.[1] In such contexts where medicine work is seamlessly woven into the fabric of daily life, the value of the altered state is contingent on the assimilation of transcendental insights back into one's community. In contrast, contemporary Western psychedelic sessions in medicalized contexts are sequestered from our everyday lives and do not provide adequate opportunities for integration nor reflection on how we might bring beneficial wisdom and ethical action back to the world around us. Western culture encourages estrangement from psychospiritual ancestors and prevents many from even noticing the lack of traditional cultural containers, so it becomes all the more necessary to specifically emphasize intentional integration practices.

Wheal stresses the moral importance of bringing something back from mystical/peak experiences to the world to make it a better place (2021). His concept of *ecstasis–catharsis–communitas* refers to his integration recommendations: appreciate and understand the value/limitations of your "mountaintop" experience; work with the received revelations; and then bring the best of yourself and the revelations *back* to the world, the community, and all of your relationships. Otherwise, self-transcendence likely stalls at the immature level of solipsistic self-indulgence, where the highest potential for transformation is diverted by our contemporary Western individualist-centered programming.

In alignment with mythologist Joseph Campbell's (1991) concept of "the hero's return," Walsh (2002) also strongly advocates that regardless of mystical path or tradition, it is a moral imperative for those who have received personal illumination "to return to the ordinary world so that all may benefit from the light that can be bestowed" (p. 80). Additionally, Sherree Godasi (2019) views psychedelics and integration as evolutionary instruments for humanity's maturation as a species by reframing the context from the singular/personal realm to the collective realm, wherein ongoing individual integration bolsters theoretical advancement of community development and growth.

Challenges to Integration

While the existing literature on psychedelic integration effectively introduces most of its benefits, this chapter will present common obstacles that can emerge, as well as the hidden therapeutic opportunities embedded in the challenges. We feel strongly that a deeper understanding of the complexities and potential pitfalls will help clinicians maximize and strengthen the durability of any potential benefits from these innovative treatments. We also believe that the maturation of our field is dependent upon increasing awareness of the impediments that inevitably appear on the path and ongoing training in the sophisticated navigation of such stumbling blocks.

Zigzagging

Despite our most fervent wishes for the instant cure, healing generally does not follow a simple, linear progression. A pattern of inconsistent and unpredictable gains and losses may induce waves of hope and disappointment, revealing deep-rooted expectations about how treatment is *supposed* to unfold. Some are prone

HEALING
(OF THE HEART, BODY, MIND, OR SOUL)

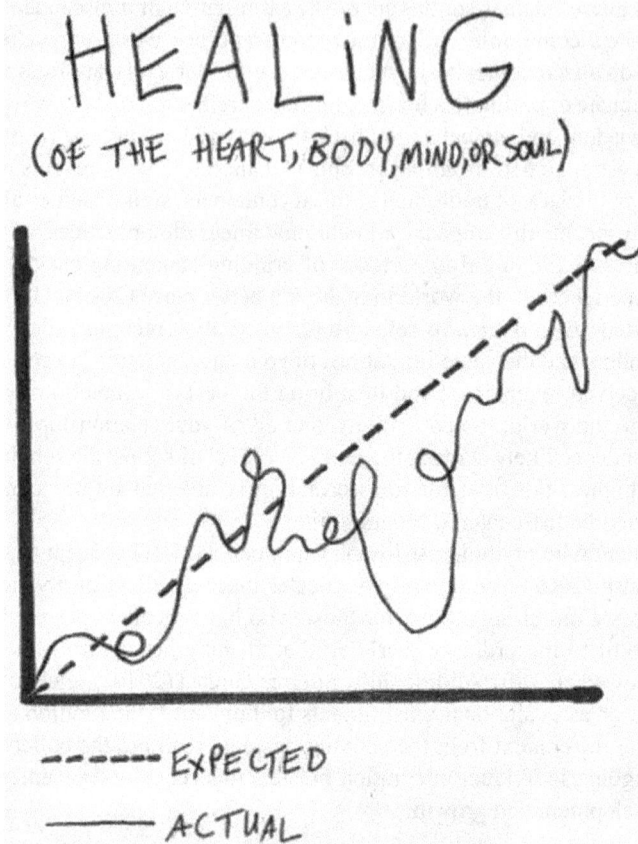

------- EXPECTED

——— ACTUAL

Figure 14.1 The zigzagging nature of the healing process

to misconstruing any form of instability in this process as a sign of personal or treatment failure, triggering potential shame and/or blame. Navigating these switchbacks and potholes on the path to recovery is key to making the most out of psychedelic therapy; these zigzags may be loaded with growth potential when negotiated with creativity, mutuality, and wisdom.

Providers can help hold the larger picture of the healing arc, predicting and normalizing the wiggly curve toward wellness, and depathologizing any perceived setbacks. Because the preparation phase often invites clients to set intentions for each medicine session, we can use these moments to inquire about expectations and gently suggest that the journey toward treatment goals may not be as straightforward as mainstream media lead us to believe. This may inspire an inventory of various healthy coping strategies to help manage the current moment while staying the course over the potential ups and downs, which is crucial in reducing excess distress and treatment dropout.

Surprising swings during psychedelic treatment can manifest in challenges to sustainable benefits. We will consider the unintended consequences of both the zigs and the zags separately here.

Rapid Relapse ("the Downswing")

Rapid relapse may be one of the most problematic setbacks in this collection of obstacles. This sudden, unexpected loss of therapeutic benefits (such as symptom relief or positive perspective shifts) following a psychedelic-assisted therapy session may even present as an amplification of the initial pretreatment symptomatology. This type of regressive shift often occurs in the hours or days immediately after a session, following a brief (or even extended) period of symptom relief; however, it can manifest at any time along the long arc of recovery and transformation.

Because many who seek these newer unconventional therapy modalities (particularly those struggling with depression or PTSD) do so after multiple failed treatment attempts with other medications and methods, rapid relapse requires more careful processing than most other challenges. Clients attempting a last-ditch intervention frequently enter with elevated personal stakes and an exaggerated reliance on blind hopefulness. When expectations of a miracle cure (and/or fear of yet another failure) are present, any impression of a setback can precipitate a significant disruption.

These reversals can occur *despite* a thorough preparation phase that covers the importance of expectation management, along with psychoeducation that anticipates the inevitable uncertainties in treatment and communicates the potential value of regression as part of the healing process. When a client starts to first feel relief from intractable dark moods and anxiety—sometimes after decades of depression—a sudden loss of these briefly attained benefits may cause reactions of futility and despair. Optimism seems illusory, and this justifiably may feel overwhelming, alarming, and irreparable.

Rapid relapse may result from—or be exacerbated by—a wide range of factors:

- Incomplete or inaccurate medical and/or psychological intake evaluations
- Inadequate preparation
- Dosing errors or inaccuracies
- Onset of biological/medical conditions
- Unanticipated mixed drug reactions (drug mitigators and interactions)
- Substance misuse
- New or continuing interpersonal stressors
- Vocational crises
- Traumatic events, such as car accidents, fires, or housing crises
- Family crises (including with pets)
- Unexpected stressful political and societal (non-personal) events
- Unexpected side effects of the treatments

Other important factors (discussed at greater length in later sections) to consider may include:

- Intrapsychic dynamics between the therapist and client; problems in the therapeutic alliance
- Reactions to incompletely processed traumatic material that emerged during the medicine session(s)
- Opposition from parts of the client's psyche that have felt displaced, overwhelmed, or disempowered by therapeutic progress

It should be noted that even in most non-problematic and positive cases, the return to ordinary consciousness following the expansiveness of a non-ordinary state of consciousness can often elicit feelings of loss, grief, disappointment, deflation, and anger. This may be expressed in a variety of ways, including troublesome rumination, self-defeating doubts, or the subtle undermining of powerful spiritual experiences and previously hopeful expectations. When not properly processed, these unexpected feelings and thought patterns can exacerbate the relapse. As already discussed, this can be experienced as a return to pretreatment symptom levels and can adversely impact attitudes toward current and future treatment.

Clinical Example (A)

A chronically anxious and depressed client arrived home following a meaningful and transcendent first KAP session to discover that a water pipe had burst in the family home, causing significant damage that required much time and attention. The unexpected crisis and the immediate stressful demands not only disrupted the new hope-inspiring sense of equanimity, but seemed to obliterate the accumulation of symptom relief, casting a cynical pall over our forward progress.

Clinical Example (B)

A client who came to treatment for PTSD (resulting from childhood sexual abuse) had a near-fatal encounter in a crosswalk with an aggressive motorist while crossing the street on foot. This incident re-traumatized them, and they collapsed back into an old victimhood-based mindset of self-blame and helplessness. This threatened to erase the positive insights, mood elevation, and optimism that had been achieved from the medicine sessions.

As with all the integration obstacles described in this chapter, rapid relapse holds both challenges and opportunities for transforming the healing process. The challenges include a fortification of the defensive system and limiting belief patterns, as well as premature foreclosure and termination from treatment.

Although initially disruptive and disturbing, this phase may present an opportunity to recalibrate our therapeutic approach, allowing for successful navigation of future pitfalls. This is an invitation for reassessment of treatment variables, including set and setting, dosing, route of administration, psychotherapy strategies, and aftercare suggestions. Additionally, the emergence of previously inaccessible traumatic feelings, memories, and beliefs that are prompted by rapid relapse may serve to inform next steps and provide valuable opportunities for working through.

This is not only an optimal time for further refinement and optimization of the entire treatment protocol but, most importantly, a prompt for strengthening the therapeutic alliance. This opportunity for the therapy dyad to problem-solve together, depathologizing and reducing shame around relapse for both client *and* provider, serves to further educate the client on the undulating, zigzagging path of successful healing. With patience and perseverance, confidence and faith can be strengthened within the therapeutic relationship.

Navigating through the difficult passage of a seemingly insurmountable setback may contribute to the client's overall sense of resilience, providing valuable lived and embodied experience, fostering a lasting sense of greater flexibility and adaptability, along with greater trust in the collaboration required for successful treatment. From this perspective, effective outcomes always include an improved ability to "surf" not only the NOSC itself but the overall nonlinearity—the ups and downs and the shadow and light—of not only psychedelic-assisted therapy but life in general.

The Therapeutic Bends ("the Upswing")

The rediscovery of psychedelics as a powerfully efficient treatment for chronic refractory mental health conditions has been hailed as a massive boon to those living with symptoms, their loved ones, and providers alike. Many welcome rapid recovery with relief and gratitude in being able to return to their lives; however, it may also be clinically relevant to explore the potential *unintended* consequences of these effective, fast-acting interventions.

Some practitioners have noticed that a small minority of clients visibly experience a period of disequilibrium and difficulty in adjusting to such positive change. On closer examination, we may discover an even larger percentage of people who present with a mixed, ambivalent picture, where happiness is interwoven with negative reactions. These reactions can range from over-reliance on older coping styles that no longer match one's current state to the distress that comes from the loss of a habituated identity and to the emergence of unexpected affective states. We have come to refer to this response metaphorically as "the therapeutic bends," as a way to suggest the effects that can occur when we ascend rapidly from great depths.

Experienced clinicians are already accustomed to a variety of ambivalent-to-negative reactions to the prospect of improvement, and many approaches provide both theoretical explanatory models and technical interventions to target the concept of "resistance." However, conventional psychotherapy generally offers recovery as a gradual process, with adequate time to adjust and be supported. The advent of these new treatments requires a shift in how we guide people through this work, as we continue to ask ourselves: what can happen when people recover from long-standing difficulties quickly? How do practitioners respond when we witness such difficulty adjusting? How can we assist those navigating this new territory?

We will discuss here some possible layers where distress can occur and interventions to consider at each level.

CONFRONTING REALITY: COGNITIVE BEHAVIORAL LAYER

Any chronic and debilitating illness takes a toll on one's life over time; as energy and focus are drawn largely toward survival and recovery, essential life tasks may be neglected. Bills go unpaid, household chores pile up, inboxes overflow, hobbies and interests atrophy, and growth opportunities are missed.

Rapid remission might indeed bring long-sought relief; however, it is not uncommon to also feel trepidation and deflation when facing the heap of tasks to be tackled to put one's life back together. People often report dread and overwhelming stress when approaching such accumulated burdens. We have commonly heard such comments as, "My depression's gone . . . but now I'm anxious, because I have to figure out what to do with my life!" This may perpetuate a reflexive return of symptoms that form a protective layer against having to fully engage in life, providing an escape from making difficult choices or confronting painful realities.

Clinical Example

Those accustomed to very brief respites from symptoms may have a habitual tendency to throw themselves headlong into intense task completion mode the moment remission begins. We worked with a high achiever who struggled with lifelong depressive episodes prior to ketamine treatment. They described a pattern of avoidance and procrastination while depressed, alternating with brief flurries of intense work when their mood lifted, in an attempt to "get everything in the pile done before the storm hits again." As ketamine provided longer windows of symptom relief, we found that this avoidance/overwork pattern was based on an assumption of a limited time window for task completion, leading to exhausted collapse. They requested support around learning new coping skills and time management habits.

Cognitive behavioral therapy models may be of use in tackling both unhelpful activity patterns and the underlying beliefs that fuel them by reframing mental approaches to task completion and teaching new ways to manage the demands of life.

Providers may want to focus here on slowing the pace down so as not to trigger overwhelm and to encourage rebuilding long-depleted energy reserves. We can remind clients that their current situation did not develop overnight, so "digging out of the pile" will also take time, reassuring them that they will have the chance to gradually repair their lives. It may be important to highlight each small success or step toward goals to help build self-esteem and self-efficacy. We can also discuss underlying beliefs about core worth as linked to work output and achievement and provide a critical lens for how modern Western culture promotes such self-estrangement.

Behaviorally, providers can support clients in developing more effective time management habits, creating structure in their schedule that balances productivity with necessary self-care. Again, it is important to emphasize a slower process of learning and practicing these behavioral shifts, rather than promoting expectations of instant change that then provoke disappointment.

We also often remind people to ask for help: if they have social resources, they may enlist family and/or extended network support; if they have financial resources, they can hire a professional organizer or coach. If neither are readily available, we might offer several good sources of self-help material addressing procrastination, time management, and organization, and can work with these in the context of our treatment. Support groups may assist in normalizing the recovery process and provide helpful perspective and encouragement from others.

Many public systems offer some type of peer and/or professional resources, including vocational training, for those looking to reenter the workforce after a period of unemployment. Ideally, this type of support should encourage autonomy, allow exploration of ability and identity, and avoid perpetuating disempowering ideas about what those with mental health concerns are able to contribute to the world.

LETTING IT OUT: EMOTIONAL LAYER

As noted earlier, rapid remission may also induce a host of emotional reactions. Dr. Raquel Bennett, founder of the KRIYA Institute and a psychologist who has worked with ketamine for many years, has astutely observed that as clients contemplate the time and opportunities lost to illness, they can become "angry at God for making them sick . . . or all the doctors that didn't help them previously. We need to think about how painful it is to just be with that, what this condition has done to one's life" (personal communication, August 12, 2018).

This can be an incredibly healing process if one is supported by those who understand such emerging emotional responses in context but can be difficult to navigate on one's own. Providers may empathically invite such expressions of regret and grief around the sense of lost opportunities as a way to begin working through these feelings and to normalize mourning as a natural part of recovery.

Additionally, we have supported clients who, once they were relieved of depressive burdens, were then able to confront and feel appropriate anger stemming from past trauma, abandonment, or loss. Classic psychoanalytic conceptualizations regarding depression as "anger turned inward" can help frame the newly externalized irritability or distress that may surface unexpectedly when symptoms remit.

Although popular conceptions formulate depression as "sadness" and recovery as "happiness," the reality is often not as simple. Depression often presents with a numbing or flattening of emotions, and the thawing process may mean regaining access to a wide range of different feeling states. Learning to navigate these states is essential and can greatly enhance one's quality of life.

Clinical Example

A client presented to KAP treatment with long-standing depression and substance misuse; a single higher-dose intramuscular administration provided substantial mood improvement. A deep anger then emerged in a manner that both startled the client and triggered a shame response, as they unconsciously linked angry feelings to a punitive, explosive caregiver. They also expressed concerns around how uncontrolled anger might threaten their current relationship stability. This initiated deeper exploration of early relationships and how they shaped the client's internal emotional templates. We also discussed cultural constructs regarding the appropriateness of anger expression within this client's intersections of ethnic and gender identities.

It is vitally important to set expectations for all involved that recovery may involve unearthing unanticipated feelings, and to suggest making space for this process in a way that depathologizes the wide range of human emotional responses. It may help to reframe this as *eustress*—or how the nervous system can react initially to even positive changes (such as new jobs, weddings, or other major life milestones) with increased activation—and to normalize the surprising psychosomatic reactions that may result.

Providers can encourage expression of affect in session, helping clients to metabolize and understand these new feeling states; many conventional psychotherapy models provide applicable frameworks. We may use IFS or other parts work to witness, validate, unburden, and reintegrate the exiled fragments of the psyche holding such feelings (see Chapter 11).

Dialectical behavior therapy provides tools for emotional regulation (such as opposite action or positive self-talk) and distress tolerance (such as self-soothing or improving the moment). Acceptance and commitment therapy blends acceptance and mindfulness with behavior change strategies (such as cognitive defusion or self as context) to increase psychological flexibility. Anger management psychoeducation may also be helpful in reducing the stigma around anger and increasing self-regulation efficacy with techniques, such as taking a time-out or assertiveness training.

Because our emotions are, in essence, deeply *embodied* experiences, somatic therapy modalities (such as Hakomi, Somatic Experiencing, Sensorimotor Psychotherapy, and Organic Intelligence) and techniques can assist us in gently exploring our moment-to-moment reactions (see Chapter 6). Teaching and practicing grounding exercises can help clients to re-regulate when distressed, develop internal and external resources, and discover (and potentially widen) their window of tolerance.

All techniques and approaches should serve to broaden our ideas about how a more balanced emotional life is not one that grasps for simplistic, idealized versions of "happiness" but instead includes a wide range of emotional experience, builds resiliency for facing future challenges, and helps us navigate toward a life that feels more meaningful.

EXPLORING IDENTITY: PERSONAL IDENTITY LAYER

Paired with the deep human longing for growth/change is the equally strong need for stability/security. This paradoxical tension can show up as an expectation in the continuity of the *self*. We become habituated to our capacities for activity and relating and depend on the ability to predict how we might think and feel in any given situation. It can be incredibly disorienting when a cluster of everyday experiences disappears overnight, and it can foster a sense of "not knowing myself" anymore. This sense of dislocation may also manifest more subtly as confusion.

When one has lived with a longer-term condition, it can become quietly woven into one's own identity. Participation in online forums and support groups can provide invaluable insight and camaraderie. This sense of belonging and community can be extremely helpful *and* may also reify one's social role as a fellow sufferer. We come to define ourselves as a depressed person, as someone struggling with fibromyalgia, or as a recipient of Social Security or disability benefits. What may then happen to our self-representation when suffering ceases?

Clinical Example

A client who experienced a particularly rapid and dramatic remission in long-standing mood symptoms during a course of ketamine treatment displayed enthusiastic gratitude to the prescribing medical staff, yet self-consciously expressed a growing sense of bewilderment in psychotherapy sessions, often stated as a sense of "being lost." With ongoing encouragement and space made to explore these reactions, they were finally able to articulate, "I don't know who I am anymore, without my old buddy, Depression," and began exploring the nuances of this ambivalent "love affair." This initiated a meaningful phase of inner dialogue between the client and this lifelong companion, negotiating possibilities for collaboration on the new path that lay ahead.

Just as we would allow space for someone to discover new aspects of their being during a coming-out process around sexual orientation or gender identity, so may we extend this spaciousness in our healing relationships during recovery from long-standing mental health concerns. The identity-making process is an ongoing conversation with the self over a lifetime, and the remission period—if navigated skillfully—can be a particularly rich and fruitful phase of exploration.

Practitioners may wish to acknowledge that with every new gain made, there are losses and parts of our lives and selves that we are saying goodbye to. We can invite people to share whatever old beliefs may be surfacing and gently question their accuracy, aiming toward an expanded sense of self.

We may also draw upon IFS techniques to help clients have non-judgmental, productive conversations with different parts of the psyche and discover the meaning underlying attachments to an identity constructed around illness. It can be helpful to explore the relationship someone has with their depression and how that relationship has changed over time. Relational psychodynamic/psychoanalytic frameworks are fundamental to understanding the operation of these deep templates, as well as their source in our earliest interactions; these templates may be best addressed by working directly within transference–countertransference enactments (see Chapter 5). Narrative therapy ideas and practices (such as externalization or deconstruction) can assist people in rewriting the stories of their lives into a more integrated personal mythology.

READJUSTING ROLES: INTERPERSONAL LAYER

Self-expectations are intertwined with social roles, which reveal the *relational* expectations for personal continuity over time. Others around us have adapted to how we typically act and express ourselves and may react with surprise when that changes. Such reactions can subtly encourage return to one's previous baseline. This is rarely intentional but is extremely important to recognize. Family and other intimate relationships may provide essential, life-sustaining support for those with severe and chronic mental health conditions. These ongoing relationships can become organized around such caregiving dynamics. An unexpected outcome of symptom remission may be a shift in these dynamics, especially around life functioning; others might come to expect more out of someone who has recovered.

From a family therapy perspective, the person presenting to treatment may sometimes be viewed as the "identified patient" (also "symptom bearer" or "scapegoat"). This term refers to a member of a dysfunctional system that has been unconsciously selected to express the distress of that system (such as when a child misbehaves at school as a way to distract attention from parental conflict at home). Other members of the system may profess concern for the identified patient but may also react instinctively (and unintentionally) to any improvement by working to reinstate the status quo.

What once seemed like an entirely biochemical illness can often be revealed as multiply determined when we notice loved ones' discomfort with their ward slipping out of their "sick role." We have often felt concern for those who achieve remission but then return to the same stressful environment and interpersonal relationships in which the initial issues flourished and which provide little space for new growth and change.

Clinical Example

An adult client struggling with a long history of depression described their family role as a dependent child, living with caretaker parents, and also referred to their partner as their "emotional service dog." Their partner expressed fear that the client would leave if the depression lifted, no longer needing ongoing support. During a brief remission, the client felt some unspoken distance and disappointment in the relationship and experienced this as "celebrating recovery alone, which felt bittersweet." The relational dynamics that unfolded seemed to have a homeostatic pull, as "I soon went back to being depressed, and [my partner] went back to being my service dog."

Initial phases of treatment and recovery might include referrals to family or couples therapy, alongside individual treatment, as supplemental support for the entire system. Individual providers can additionally offer psychoeducation on the nature of family/group dynamics. We can invite clients to talk through how their relationships might change if their symptoms improve or any fears of what could be expected of them if their condition shifts.

We can support clients to set appropriate boundaries and have difficult conversations with loved ones; this may involve teaching and practicing non-violent communication or other conflict resolution strategies, or psychoeducation around appropriate assertiveness and anger management techniques as indicated. We may also encourage people to make more intentional and conscious choices about their relationships and support networks, and move toward those who nourish their growth. Simultaneously, relational psychodynamic/psychoanalytic approaches may help deepen understanding of their interpersonal templates and bring more awareness to how childhood themes continue to replay in adult interactions.

DIGGING DEEPER: UNCONSCIOUS LAYER

Above all, we must make space for the deeply personal and idiosyncratic responses people have to both their symptoms *and* the remission of those symptoms. We cannot assume that this process has identical meaning for all. Honoring the uniqueness of the self and its adaptations to life's challenges is part of what gives our work beauty and depth.

Furthermore, meaning is held both consciously and unconsciously. Deep structures of the self are laid down early in life, in the interactions between temperament and environment, and are rarely available for immediate reflection. Ongoing inquiry within the therapeutic relationship aims to bring these templates into awareness. Psychedelic therapy may more rapidly ameliorate the constellation of symptoms that mask and/or express our deeply rooted psychic wounds, bringing these wounds to the surface for closer examination. Hill (2013) cautions that quickly releasing disturbing unconscious material during psychedelic experiences can have a dangerous and overwhelming effect on the ego, especially when there has been considerable effort to keep this material out of awareness.

Clinical Example

As a client's long-standing depression began to lift during ketamine treatment, we noticed a panic reaction emerging, and the medical providers wondered about adverse pharmacological reactions. However, during integration sessions, we explored the client's sense of terror around mood improvement. We discovered together that sadness felt like the only remaining link to a beloved sibling who had died young of a drug overdose, and that these symptoms served as a tribute to the depth of their connection. The client articulated a fear of leaving this loved one behind during recovery. We suggested slowing the treatment process down, creating enough space to process their responses of grief, loss, and abandonment, and to reconfigure early attachment templates within the therapeutic relationship that might allow for the possibility of healing.

Many generations of psychodynamically trained analysts have prized access to the unconscious (especially via fantasy and dreams) as the pathway toward greater wholeness and wellness. A wide variety of psychoanalytic approaches are therefore well suited to work with the material that arises in psychedelic sessions, as most offer robust frameworks for interpretation of unconscious meaning and analysis of the transference–countertransference dynamics. Jungian and other depth psychology dreamwork techniques offer creative methods (such as amplification of personal, cultural, and archetypal symbolic meanings) to work with the symbols that arise as expressions of unknown parts of the Self (See Chapter 8).

Generally, clients and therapists alike are encouraged to curiously follow whatever emerges without judgment or discrimination and to trust that the inner healing intelligence is capable of revealing previously uncharted obstacles embedded in the unconscious, as well as unexpected insights and passageways toward emotional resolution. Cultivating this larger faith in the process during preparation sessions will pay massive dividends during the integration phase of treatment.

Trauma Reactions

As noted earlier, altered states often open up submerged parts of the psyche. Psychedelic-assisted therapy intentionally embeds this powerful potential within a strong therapeutic frame to enhance the ability of those suffering from treatment-resistant PTSD to face and begin processing traumatic memories.[2] Clients taking psychedelics outside of psychotherapy-centered frameworks may have unacknowledged trauma and/or undiagnosed stress reactions that emerge unexpectedly during the experience itself, in the immediate aftermath, or (as previously mentioned) when depressive symptoms remit. This once-repressed material might then trigger alarm in the nervous system, potentially manifesting in fight/flight/freeze/collapse/dissociate sequences.

Those with early-onset/childhood and relational trauma might be most at risk for being pushed outside a zone of tolerance, especially when not given adequate therapeutic support. Some have shared that being left unattended while recovering from a ketamine infusion constituted a *secondary* trauma, as they felt alone in facing some of their most difficult experiences, or "shut down" by an overly medicalized environment and providers untrained to help them hold this material. However, even with prepared clients in a supportive environment, people may reflexively interrupt treatment to preemptively avoid further reexperiencing of frightening memories.

Clinical Example

A client who had experienced ongoing childhood physical and sexual abuse sought psychedelic-assisted therapy for chronic PTSD symptoms. The overwhelming nature of the traumatic material that emerged during the session precipitated a relapse, in spite of the therapist's best efforts to contain and process the painful emotions and memories that were resurfacing. The day after treatment, an internal protective part of the client's psyche responded with intensity, declaring that the treatment was "dangerous to my safety and well-being" and "a waste of time." This part, cultivated as a coping system during childhood, had felt wrongly left out of the treatment alliance, so became polarized with the therapist. When accessed, this part expressed disbelief in the transient relief the client had been experiencing and became vigilantly preoccupied with the potential danger of further sessions and ongoing processing. The client began to use alcohol to cope with these uncomfortable feelings, voiced the desire to discontinue treatment, and expressed fantasies of self-injury.

Trauma-informed care is essential when working with psychedelics. The current gold standard for treatment is a phase-oriented approach, where safety and stabilization are obtained *before* memory processing begins. The old paradigm of simple exposure can exacerbate symptoms and cause undue distress. Because trauma so often involves feeling a loss of control over one's body/psyche, it is vital to restore a sense of autonomy by moving at a more measured pace and teaching clients how to pump the brakes/re-regulate when flooded with traumatic recall.

The aforementioned somatic psychotherapy modalities allow for gentler titration of troubling material, drawing upon the provider's support to revisit frozen states while staying within a zone of tolerance. IFS aims to get protective parts' *consent* to work with wounded exiles, moving through a process of unburdening, retrieving, and integrating them into a more nurturing environment in the client's adult psyche and life. Relational psychodynamic and attachment-based approaches skillfully attend to the reopening "attachment windows" (critical developmental attachment templates) to gently reconfigure character and interpersonal patterns around early unmet needs and adverse experiences (see Chapter 5). Finally, providers informed by Grof's cartography of the psyche—which reflects early perinatal experiences and transpersonal realms—might tailor their support to help unlock previously unknown barriers and steward clients toward successful resolution of traumatic perinatal experiences.

Survivor Guilt: Virtue and Its Confusions

Given that access to these novel treatments is currently quite limited, confusion around whether one is truly *deserving* of this help may emerge. Sometimes, a client's forward progress in psychedelic-assisted therapy can unexpectedly derail when recovery begins to feel unearned or constitutes some form of betrayal to others.

Survivor guilt (also known as "survivor syndrome" or "survivor disorder") can develop following traumatic situations as a type of identity enmeshment, wherein one's happiness and freedom are held hostage to the limitations of those who did/could not survive an event, or chose not to leave a problematic system. This complex may emerge out of a variety of situations, including natural disasters, violent crimes, terrorist attacks, accidental deaths, fatal illnesses, military combat, or refugee emigration. It can also manifest after leaving dysfunctional family systems, cults, fundamentalist religions (especially if also involving drugs and physical/sexual abuse), and a variety of other sources.

We may also miss or underestimate more subtle or less dramatic circumstances that give rise to relational survivor guilt, such as when one member of a family system or community begins significant healing, while the others choose not to (or fail at their own attempts). This dynamic can span from problematic substance use to unspoken resignation around socioeconomic immobility. When survivorship is condemned by the group as heretically breaking away from tacitly agreed-upon dysfunctional practices, others still trapped within the system may unfairly judge, rebuke, or ostracize the individual who is healing (escaping/separating/surviving).

Multiple mechanisms can be at play simultaneously. When members of a survivor's system endeavor to sabotage the healing process, the survivor may concurrently—and unwittingly—enact subtle forms of self-sabotage to unconsciously mitigate guilt based on rigid identification with the group. Even without overt reactionary ostracism from significant others, survivors may feel uncomfortably estranged or obligated to rescue others from the same conditions before they feel they have the right to fulfill their own healing mission and life's potential.

At the core of survivor guilt lies a perplexing confusion of identity and conflicting feeling states that become unmanageable. Polarized allegiances between self-interest and connection are often animated by contrasting feelings of gratitude/ grief, loyalty/disloyalty, and the right to happiness/obligation to despair. Those struggling with this dynamic may not be consciously aware of conflicted feelings about surviving their ordeals; however, the client's interpretations and behaviors reveal an underlying attitude that they do not deserve to be happy, healed, healthy, or fully functional. Survivors may feel like their lives should remain painful and limited, so that their suffering embodies their loyalty and devotion to those who, unlike themselves, have not lived on.

Clinical Example (A)

One client felt that they could not continue to make progress until they rescued their self-destructive sibling from a downward spiral into alcohol dependency. This distracted them from their own recovery process, while the sense of "failure" to reach their family member led to a series of their own alcohol relapses.

Clinical Example (B)

Another client found their fundamentalist Christian family railing against the use of the psychedelic medicines that offered a vehicle for healing. The family proclaimed the use of these therapeutic agents was "against our God" and a betrayal of both the faith and the family. This bogged the client down in fruitless cycles of self-doubt, guilt, and paralyzing shame.

These strange confusions around loyalty, honor, fear, shame, guilt, and self-punishment may render remediation through rational argument or logic alone ineffective or, even worse, can unintentionally deepen bewilderment and alienation. A more promising approach begins with the therapeutic power of *naming* this seemingly illogical fusion of relief and grief and helping the client *understand* its counterintuitive stranglehold. This may be followed by a co-investigation into the survivor's core conundrum of an unbounded sense of helplessness and the drive to self-sacrifice to atone for the "crime" of surviving.

The crux of this entrapment is the well-intended mismanagement of moral virtue, so liberation aspires to a mindful *maturation* of one's understanding of moral virtue. It is extremely important to convey that this complex is a double-edged sword, forged by the survivor's commitment to their own integrity and morality in the crucible of overwhelming traumatic loss. When complete healing is experienced as a betrayal of the dead or the entrapped, then the virtue of suffering or incomplete healing may have become internalized. The organic inner healing intelligence activated by psychedelic therapy may temporarily untether the client's sovereign self from the ego's self-limiting misdirection.

Ultimately, beyond processing new understandings to help untangle confusions around identity and loyalty, opportunities may arise to repurpose sincerely-held morals and values into a healthier call to action, that is, to dedicate and devote one's complete healing to those who have departed or those who must be left behind, and/or to commit some of one's time and self to forms of charity or service to others.

Challenging Transpersonal/Archetypal Experiences

Psychedelic journeys, especially in the higher-dose range, can facilitate profound transpersonal or mystical peak experiences. From heavenly states of bliss and merger with divinity to unfathomable "hell realms," inflation/deflation/terror, or inexplicable encounters with benevolent/disturbing entities (such as dead relatives or archetypal figures), these powerful numinous experiences have the capacity to expand one's sense of self and permanently alter existential and spiritual beliefs. It can also be confusing for client and provider alike to truly and definitively differentiate personal/biographical material from collective/archetypal or spiritual content. There are a variety of potential challenges that practitioners are advised to watch for as this material unfolds.

Ontological Shock

Expanded states can be intense, overwhelming, and disorienting, *especially* without adequate preparation and understanding of where these journeys might lead. Those without a prior spiritual practice or framework to comprehend and contain such encounters may be deeply disturbed by this content and will require time and space to make sense of shifting understandings of life, the universe, and/or the self.

This may be particularly true for those raised in environments of radical atheism or scientism, wherein any references to spiritual/mystical/magical content were met with cynical contempt. Transpersonal material might then lead not only to ruptures in family alliances, but it can also catalyze a paradoxical combination of internalized shame/terror and freedom/liberation.

Clients with rigidly concrete/pragmatic beliefs may express doubt about how such experiences could possibly be of any use to the healing process. Alternatively, those not acclimated to navigating non-ordinary consciousness might incorporate this material into ego-inflated states, aligning one's personal self with God-like power and attributes.

Clinical Example

A client who identified with an atheist/hedonistic worldview presented to KAP with substance misuse and life path questions. Their first medicine session opened into an ecstatic encounter with heavenly/divinity realms. In the immediate aftermath, they suggested "we redefine the meanings of all words like love, freedom, death, life, God, and forgiveness." This profoundly benevolent yet disturbing disruption of their nihilistic prior outlook then led to deep regret about all they had missed in life. Subsequent integration sessions focused on processing the ensuing waves of grief.

The integration process of slowly digesting and metabolizing these experiences and supporting the meaning-making process helps allay anxiety and confusion, leading to more lasting benefits, discouraging excessive inflation, and decreasing the risk of premature flight from treatment.

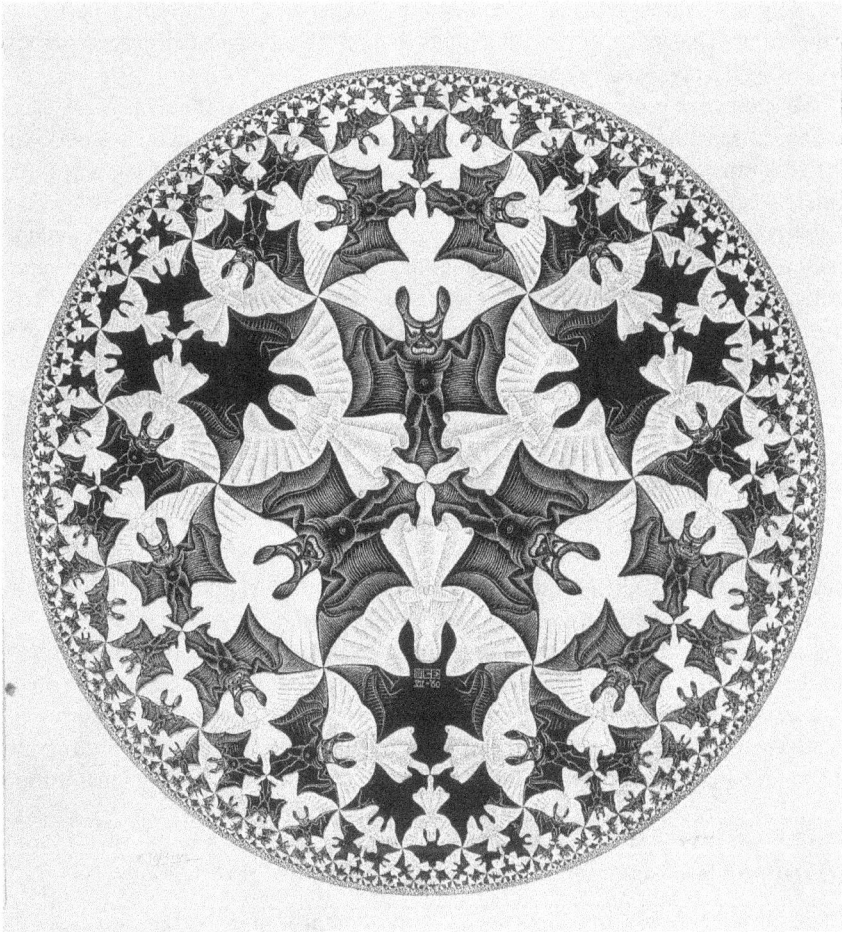

Figure 14.2 M.C. Escher's "Circle Limit IV"

Spiritual Emergence/Emergency

Psychic and spiritual content—especially during or following the use of psychedelics—can be mistaken for symptoms of psychosis in our highly secular culture. The combined forces of biases in the mental health field, the tragically misguided and oppressive War on Drugs (and resulting ignorance about psychedelic states), and countertransference anxiety have resulted in referring those perceived as having a "bad trip" to psychiatric emergency services and/or prescribed antipsychotic medications, thus derailing any potential healing in the experience. However, when held in a supportive context, these experiences can be extraordinarily meaningful to people. Organizations, like the Zendo Project, which supports festival attendees to safely work through (and even transform) challenging psychedelic experiences, have inspired a new generation of helpers to think about expanded states as survivable as well as potentially generative.

We encourage providers to differentiate between an actual illness process vs. an enhanced sensitivity to transpersonal material and to familiarize themselves with the techniques and mindset necessary for supporting someone during a spiritual emergence or crisis process in non-pathologizing ways. Stan and Christina Grof (1989) offer the seminal text on this subject. Various alternatives to hospitalization, such as the Soteria paradigm (Calton et al., 2008), may provide models for more holistic care. Most of these models emphasize providing external structure for containment/safety, helping clients depathologize and understand their experiences via a psychospiritual framework, and creating authentic human connection.

We cannot emphasize strongly enough that a thorough intake process for psychedelic-assisted therapy *must* include conversations about the client's existential concerns, metaphysical encounters, religious background, spiritual development, and beliefs about the nature of reality or the universe. It is similarly essential to prepare clients for experiences that may lead them far outside their ontological comfort zones and to provide for adequate time to metabolize and make meaning out of this material. Clients may also want to seek spiritual guidance within organized or informal traditions (whether Western, Eastern, Indigenous, or other).

Additionally, clinicians should be attuned to their *own* psychospiritual process while working to bracket their belief systems to allow for free expression of the unexpected, and tailor the ritual/ceremonial context to respect clients' histories and preferences. Successful integration of psychedelic therapy begins with *both* careful client preparation and provider familiarity with potential maps of the inner terrain.

Flight Into Health and Spiritual Bypass: Setbacks Disguised as Success

Both spiritual bypass and flight into health attempt to prematurely foreclose the therapeutic process by skipping over the "hard stuff" of distressing emotional processing, painstaking self-inquiry, and authentic individuation. These similar (and potentially overlapping) obstacles threaten to derail healing and decrease the likelihood of sustainable improvements.

These processes are fueled by hypomanic defenses and evasion strategies (such as omnipotence, avoidance, intellectualization, minimization, denial, rationalization, and deflection). Although these defenses emerge in all clinical settings, the NOSC that are foundational to psychedelics—and the attendant feelings of transcendence, personal liberation, merger with the cosmos/divine, universal love, and empathy for our transgressors—can greatly potentiate the "realness" of the belief that one no longer needs to process the conflicts that inspired treatment.

Ecstatic and mystical experiences have been related to important innovations in science, art, and religion, as well as breakthroughs in psychological healing. However, the shadow side of such experiences arises when clients are carried away by magical thinking, such that what feels true is believed as ultimate truth. These states of inflation may encourage narcissistic fantasies of omnipotence, imbue a sense of specialness, or suggest that one has figured out the secrets of existence.

These challenges tend to occur when initial psychedelic work has gone extremely well; such impactful early sessions may lead one to believe overt symptoms have been magically vanquished. One might then conclude that there is no further need to work on the internal/interpersonal root causes of difficulty, which subverts sustainable, long-term healing.

Flight Into Health

Flight into health lacks the divine philosophical narratives of spiritual bypass and is most often based on incomplete or false interpretations of the felt experience of spontaneous healing. In these instances, by celebrating a "full recovery," one is essentially evading further exploration or uncertainty.

Flight into health has historically been referred to in the psychotherapeutic lexicon as a "transference cure" or a "transference remission" for the better part of a century (although its specific origins remain obscure). The traditional psychoanalytic use of the term refers to sudden, global massive repressions and suppressions of pathological feelings and actions often occurring very early in a treatment and understood to be the result of splitting, denial, and projection (Oremland, 1972).

As Masters (2010) explains, fear of painful emotions—such as anger, fear, shame, doubt, terror, hatred, ambivalence, disgust, self-doubt, loneliness, and grief—keeps us superficial and emotionally anemic, addicted to whatever helps to numb negativity, and hooked on the inflation of an alternative (yet inauthentic) identity that requires no further discomfort. A reactive flight into health may result from conscious manipulation or may occur unconsciously without any self-awareness.

Clinical Example

A client who had been suffering from decades of depression had two initial KAP sessions that featured complete ego dissolution (without spiritual content). This experience convinced them that all prior worries were so miniscule and irrelevant to the universe's bigger picture; all problematic symptoms would be resolved through this profound perspective shift and forever mitigated by merely recalling this ecstatic experience at will. They felt this two-session treatment was total and complete, without the need for any additional investigation, nuanced integration, or maintenance support. Although much of this new optimistic perspective was valid, the combination of ecstatic conversion and staunch avoidance elevated the alienation and estrangement in their very troubled marriage. This led to further marital conflict and derailed the initial "high" and its symptom-alleviating benefits. The client responded by dropping out of treatment prematurely.

Spiritual Bypass

Spiritual bypass can be framed as an escapist defense dressed up as spiritual awakening. In some cases, this inflation extends to a belief in unearned transcendence and enlightenment (Welwood, 2002). This poses a more complex and elaborate obstacle, as it involves the misappropriation of valid spiritual doctrines into a labyrinthine tangle of philosophical truths and personal self-deceptions that often reach beyond short-term psychotherapeutic discourse.

The term *spiritual bypass* was initially used in the early 1980s by Buddhist teacher and psychotherapist John Welwood, who defined it as a defense used to turn away from pain; minimize challenges; embrace superficiality; surrender to magical thinking; and outright deny/negate any inner conflict, suffering, shame, or other shadow sides of one's psychological and life experiences (as noted earlier with flight into health). Rather than investigating a wide range of challenging feelings, the client takes a euphoric detour, passing through a landscape of familiar spiritualized lingo.

This may result from a client feeling manically liberated by the altered state, erroneously conflating the journey into awe with a permanent release from fear and pain, and resolving the unbound vertiginous sense of the NOSC by clinging to the highly popularized (yet false) notion of psychedelic therapy as a panacea. One may be so relieved at the transient disappearance of symptoms that the preparatory cautions around "psychedelics are not silver bullets" are willfully overridden.[3]

Some respond to exceptional peak experiences by grabbing onto facile platitudes, unsupported beliefs, and/or saccharine positivity in an attempt to make sense of the expansive state. This may prompt a retreat to rote spiritual doctrines—from the concretely fundamentalist to the vapory New Age—to explain away unwanted intrusive thoughts/sensations, such as unease, uncertainty, and internal inconsistencies.

In discussing the potential pitfalls of ecstatic states (including psychedelics), author Jamie Wheal (2021) points out the risks of ontological addiction or the tendency to chase peak states for their own sake, without integrating the resulting wisdom and inspiration back into everyday life and relationships—and often with a justifying spiritual or philosophical cover narrative.

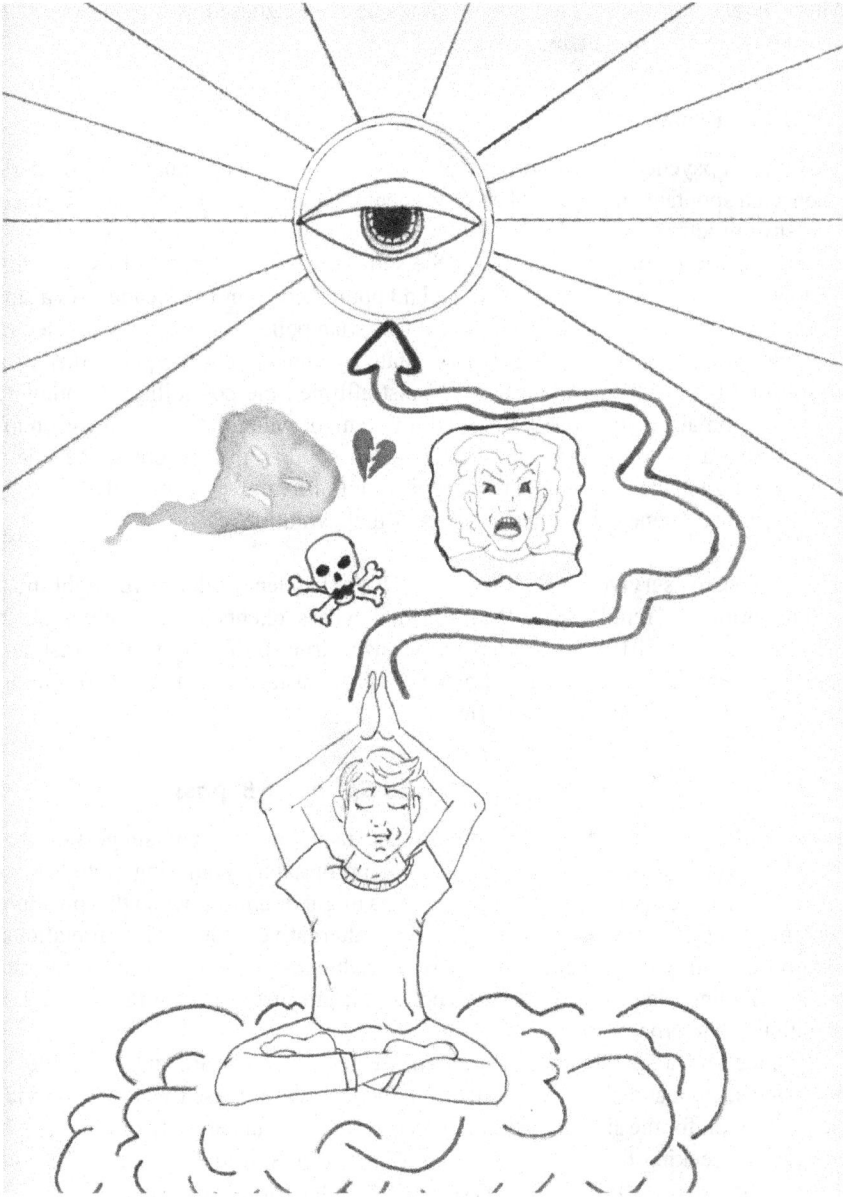

Figure 14.3 Spiritual bypass

This bypass may sometimes arise from the perturbations of a narcissistic personality, staving off a more serious breakdown following a demeaning disappointment or clinging to the ego inflation associated with a peak experience. This maneuver may also be used to compartmentalize and repress a potential spiritual emergency.

Alternatively, spiritual bypass may at times be misdiagnosed as bipolar disorder, reactive psychosis, or a manic episode.

Clinical Example

During a psychedelic session, a survivor of physical and sexual abuse experienced a spontaneous mystical spiritual healing, expressing forgiveness for their many perpetrators. This led them to believe they no longer needed to spend any time processing trauma, shame, or the self-defeating catechism of psychically downloaded pathological beliefs that had oppressed them for decades. As a student of various New Age and mystical Christian belief systems, they refused to compromise their newly "awakened" state by considering the possibility of a spiritual bypass. Even when the therapist affirmed the possibility of complete and legitimate trauma resolution and awakening, yet still advocated for ongoing integration to support, consolidate, and solidify this progress, the client expressed feeling undercut. They dropped out of treatment, stating that therapy was an interference in further psychospiritual evolution.

As Holocaust survivor and writer Viktor Frankl stated, "What gives light must endure burning" (Frankl, 2000). With spiritual bypass, clients like the light but hate the heat (Masters, 2010). As Masters emphasizes, true spirituality is not a rush nor just a transient blast into an exalted plane of consciousness, nor a bubble of immunity from life's challenges and injuries.

Working With Flight Into Health and Spiritual Bypass

Those in the grip of such patterns often react suspiciously to any suggestion that they are being naively self-deceptive or inappropriately conjuring pseudo-successes. When questioned or challenged, clients might double down on this position, becoming rigidly inflexible to investigating alternative/multiple interpretations. This intractability can escalate into extreme righteousness and indignation to the point of feeling victimized by those who do not fall into line with their misinterpretation of the process.

Patience and a shared commitment to seeking the truth are indispensable in assessing such nuanced ambiguities. When evaluating for these dynamics, providers might look for the signs of skipping over the inherent uncertainty of inner work, and instead seeking the unearned refuge of contrived spiritual maturity. This can manifest as patterns of fearing one's own anger/aggression, rationalizing/minimizing traumatic history, blind compassion, and premature or affected expressions of forgiveness.

Front-loading the initial intake and preparatory sessions with cautionary information about the concerns and causes of spiritual bypass and flight into health may help clinicians navigate these challenges. The therapeutic dyad may collaboratively evaluate the limitations of these dynamics by bravely surveying the otherwise disowned aspects of the psyche: the painful, the disfigured, the ostracized, and the unwanted. The essential clinical task here is to help clients learn to hold the paradoxical nature of psychological and spiritual healing—the tension between expansive new perspectives and the earthly challenges of human relating, without collapsing one or the other.

Splitting the Clinical Team: Conquering the Divide

Rigorous research protocols for psychedelic-assisted therapy clinical trials have required two therapists to work simultaneously with the participant, and some clinical practices also choose to use this treatment model. This triadic[4] approach provides some advantages over a more traditional one-to-one individual therapy model, such as greater capacity to manage medical/psychiatric difficulties across long sessions, as well as providing potentially reparative experiences by allowing a client to feel supported by a symbolic family/social system. Ideally, all professionals in a team commit to supporting each other with the psychological stresses of the work, including open communication about vulnerabilities and blind spots; this also serves to model healthy relating for the client.

However, this triadic model also presents some unique risks and challenges, such as when the client "splits" the clinical team, assigning one therapist the safe/good role, and casting the other as the dangerous/bad one. These splits can divide along lines of gender identity, race/ethnicity, sexual orientation, age, and/or the client's general rapport and ease with one therapist in contrast to the other. Differences in interpersonal mannerisms, level of emotional availability, or surface reactions to a client's challenging dynamics may also amplify splitting potential.

The concept of splitting was originally described in the psychoanalytic literature as a primitive defense mechanism, which unconsciously attempts to protect against intense negative feelings (such as abandonment, rejection, intrusion, or loneliness) by polarizing complex realities into a simple good/bad binary, then discarding and rejecting the "bad" and idealizing the "good." This hyperpolarizing dynamic may represent the client's evasion of emerging unconscious difficult/traumatic material or even an unconscious attempt to stress test the therapeutic container.

Splitting is also a common family/group dynamic, in which someone is drawn into siding with one member against another. Clients may reenact this dynamic from their early home environment by idealizing one therapist as a golden savior, while seeing the other as a malevolent threat to be held at bay. Psychedelic medicines may intensify such dynamics.

Splitting can also arise from within the clinician team, most often due to inadequate communication or incongruencies of professional worldview between members of the treatment team. The multidisciplinary teams needed to properly support psychedelic-assisted therapy offer valuable multiple perspectives but may also highlight clashing clinical approaches and can result in "turf" competitions. More problematically, some providers tend to dominate relationships and/or have such

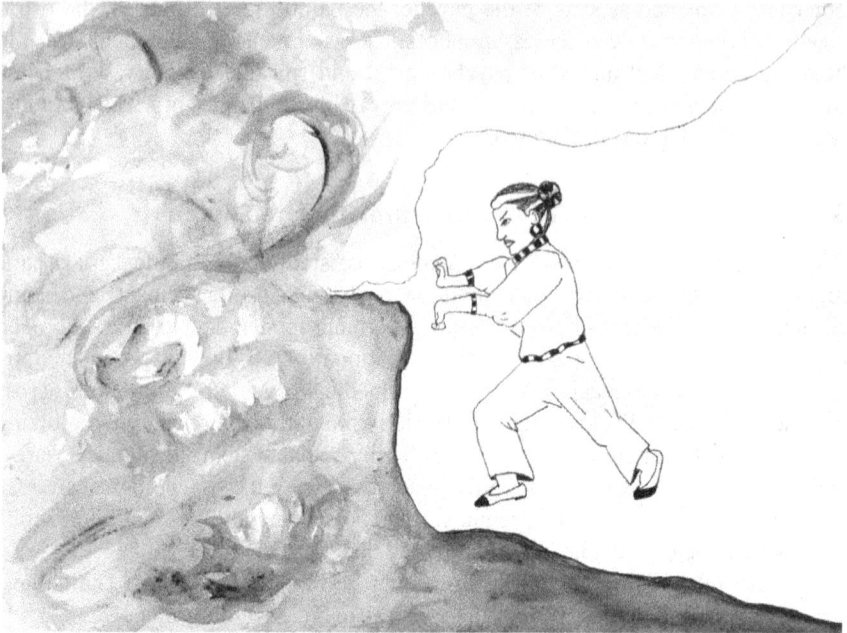

Figure 14.4 Splitting

an inordinate need for control that they inherently create imbalance in a therapy team.

The client's significant others may also express biases or doubts that amplify spitting of the clinical team as well as aggravate internal conflict in the client about the treatment process. Outside psychotherapists or psychiatrists can draw the client into the difficult position of feeling ineffectively suspended between two sets of well-meaning helpers.

Clinical Example

A female-identified sexual abuse survivor refused to look at the male-identified member of the therapy team for quite some time. The flexibility of the team to make space for her difficulties and initial preferences helped her to feel respected and validated. She was eventually able to lovingly engage with both therapists as her healing progressed and her internal world felt more integrated. Additionally, developing supportive relationships with both members of the therapy team helped foster a sense of success and mastery.

As with all obstacles discussed in this chapter, splitting holds the potential to derail treatment while simultaneously providing an opportunity to restore psychic balance. Medicine and integration sessions may offer deeper reflection on one's relational templates via unintentionally reenacting old biographical splitting defenses, reworking earlier attachment traumas, and exploring more inclusive relational experiences. This is contingent on the co-therapists remaining steadfast in their alliance and not unconsciously colluding with a client's projections or polarizations, or falling prey to their own biases. There must be a shared staunch commitment to open-minded curiosity while vigilantly working together to process the unfolding splitting dynamics.

While discussing all potential complications of working with outside therapists is beyond the scope of this chapter, emphasizing preparatory work and collaboration (with consent to speak with other providers) in aligning expectations and goals helps preempt possible professional discordance that could place the client's progress in jeopardy. Additionally, weaving together the ongoing psychotherapy and adjunctive psychedelic treatment—via generous inclusivity with the outside therapist and referring to them specifically in dialogues during sessions—can optimally provide the client with a sense of being held by a team.

Finally, all parties must feel encouraged to speak out about their perceptions of the therapy triad. These group explorations should expressly establish permission to discuss the permutations of splitting, including how (consciously or unconsciously) someone might benefit from the misalignment. The more attuned the clinical team is to the treatment dynamics, the more reflective each member can be about their own role in the process. The origin of splitting may emerge from anyone in the field, and we would do well to always consider ourselves as potential contributors to this process.

Negative Transferences and Clinical Errors: Seeking a Lotus Under the Mud

Negative transferences and clinical errors may also present as obstacles in psychedelic treatment. Common transference challenges can arise when clients have difficulty processing negative feelings about the therapeutic relationship, such as disappointment, frustration, rage, abandonment, shame, and/or betrayal. On the flip side of the coin, intense positive feelings (such as attraction, emotional dependency, romantic infatuation, or impulses to cross therapeutic boundaries) also present transference issues that require careful processing.

Because psychedelics non-specifically amplify all psychological content—including challenging experiences—they may also add to the complexity of clinical relationships and potentiate difficulties. Psychedelic therapy holds higher potential for re-traumatization in the dyad/triad, bubbling up out of minor misunderstandings or empathic failures, and may even escalate to full-blown impasses with threats of litigation.

While it is clinically accepted that people project unresolved inner conflicts and traumatic experiences onto their therapists, they may also accurately perceive relational nuances that lie outside the therapist's awareness. Providers may fail to skillfully navigate their own negative countertransference contributions to the psychedelically enhanced intensity of the interpersonal dynamics in the treatment.

Even the most mindful clinicians can become overwhelmed, detached, forgetful, and/or frustrated. They may have crises of faith in themselves or in their clinical work. Unbeknownst to them, these feelings can leak into the therapeutic relationship, at times in overt or clumsy expressions (such as coming late, missing appointments, and inattentive listening) or with more subtle yet insidious expressions (persistent unresponsiveness, pathologizing, dismissiveness, or veiled hostile/seductive remarks).

Clients may perceive (accurately or inaccurately) their providers as reproducing the oppressive behaviors of early caretakers and family members, such as dominating, manipulating, betraying, dysfunctionally enabling, or passively abandoning them. When confronted by these perceptions, therapists may be reflexively defensive, regardless of the legitimacy of such claims. Unfortunately, many practitioners have not been trained to authentically repair and reset the course of treatment following a difficult relational passage. Therapists vary widely in approaches to therapeutic disruptions, and some may not appreciate the value in mutual inquiry and analysis in the collaborative untangling of misunderstandings and conflicts.

Additionally, providers that hail from more dominant/privileged groups may be ill-prepared for this work without enough exposure to people from communities outside of their own. A client may accurately pick up on a therapist's insensitivity or biases regarding the client's gender identity, sexual orientation, race/ethnicity, or culture. Some clients from routinely marginalized communities may sense their practitioners are aligned with attitudes and values that reinforce alienation and estrangement. A therapist's anxiety around cultural sensitivity may also result in counterproductive withholding, out of fear of making mistakes or encountering issues they are unprepared to process. Far too often, the therapist's default defensive posture forms a self-serving, impenetrable aura of professionalism and clinical authority. A practitioner's unconscious insensitivities in these areas often fly under their own radar, as these tropes are regularly reinforced by a non-inclusive mainstream culture.

All therapists can (and will) make a variety of clinical errors, including projecting biased beliefs and inaccurate preconceptions onto their clients. The intensity of the psychedelic-enhanced process can throw us further off-balance, leading to additional missteps. Therapists and clients can activate each other's previously unprocessed and dissociated experiences, and this can leave the relationship open to a variety of enactments.[5]

The key to successful navigation of such challenges is recognizing, understanding, and valuing the patterns of "rupture and repair" that lie at the core of all developmental processes, including psychotherapy. Kohut (1971, 1977) was the first psychoanalyst to emphasize that beyond empathic resonance/understanding lies the transformative potential—and essential clinical value—of the inevitable therapeutic missteps and disruptions of emotional attunement. Kohut saw these rupture–repair sequences as therapeutically foundational, strengthening the client's sense of self through the process of ongoing "optimal frustration" and "transmuting internalizations," wherein the therapist's focus on empathic understanding of the client's developmental needs and upsets leads to an expanded capacity to tolerate the mixed bag of challenges and disappointments that life presents.

Through Kohut's lens, these unforeseen and unpredictable misunderstandings and ruptures provide access to vulnerabilities and split-off traumatic experiences that might not otherwise be possible. Therapists who work thoughtfully with these disruptions can cultivate rare opportunities to repair fundamental underlying psychological damage; however, from a relational psychoanalytic perspective, transformative potential emerges only when *both* the therapist and the client share their contributions to/participation in enactments and injuries (Stern, 2010).

Although psychedelics can helpfully reduce fear and distrust, enabling a quicker pace for relational resolution, the essence of effective integration work with both negative transferences and clinical errors lies in a strong commitment to *shared* inquiry and understanding the value of these rupture–repair sequences. Integration provides the ongoing relational space where all tensions between rupture and repair become grist for the mill, ultimately building deeper intimacy and trust and aiding the development of a flexible, resilient, and cohesive sense of self.

Preventing Premature Life Decisions

The aforementioned mystical and/or peak experiences often impart revelatory insights about one's life path, and at times they even provide a sense of tapping into deep spiritual guidance from something larger than the personal self. This quality may be of immense value for the long-term change process. However, bumps in the integration path can occur when a client acts on strong urges for change by making rash decisions (e.g., starting or ending a significant relationship, signing a binding contract, quitting a job, making a large purchase, and leaving the country) following a medicine session, without taking time and space to consider all the larger ramifications.

We generally advise clients to not make any unplanned major and consequential life changes for the first few weeks after a journey and to take time to reflect and explore these desires with trusted advisors and professionals who can help place them in context of their life's overall trajectory. This caution can become a thorny transference–countertransference dilemma if clients perceive us as holding them back or not having trust in their unfolding process. We emphasize that these experiences might indeed plant seeds for lasting change, but time and support help these seeds germinate and flower in more sustainable ways.

Insufficient Follow-Up: Dropping the Ball

As integration-focused providers, we routinely provide both in-session encouragement for clients to bring psychedelic session wisdom and experiences back into daily practices, as well as a written set of preparation/aftercare instructions that include tips for skillful integration. These tips typically include such suggestions as:

- Taking adequate time and space after the journey to rest and reflect
- Avoiding post-session stressors (including troubled relational interactions) where possible
- Spending time in nature
- Limiting screen/devices time
- Capturing one's experience (via journaling and artistic expression)
- Connecting with supportive others who are able to effectively hold vulnerable psychedelic experiences
- Cultivating meditation/mindfulness practices
- Paying attention to the needs of the body (activity, sleep, and nourishment)
- Exploring new possibilities (other healing modalities, hobbies, and interests)
- Shifting old patterns and habits (substance misuse, decluttering, and addressing relationship issues)

We strongly encourage clients to commit to a series of integration therapy sessions to help in unpacking their experiences and experimenting with the mentioned ideas. Many providers also require daily mood monitoring/journaling (via apps or other modalities) to help track potential changes and treatment efficacy.

However, despite these oft-repeated recommendations for best results, most providers still struggle with poor post-medicine treatment compliance and insufficient follow-up. Frustration often emerges in provider countertransference as a result of clients not completing tracking/journaling requests, canceling follow-up integration therapy sessions, ignoring aftercare tips—and then declaring psychedelic treatment itself a failure.

Again, curious exploration of this so-called resistance may reveal a rich treasure trove of material that then fruitfully informs the therapeutic process. We often begin with clarifying beliefs about what integration is and how the post-treatment process is expected to unfold. It is often necessary, especially within Western medicalized contexts, to replace the *passive* client model (where the client is expected merely to show up for treatment and let the medicine's molecular action does all the work) with an *active* client model, in which the client actively *participates* in using the altered state experiences and insights to make substantive change in their lives (Bennett, 2019).

However, we may also discover a variety of previously hidden barriers, ranging from the concrete (e.g., lack of financial resources for follow-up sessions) to the relational (e.g., the aforementioned transference enactments that rupture provider/client connection) to the intrapsychic (e.g., perfectionistic tendencies that disrupt gradual changes).

When a client "drops the ball" during the integration process, any of the challenges mentioned in this chapter may be a possible root cause, and practitioners are advised to inquire with compassion, staying open to what might emerge in this co-creative process. In-depth inquiry of the motivation underlying these behaviors may reveal essential information and expose important dynamics that might have otherwise gone undiscovered, and thus unprocessed.

Theoretical Models and Interventions That Support Integration

We are often asked to identify *the best* therapeutic approach for psychedelic-assisted therapy. We believe that skillfully addressing these myriad potential challenges calls for professional flexibility and an integrative approach, as dogmatic adherence to any one theoretical system forecloses the open exploration of individualized responses.

Curious inquiry, a desire to hear about any emerging meanings, and a willingness to experiment with potential interventions all go much further than the most brilliant textbook formulation or manualized protocol. "*I don't know*" is a remarkably underutilized intervention; the invitation to be in *not knowing* together may be the key that opens generative conversations, stewarding us through such vital moments of grappling with uncertainty. Empathic witnessing and non-intrusive stewardship help us follow the client's own sovereign self-direction and healing instincts—even when these seem to lead down counterintuitive, circuitous, or dead-end paths.

The preceding sections offer some frameworks that match techniques to the perceived barriers and/or layers of functioning (while simultaneously acknowledging that truly sharp delineations between levels of human functioning are illusory). We also find consensus with Dubouchet and Fiévet (2020), who insist on the polysemic nature of psychedelic visions, and encourage providers to explore this material on multiple levels *simultaneously* "so that interpretations can be broken down and not rushed through too quickly, for the sake of an immediate 'aha' moment that would obscure and eliminate all other possibilities."

We previously emphasized the value of both relational psychoanalytic/dynamic theory (to address transference/countertransference and attachment issues with mutuality) and explicit parts work (to skillfully navigate the inherent multiplicity of the mind); we will now further explore some other potentially helpful theoretical models and general approaches to integration. Each of these systems offers diverse ways of making sense of the presenting issues, as well as possible responses to realign the treatment when a challenge appears. Our suggestions are not meant to be exhaustive or instructive, but they rather seek to model openness in adapting our interventions to the variety of issues that may emerge in our work.

Somatic

Psychotherapy systems, such as Hakomi, Somatic Experiencing, Sensorimotor Psychotherapy, and Organic Intelligence, offer not only techniques for grounding and emotional regulation during phases of distress, but they can aid the integration process immensely. These models often encourage developing a somatic *anchor*—a posture, gesture, image, or targeted sensory awareness—during key moments during the session that one can then return to in the following days as a way to revisit the lessons from the expanded state and intentionally fold them into one's embodied daily existence as a form of "muscle memory."

We have found that encouraging clients to recall and practice these anchors a few hours after the session, as well as regularly during the following week, allows for deeper shifts than mere reflection on verbal insights. This is similar to/can be combined with the IFS suggestion of reconnecting with a newly encountered/retrieved exile regularly, making sure this part continues to feel invited into the system and/ or does not feel re-abandoned.

Additionally, altered states of consciousness often manifest as *body-centered* experiences, such as contraction, pain, cathartic release, or vital embodiment. Integration work can then support further healing with specific practices tailored to the process initiated by the journey (such as ongoing release of tension, purification rituals, engagement of the senses, reconnection with nature, rest/relaxation, or other bodily self-care habits).

Intense energetic/somatic experiences can leave people feeling overwhelmed, overstimulated, or exhausted. Gentle grounding and stabilization techniques (such as restorative yoga or spending quiet time in nature) are often suggested to allow the system to come back into balance. Therapists may want to work collaboratively with somatic bodyworkers, acupuncturists, and/or other complementary care providers that specifically address bodily imbalances.

Jungian and Depth Psychology

As mentioned previously, Hill (2013) offers a Jungian approach to psychedelic integration, in part inspired by depth psychology dreamwork, which holds the emerging symbols as potent expressions of complexities not yet clearly apprehended by the conscious mind. This model suggests that the disturbing content arising from the unconscious offers consciousness the very medicine it needs. Hill emphasizes the mediating role the practitioner plays in supporting the ego during this potentially disruptive confrontation with the unconscious, providing a useful bridge between that realm and default reality.

Jung advocated that both *creative formulation* (such as artistic, symbolic, or imaginal expression) and *understanding of meaning* supplement each other, wherein fantasy content is first freely given shape and then actively interpreted. Creative formulation alone may sidetrack therapy by allowing purely artistic concerns to dominate, while mere intellectual analysis is not entirely reliable and may miss vital feeling-toned qualities that one cannot fully grasp cognitively. This approach is congruent for working with both the rich imagery and noetic, piercing insights that can occur in altered states (see Chapter 8 for further elaboration).

Ecopsychology/Ecotherapy

Integration tips commonly prompt one to spend time in nature, and many providers feel this to be one of the *most* effective suggestions for maintaining treatment benefits, providing a readily available resource for support and ongoing self-expansion. Additionally, Western enthusiasts of psychedelics tend to highlight their capacity to reconnect our increasingly alienated and technology-saturated species to our ecological environment.

A recent article (Gandy et al., 2020) summarizes the similar benefits of psychedelic-assisted therapy and contact with nature (decreased rumination and negative affect, enhanced psychological connectedness and mindfulness-related capacities, and heightened states of awe and transcendent experiences). The authors suggest that nature-based settings may complement the preparation and integration phases, and then consider how a more specific model of nature-focused psychedelic work (including outdoor medicine sessions) could be developed, with the goal of enhancing nature relatedness.

Nature relatedness is not only linked to individual mental health improvements, but it is also a strong predictor of pro-environmental attitudes and behavior (Diessner et al., 2018). Given the notable lack of effective interventions for reversing environmentally damaging human activities, this potential set of benefits might be the most salient for helping address the current climate/ecological crises that lie beyond the therapeutic consulting room.

Takeaways and Summary Ideas

We hope that the preceding sections illustrate how setbacks, detours, and zigzags are loaded with healing potential when navigated with creativity, mutuality, and wisdom. Perhaps the most key takeaway here is that when healing energy rises—as powerfully boosted by the medicine/therapy combination—the energy of resistance *also* rises. The human psyche constantly moves through such polarities as it matures, with growing ability to hold the essential paradoxes of life (such as stability/change, shadow/light, progression/regression, competition/collaboration, ego/Self, activity/passivity, and individuation/connection). Providers are encouraged to both familiarize themselves with these psychological phenomena to normalize and de-pathologize such oscillations and to work within the therapeutic relationship to navigate and explore these bumps in the road together.

Ideally, our end goal in the integration phase is to uncover or evoke something *new* (skills, self-understanding, emotional insight, and resilience) that people can take with them when they ultimately complete treatment, discouraging unnecessary dependencies on the medicine/healers. Assisting people to connect to their own organic inner healing intelligence (a stance we often refer to as "the magic was in you all along") is what makes this type of treatment more sustainable in the long run.

In closing, when integration proceeds optimally, we are:

- Not *chasing* the high
- Not *forgetting* the high/journey or insights
- Not *running from* the shadow/challenging material

- Not *throwing away* the lessons/revelations of the journey
- *Living the revelations of the journey* in real life/real time

"[A]fter having a glimpse of the top of the mountain, it is easier for many to maintain the motivation to struggle through the swamps, thickets and rocky terrain on the path that leads to the summit" (Richards, 2016).

Notes

1   A full review of all shamanic and/or Indigenous traditions and practices lies outside the scope of this chapter; yet, we still seek to respectfully honor and pay homage to the ancestral lineage of deep wisdom that illuminates the gaps in our modern understanding of expanded states (see Chapter 3).
2   Additionally, Stanislav Grof (1979) observed during his extensive history of LSD sessions that intense/traumatic perinatal events (the fetus's experiences while in the womb or during labor/delivery) held outside of conscious awareness were often evoked by the medicine and provided a model for supporting each stage of this process.
3   An important caveat for exceptional outliers: there have been validated cases of authentic spontaneous recovery following either a limited number of treatments or even a single medicine session. After years of pathologizing clients under the term flight into health, Frick (1999) has cautioned that some cases can indeed represent genuine expressions of emerging health and are not always the product of self-deception or retreat from therapeutic progress; knee-jerk skepticism against the validity of all spontaneous recovery phenomena may undercut genuine progress and autonomy. In psychedelic-assisted therapy research, there has been considerable documentation of those claiming durable life-changing experiences after only a single ingestion of the medicine, and for many of these rare individuals, the perspective shifts remain consistent through time (Lattin, 2017; Pollan, 2019).
4   The term "therapy triad" is used here to indicate the relational arrangement of two therapists who work alongside each other with the client. We will also refer to the two therapists in this configuration as the *clinical team*, *treatment team*, or *therapy team* to avoid confusion with the traditional use of the term "therapy dyad" (which generally indicates the therapist/client relationship).
5   The term *enactment* was first used by Jacobs (1986) to refer to unconscious patterns of dyadic interaction and the non-reflective reactualization of unsymbolized emotional experiences and relational templates within the treatment. Although clinical lore frames this process as being initiated by the client, Jacobs specifically referred to *countertransference* enactments, highlighting the impact of the therapist's personality characteristics, affective frame, mental representations, and inner conflicts on the therapy relationship. Often involving mutual projective identification and dissociation, enactments reflect the loss of perspective in the therapy, leading to potential rupture. However, when discovered and mindfully processed, enactments hold great potential to access dissociated aspects of the client's (and the therapist's) self- and object representations (Bromberg, 2011).

References

Bennett, R. (2019, Spring). Multidisciplinary Association for Psychedelic Studies (MAPS) special edition bulletin. In *Paradigms of ketamine treatment* (Vols. 29, Issue 1, pp. 48–49). 2019 Multidisciplinary Association for Psychedelic Studies, Inc. (MAPS).

https://maps.org/news/bulletin/articles/436-maps-bulletin-spring-2019-vol-29,-no-1/7718-paradigms-of-ketamine-treatment-spring-2019

Bromberg, P. M. (2011). *The shadow of the tsunami and the growth of the relational mind.* Routledge Taylor and Francis Group.

Calton, T., Ferriter, M., Huband, N., & Spandler, H. (2008, January). Schizophrenia bulletin. In *A systematic review of the Soteria paradigm for the treatment of people diagnosed with schizophrenia* (Vol. 34, Issue 1, pp. 181–192). Oxford University Press on behalf of the Maryland Psychiatric Research Center. https://doi.org/10.1093/schbul/sbm047

Campbell, J. (1991). *The power of myth.* Anchor Books.

Coder, K. E. (2017). *After the ceremony ends: A companion guide to help you integrate visionary plant medicine experiences.* Casa de Raices y Alas Books.

Diessner, R., Genthôs, R., Praest, K., & Pohling, R. (2018). Identifying with nature mediates the influence of valuing nature's beauty on proenvironmental behaviors. *Ecopsychology, 10*(2), 97–105. http://doi.org/10.1089/eco.2017.0040

Dubouchet, D., & Fiévet, R. (2020, November 16). Keys for integrating psychedelic experiences. *Psychedelics Today.* https://www.psychedelicstoday.com/2020/11/16/keys-for-integrating-psychedelic-experiences/

Frankl, V. (2000). *Yes to life in spite of everything.* Beacon Press.

Frick, W. B. (1999). Flight into health: A new interpretation. *Journal of Humanistic Psychology, 39*(4), 58–81.

Gandy, S., Forstmann, M., Carhart-Harris, R. L., Timmermann, C., Luke, D., & Watts, R. (2020). SAGE journals, health psychology open. In *The potential synergistic effects between psychedelic administration and nature contact for the improvement of mental health* (Vol. 7, Issue 2). SAGE Publications. https://doi.org/10.1177/2055102920978123

Godasi, S. M. (2019, March 3). *Reframing psychedelic integration into a continuum with community.* Psychedelic Support Resources, Association Division on Addiction Conference, New York.

Grof, S. (1979). *Realms of the human unconscious: Observations from LSD research* (1st ed.). Viking Adult.

Grof, S., & Grof, C. (1989). *Spiritual emergency: When personal transformation becomes a crisis.* Tarcher/Perigee.

Hill, S. J. (2013/2019). *Confrontation with the unconscious: Jungian depth psychology and psychedelic experience.* Aeon Press.

House, S. G. (2007). Common processes in psychedelic-induced psychospiritual change. In M. J. Winkelman & T. B. Roberts (Eds.), *Psychedelic medicine: New evidence for hallucinogenic substances and treatments* (pp. 163–191). Praeger.

Jacobs, T. (1986). On countertransference enactments. *Journal of the American Psychoanalytic Association, 34,* 289–307.

Jung, C. G. (1969). The transcendent function. In *Collected works of C. G. Jung* (Vol. 8, pp. 67–91). (Original work published 1916 and considerably revised 1958).

Kohut, H. (1971). *The analysis of the self.* International Universities Press.

Kohut, H. (1977). *The restoration of the self.* International Universities Press.

Kotler, S., & Wheal, J. (2019). *Stealing fire: How Silicon Valley, the Navy SEALs, and maverick scientists are revolutionizing the way we live and work.* Dey Street Books.

Lattin, D. (2017). *Changing our minds: Psychedelic sacraments and the new psychotherapy.* Synergetic Press.

Marsden, R., & Lukoff, D. (2007). Transpersonal healing with hallucinogens. In M. J. Winkelman & T. B. Roberts (Eds.), *Psychedelic medicine: New evidence for hallucinogenic substances and treatments* (pp. 287–305). Praeger.

Masters, R. A. (2010). *Spiritual bypassing: When spirituality disconnects us from what really matters*. North Atlantic Books.

Miller, J. C. (2004). *The transcendent function: Jung's model of psychological growth through dialogue with the unconscious*. State University of New York Press. Randomized controlled pilot study. *Journal of Psychopharmacology, 25*, 439–452.

Oremland, J. (1972). Transference cure and flight into health. *International Journal of Psychoanalytic Psychotherapy, 1*(1), 61–75.

Pollan, M. (2019). *How to change your mind: What the new science of psychedelics teaches us about consciousness, dying, addiction, depression, and transcendence*. Penguin.

Richards, W. (2016). *Sacred knowledge: Psychedelics and religious experience*. Columbia University Press.

Smith, H. (1992). *Forgotten truth: The common vision of the world's religions*. Harper.

Stern, D. S. (2010). *Partners in thought: Working with unformulated experiences, dissociation, and enactment*. Routledge Taylor and Francis Group.

Walsh, R. (2002). Chemical and contemplative ecstasy. In C. Grob (Ed.), *Hallucinogens: A reader* (pp. 72–81). Tarcher.

Walsh, R. (2012). From state to trait: The challenge of transforming transient insights into enduring change. In T. B. Roberts (Ed.), *Spiritual growth with entheogens: Psychoactive sacramentals and human transformation* (pp. 24–30). Park Street Press.

Welwood, J. (2002). *Toward a psychology of awakening: Buddhism, psychotherapy, and the path of personal and spiritual transformation*. Shambhala.

Wheal, J. (2021). *Recapture the rapture: Rethinking god, sex and death in a world that's lost its mind*. Harper Wave.

Index

Note: Page locators in *italics* indicate a figure on the corresponding page.

For Product Safety Concerns and Information please contact our EU
representative GPSR@taylorandfrancis.com
Taylor & Francis Verlag GmbH, Kaufingerstraße 24, 80331 München, Germany

www.ingramcontent.com/pod-product-compliance
Lightning Source LLC
Chambersburg PA
CBHW050333270326
41926CB00016B/3443